Approach to Practical Pediatrics

Approach to Practical Pediatrics

SECOND EDITION

Manish Narang MBBS MD (Pediatrics)
Lecturer
Department of Pediatrics
University College of Medical Sciences and GTB Hospital
New Delhi, India

JAYPEE

JAYPEE BROTHERS MEDICAL PUBLISHERS

The Health Sciences Publisher

New Delhi | London

JAYPEE **Jaypee Brothers Medical Publishers (P) Ltd**

Headquarters
EMCA House
23/23-B, Ansari Road, Daryaganj
New Delhi 110 002, India
Landline: +91-11-23272143, +91-11-23272703
+91-11-23282021, +91-11-23245672
E-mail: jaypee@jaypeebrothers.com

Corporate Office
4838/24, Ansari Road, Daryaganj
New Delhi 110 002, India
Phone: +91-11-43574357
Fax: +91-11-43574314
E-mail: jaypee@jaypeebrothers.com

Overseas Office
J.P. Medical Ltd
83 Victoria Street, London
SW1H 0HW (UK)
Phone: +44 20 3170 8910
E-mail: info@jpmedpub.com

EU GPSR Authorised Representative
Logos Europe, 9 rue Nicolas Poussin
17000, La Rochelle, France
Phone: +33 (0) 6 67 93 73 78
E-mail: contact@logoseurope.eu

Website: www.jaypeebrothers.com
Website: www.jaypeedigital.com

Approach to Practical Pediatrics

First Edition: 2007
Second Edition: 2011
Reprint: **2026**
ISBN 978-93-5025-093-8
Printed in India

Dedicated

to

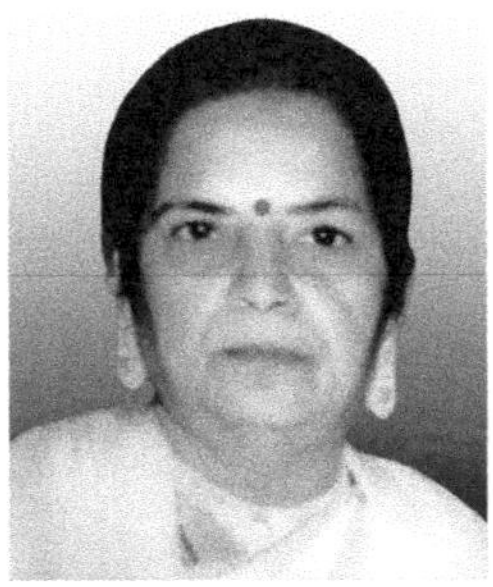

MY MOTHER

Late Dr (Mrs) CK NARANG

All that I am and ever hope to be, I owe to my angel Mother

Preface to the Second Edition

You can score 75% marks by reading just 25% but the question is which 25%. It is with the concept of finding this 25% that this book was written. I have written, what I would have loved to read as an undergraduate and postgraduate student in pediatrics. This book reflects a simplified approach to clinical cases in pediatrics.

New chapters packed with information and practical tips have been added on Anthropometry, Health Indicators, High-risk Newborns, and Leukemia. Detailed and updated information have been added about asthma devices in chapter on Instruments while vaccine controversies and newer vaccines have been discussed in chapter on Immunization. This book also covers new ground about differential diagnosis of hepatosplenomegaly, management of thalassemia and simplified approach to paraplegia. Chapter on Protein Energy Malnutrition (PEM) includes recent IAP/WHO guidelines on management of severely malnourished child while chapter on Cardiovascular System includes simplified approach for diagnosis of congenital heart diseases (CHD), recent guidelines on management of CHD and rheumatic heart disease in children.

This book is an outcome of my personal difficulties encountered during case presentations. I hope this book helps readers to achieve my goal of learning maximum without wasting time in searching answers from different sources.

I would like to hear from my readers regarding additions, omissions or just good ideas for further inclusion. These may be e-mailed to *manish_2710@yahoo.com*

Manish Narang

Preface to the First Edition

This text approaches diagnosis the way clinicians do—by symptom rather than disease entity. There is no well-structured or standardized textbook on Practical Pediatrics. Practical material of pediatrics is often scanty and theoretical. It is in this background that I decided to translate the agreed contents of bedside clinics in pediatrics into an easily readable material. It combines clinical experience and evidence-based strategies to guide clinicians through differential diagnoses and then to a specific diagnosis, then to appropriate therapy for common pediatric ailments.

Special skills required in taking Birth history/Dietary history/Developmental history/Immunization history are discussed in separate chapters. The book covers much new ground and reflects the approach of pediatrics while taking clinical cases. Chapters on Antibiotic Therapy/Legal Aspects/Newer Guidelines of American Academy of Pediatrics—2005 for neonatal resuscitation have been written keeping in mind the needs of postgraduates while chapters like Instruments/Drug Therapy/Various Cases have been written keeping in mind both postgraduates and undergraduates.

This book is an outcome of personal experience and is a vital presentation from which a student can learn maximum without wasting time in searching answers from different books. It is the next best thing to attending ward teaching rounds!

I welcome comments concerning errors, contents and critical thoughts for future editions. These may be e-mailed to *manish_2710@yahoo.com*

Manish Narang

Acknowledgments

This is a befitting occasion for me to thank my mother Late Dr CK Narang and Late Mrs and Mr RK Virmani for their immeasurable contribution to my life.

I sincerely wish to acknowledge the constant source of inspiration I have received from my teachers who have been instrumental in teaching me various aspects of pediatrics. It gives me immense pleasure to express my gratitude to Dr MMA Faridi, Professor and Head, Department of Pediatrics, UCMS and GTBH for giving me stimulating suggestions. I would like to asseverate my gratitude for Dr OP Kalra (Principal, UCMS); Dr Sunil Gomber (Professor, UCMS); Dr Piyush Gupta (Professor, UCMS), Dr Anup Mohta (Professor and Head, CNBC) and Dr. Dheeraj Shah (Reader, UCMS) for their untiring support. I feel honored and privileged to have worked under their able guidance.

I must thank all my patients without whom this work would not have been possible. I wish to express my sincere and heartful thanks to Chaitanya Das and Rahul Dhaneja, ND Comm services in their meticulous computerized paging out of this book.

Special thanks are due to my family—my grandmother Smt Kaushalya Devi Narang; my father Dr Keshav Kumar Narang; my beloved wife Dr Shiva and loving daughter Maanya; and gems of my family, my sisters Dr Sheetal and Dr Rashim; brother-in-laws Dr Peeyush and Dr Vishal; for their forbearance and whose share of time I selfishly usurped during preparation of manuscript. I also sincerely wish to express my appreciation to my dear ones, Dr BK Mehrotra, Mrs Seema and Mr Rajiv Mehrotra and Late Dr Harsh Narang.

Contents

Section - I

BASICS OF PRACTICAL PEDIATRICS

PLATE 1

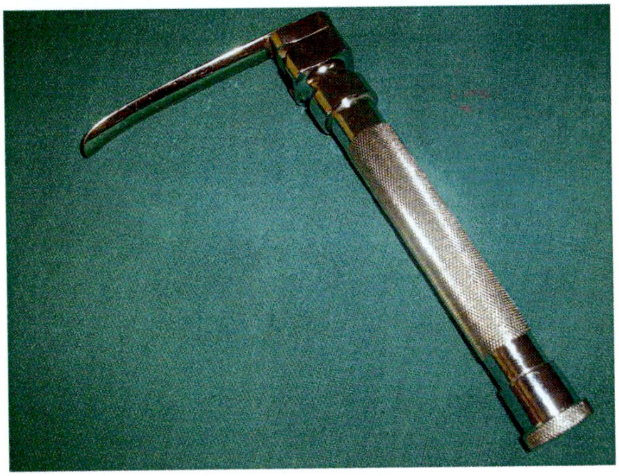

Fig. 1.1: Laryngoscope

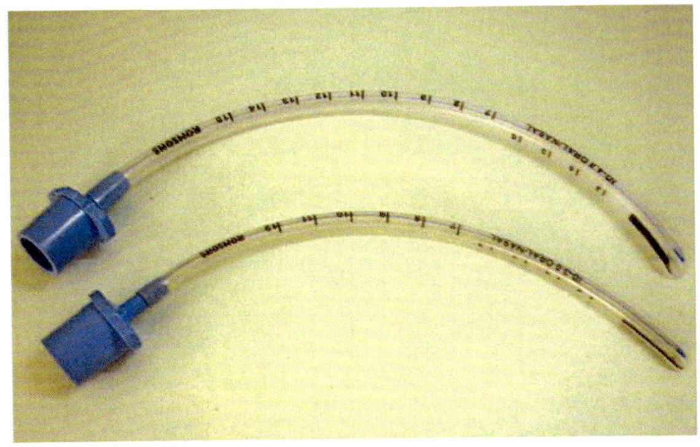

Fig. 1.2: Endotracheal tube

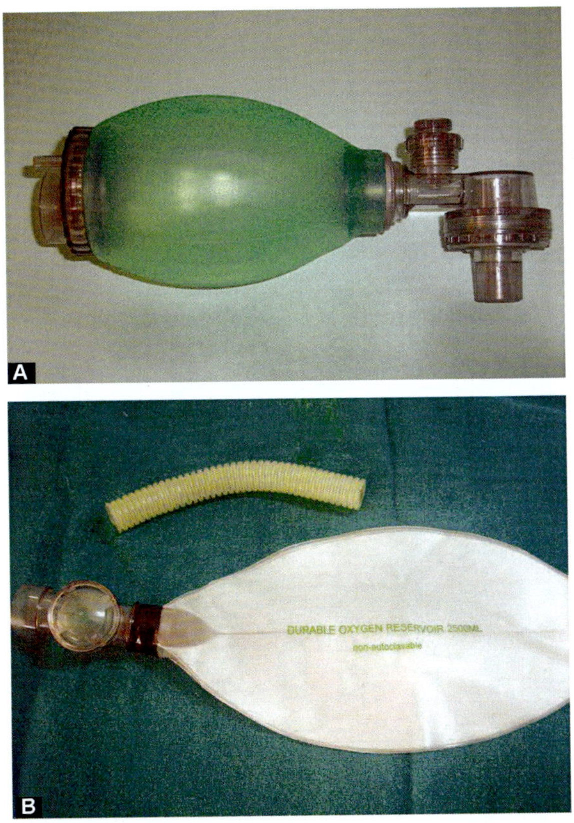

Figs 1.3A and B: Self-inflating bag with oxygen reservior

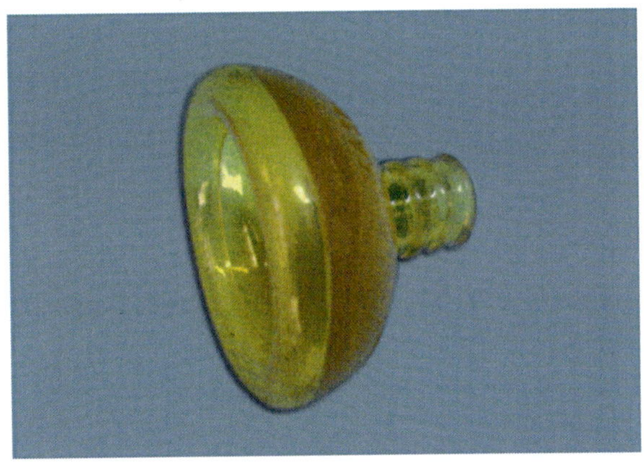

Fig. 1.4: Face mask

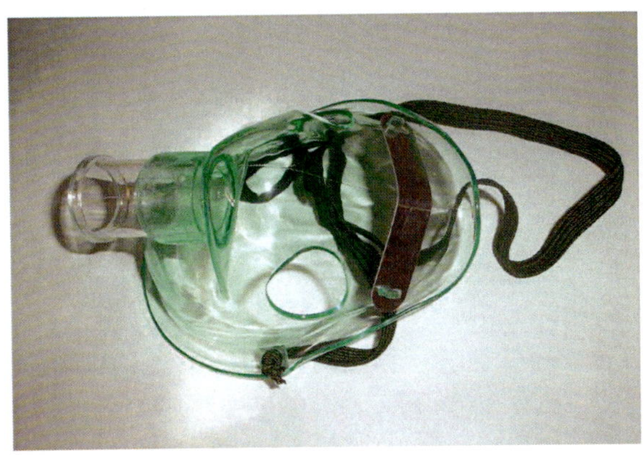

Fig. 1.5: Oxygen mask

PLATE 2

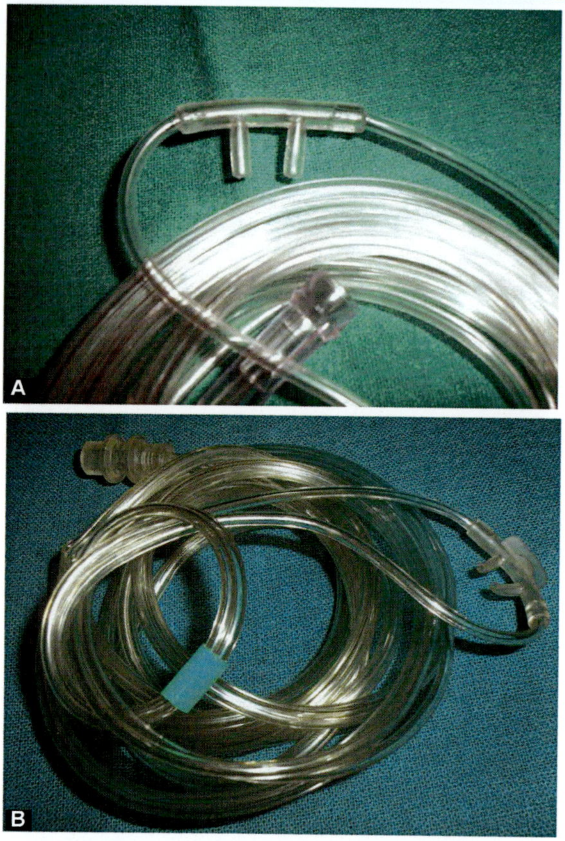

Figs 1.6A and B: Nasal oxygen catheter

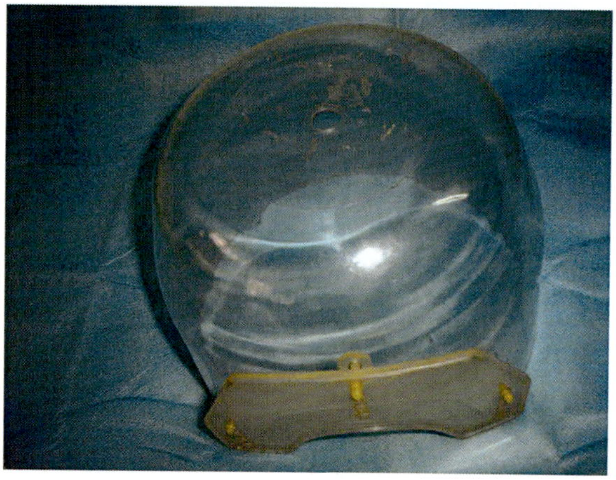

Fig. 1.7: Acrylic oxygen hood

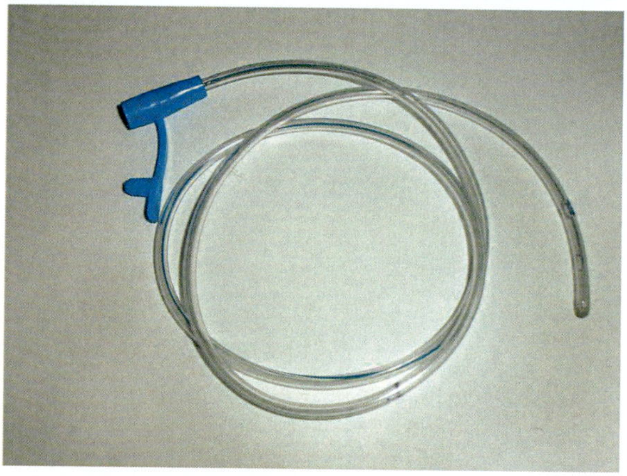

Fig. 1.8: Infant feeding tube

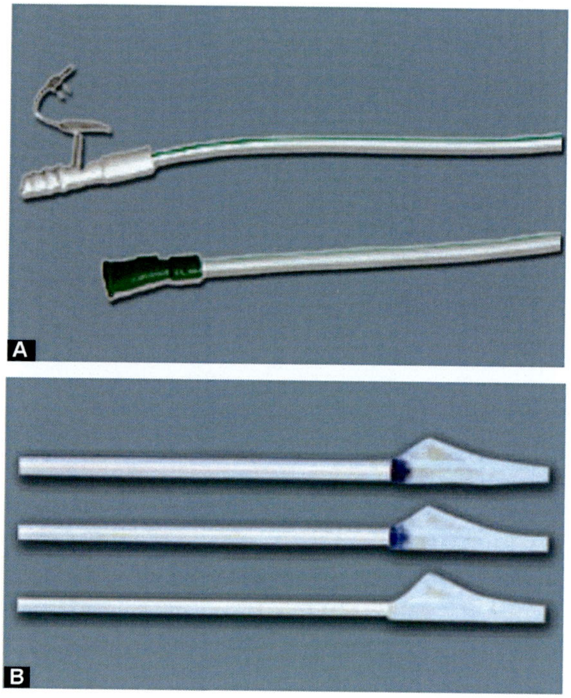

Figs 1.9A and B: Suction catheter

PLATE 3

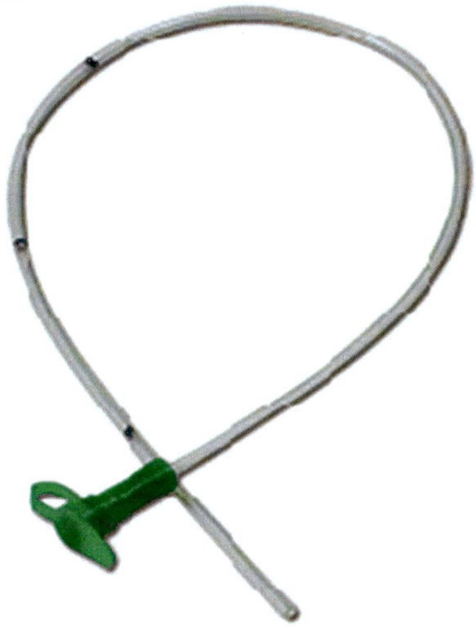

Fig. 1.10: Umbilical catheter

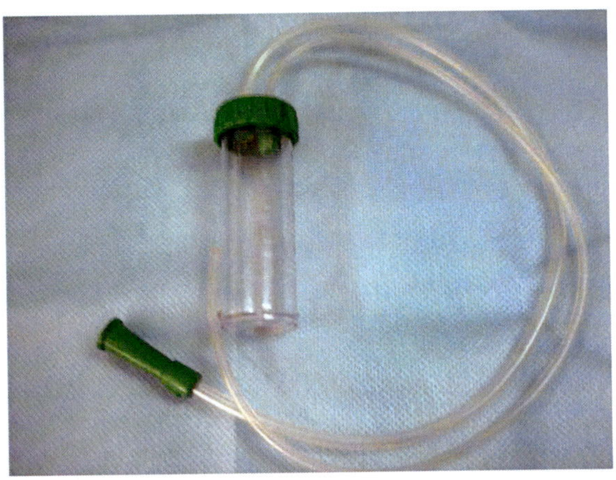

Fig. 1.11: Dileys mucus extractor

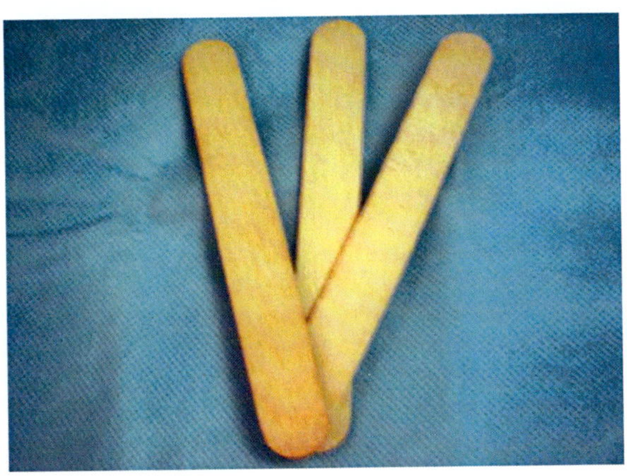

Fig. 1.12: Tongue depressor

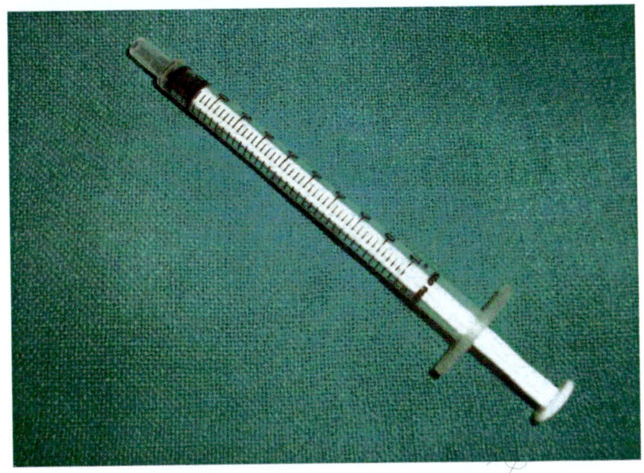

Fig. 1.13: Tuberculin syringe

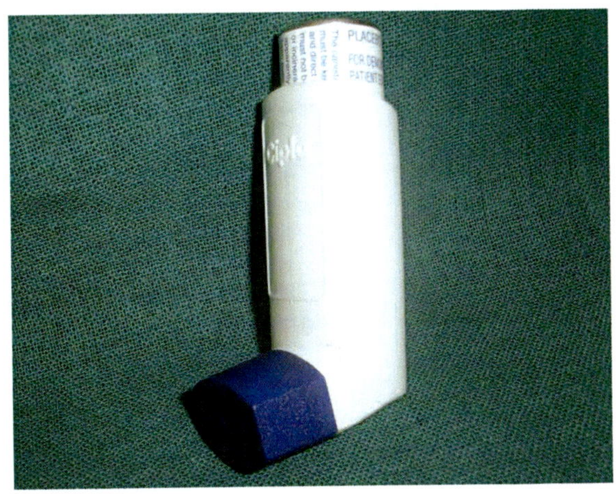

Fig. 1.14A: Metered dose inhaler

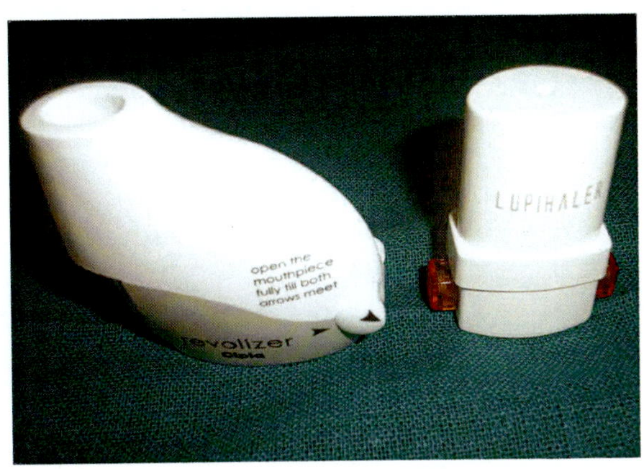

Fig. 1.16: Dry powder inhaler (DPI)

PLATE 4

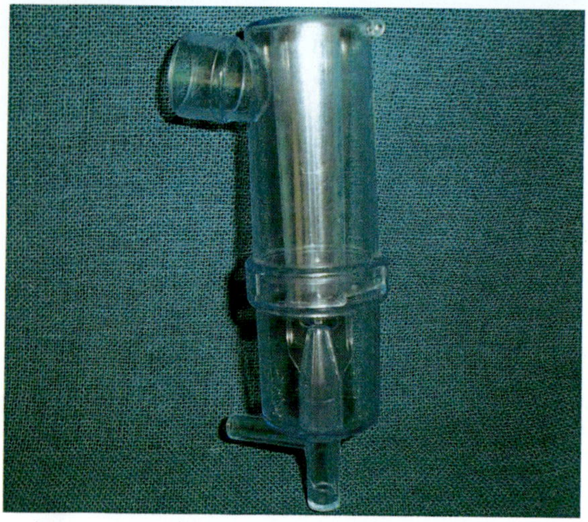

Fig. 1.17: Nebulizer chamber

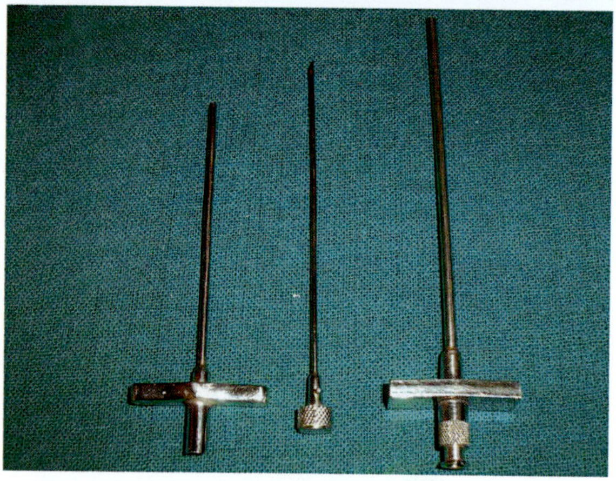

Fig. 1.20: Bone trephine biopsy

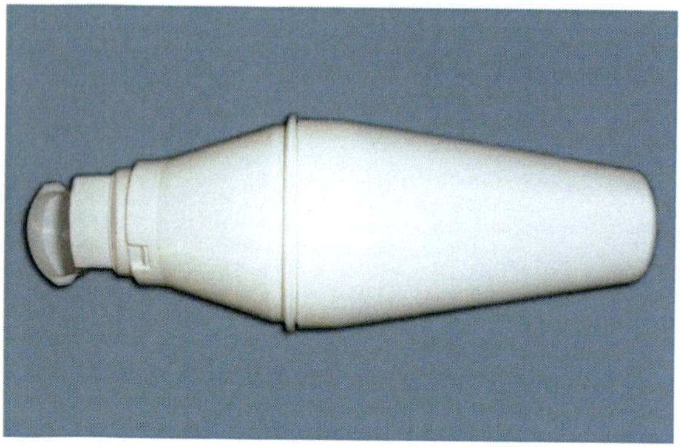

Fig. 1.18: Volume spacer

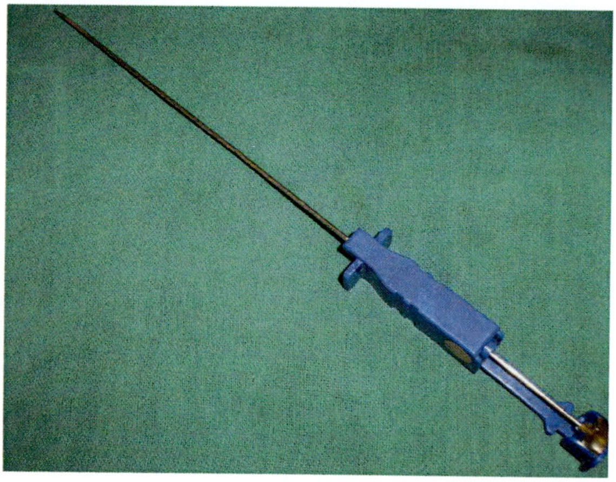

Fig. 1.23: Trucut biopsy needle

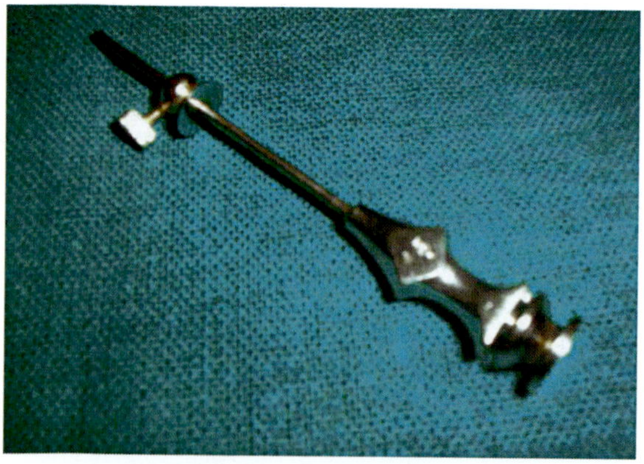

Fig. 1.19: Bone marrow aspiration needle

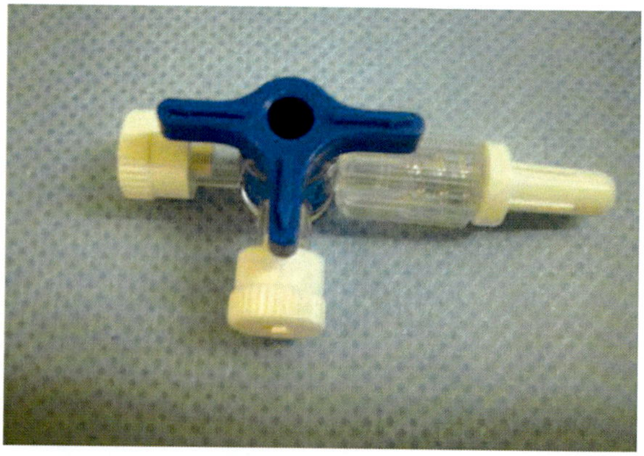

Fig. 1.24: Three way

PLATE 5

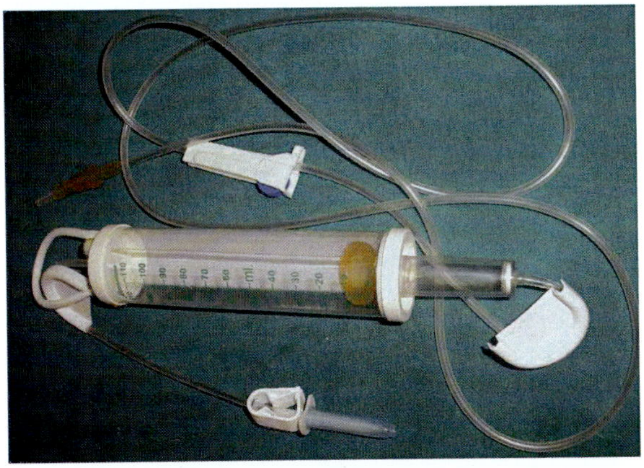

Fig. 1.25: Microdrip set

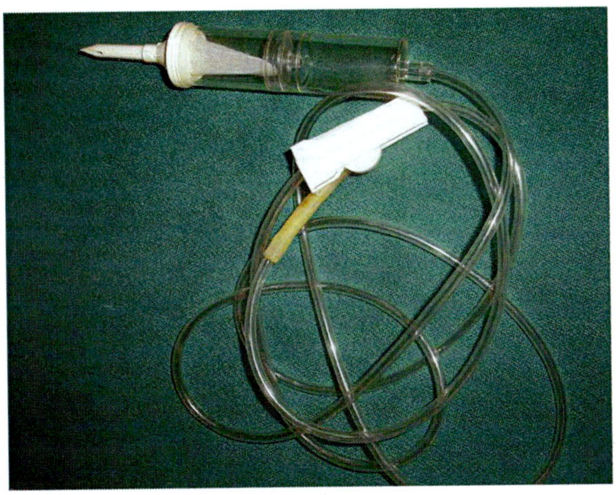

Fig. 1.26: Blood set

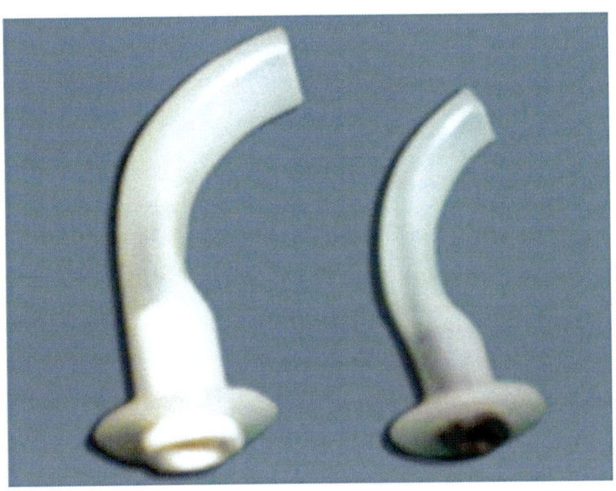

Fig. 1.27: Guedel airway

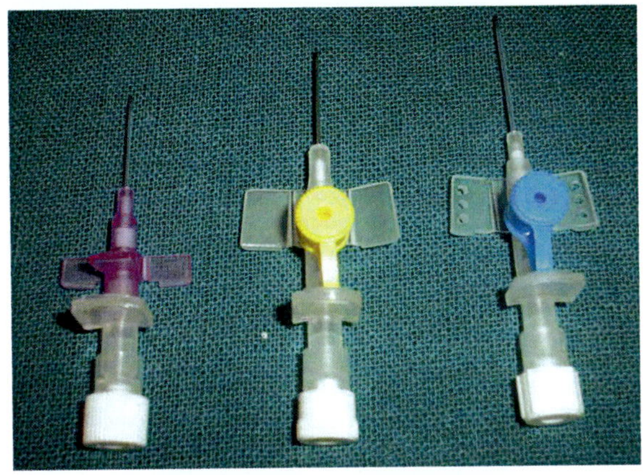

Fig. 1.28: Intravenous cannula

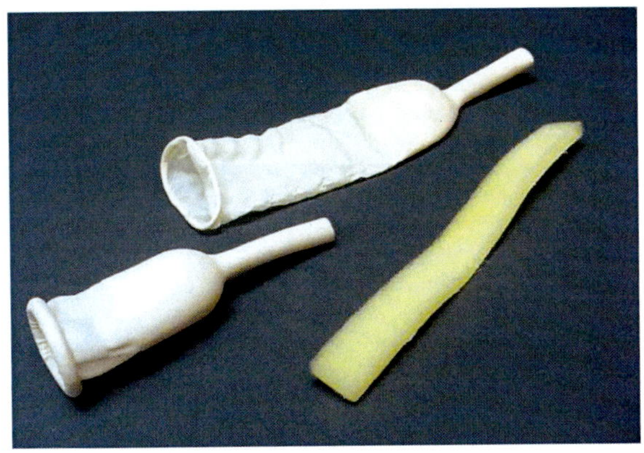

Fig. 1.29: Condom catheter

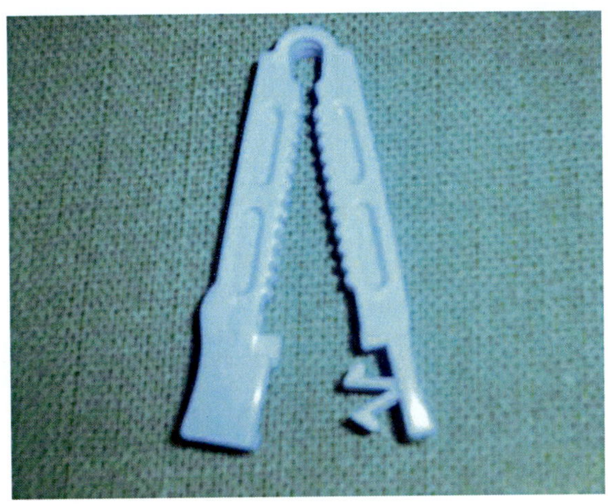

Fig. 1.30: Cord clamp

PLATE 6

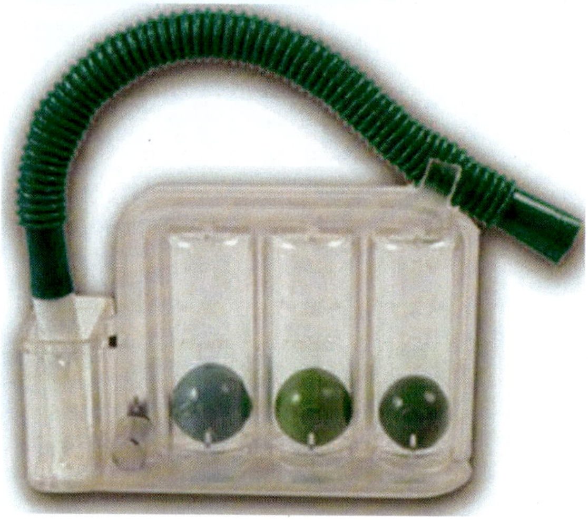

Fig. 1.31: Respiratory exerciser

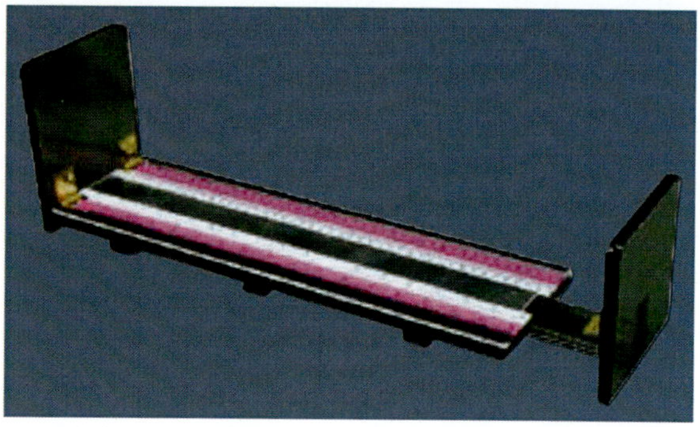

Fig. 1.33: Infantometer

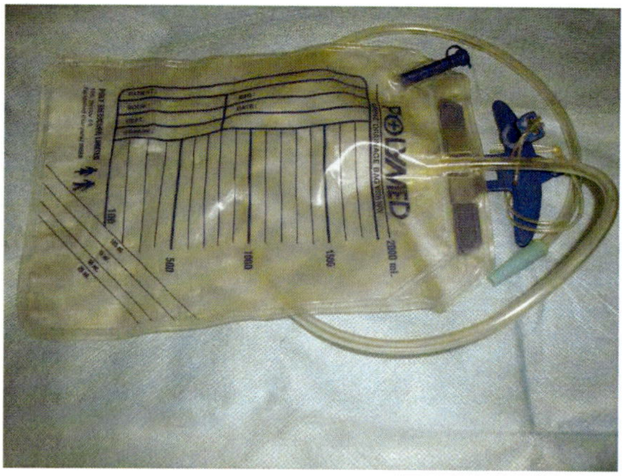

Fig. 1.32: Urine collecting bag

SECTION–I

BASICS OF PRACTICAL PEDIATRICS

CHAPTER 1

INSTRUMENTS

LARYNGOSCOPE (FIG. 1.1)

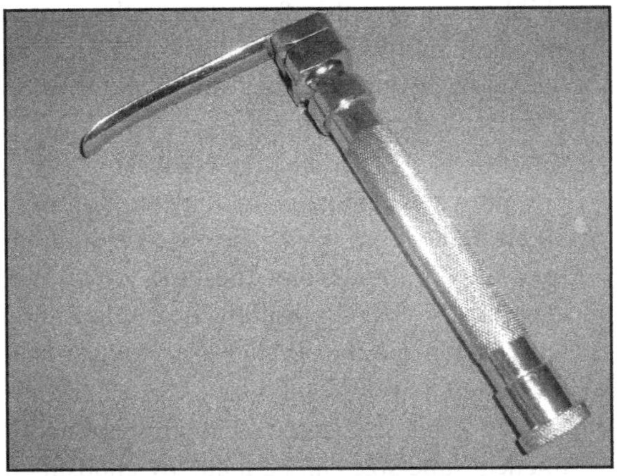

Fig. 1.1: Laryngoscope
(For color version, see Plate 1)

- The laryngoscope consists of a handle (which also contains the batteries), blade and light source.
- The blade can be either a straight blade (Miller) or a curved blade (Macintosh).
- Straight blade is preferred for infants and toddlers since it provides better visualization of glottis but a curved blade is preferred for older children since its broader blade facilities displacement of tongue and visualization of the glottis.
- Laryngoscope is designed to be held in left hand – by both right and left handed persons. If held in right hand, the closed covered part of blade will block your view of glottis, as well as make insertion of ET tube impossible.
- Turn on the laryngoscope light and hold the Laryngoscope in your left hand, between your thumb and first two or three fingers, with the blade pointing away from you. One or two fingers should be left free to rest on baby's face to provide stability.

SIZES

- Zero (Preterm neonate)
- One (Term neonate and infant)
- Two (Children)
- Three (Adolescent)

USES

Therapeutic

- Endotracheal intubation
- Suction catheter placement
- Magill forceps placement for foreign body removal

Diagnostic

- Direct Laryngoscopy in papilloma, diphtheria

STERILIZATION

- Autoclaving

COMPLICATIONS

- Injury like dislodgement of tooth
- Bradycardia
- Hypoxia

ENDOTRACHEAL TUBE (FIG.1.2)

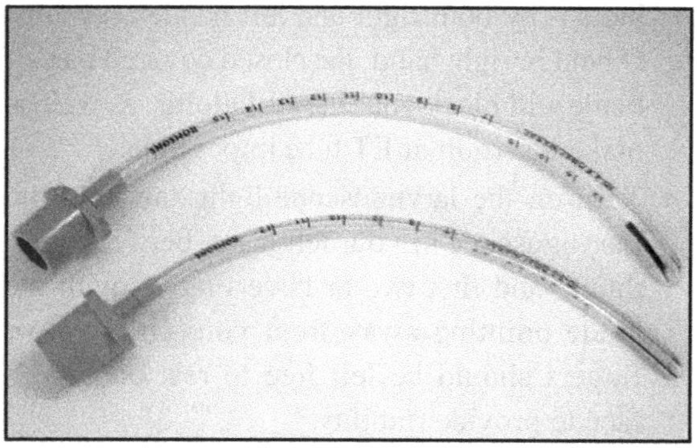

Fig. 1.2: Endotracheal tube
(For color version, see Plate 1)

The endotracheal tube should be sterile, disposable and constructed of translucent polyvinyl chloride with a radiopaque marker.

- An endotracheal tube of uniform internal diameter is preferrable to a tapered tube.
- 15 mm adapter is firmly affixed to the proximal end for attachment to a ventilating device.
- The distal end of the endotracheal tube may provide an opening in the sidewall (*Murphy eye*) to reduce the risk of right-upper-lobe atelectasis. The Murphy eye also reduces the likelihood of complete endotracheal tube obstruction if the end opening is occluded.
- The endotracheal tube should have distance markers (in centimeter) for use as reference points during placement and to facilitate detection of unintentional endotracheal tube movement. 1 cm graduation markings are to ascertain insertion depth while 2 cm indicator mark assists positioning of tube past the vocal cord.
- *Vocal cord guide:* Most ET tubes for neonates have a heavy black line set back from the tip which is meant to be aligned with the vocal cords during tube insertion. This should position the tip of the tube above the bifurcation of the trachea.
- A cuffed endotracheal tube is generally indicated for children aged 8 to 10 years or older. In children younger than 8 to 10 years the normal anatomic narrowing at the level of the cricoid cartilage provides a functional cuff and so uncuffed tube is indicated.
- Inflation is appropriate if an audible air leak is present when ventilation to a pressure of 20 to 30 cm H_2O is provided. The absence of an air leak may indicate that the cuff is inflated excessively, that the endotracheal tube is too large, or that laryngospasm is occurring around the endotracheal tube.
- Simple visual estimates of appropriate endotracheal tube size can be made by choosing a tube with an outside diameter approximating the diameter of the child's little finger (Table 1.1.)

Table 1.1: Size of ET tube

Tube size (mm)	*Weight (gm)*	*Gestation Age (weeks)*
2.5	<1000	Below 28
3.0	1,000-2,000	28-34
3.5	2,000-3,000	34-38
3.5-4.0	Above 3,000	Above 38

$$\text{Size of ET in Age} > 2 \text{ yrs} = \frac{\text{Age in years}}{4} + 4$$

- Depth of insertion in cm (alveolar ridge to midtrachea) for children older than 2 years can be approximated by:

$$\frac{\text{Age in years}}{4}+12$$

Alternatively, the distance of insertion (in cm) can be estimated by multiplying the internal diameter of the tube by 3. For example if i.d. = 4 mm

Depth of insertion = 4 × 3 = 12 cm

USES

General

- Mechanical ventilation
- Intermittent position pressure ventilation (IPPV)
- Direct suctioning of trachea in meconium aspiration
- Epiglottitis and life-threatening croup
- Tetanus (for long-term basis, tracheostomy is preferable)
- Diphtheria
- Angioneurotic edema.

Neonatal Resuscitation

- Prolonged bag and mask ventilation
- Ineffective bag and mask ventilation
- Diaphragmatic hernia.
- Meconium aspiration syndrome.

DRUGS GIVEN THROUGH ENDOTRACHEAL TUBE

- Epinephrine
- Atropine
- Naloxone
- Isoproteronol
- Lignocaine

COMPLICATIONS

- Hypoxia/apnea
- Injury
- Pneumothorax
- Bradycardia
- Obstruction

SELF-INFLATING BAG (FIGS 1.3A AND B)

There are seven basic parts to a self-inflating bag:

1. Air inlet and attachment site for oxygen reservoir
2. Oxygen inlet
3. Patient outlet
4. Valve assembly
5. Oxygen reservoir
6. Pressure release (pop-off) valve
7. Pressure manometer attachment site

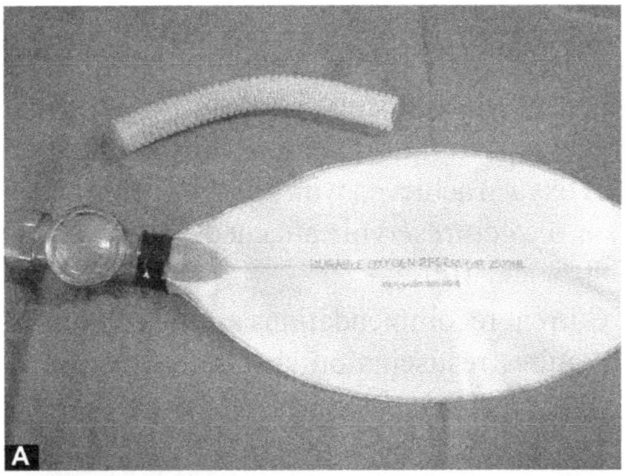

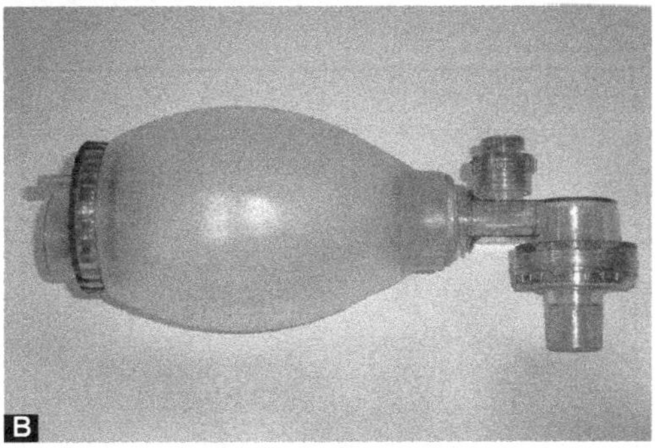

Figs 1.3A and B: Self-inflating bag with oxygen reservior
(For color version, see Plate 1)

- As the bag re-expands following compression, gas is drawn into the bag through a one way valve called *air inlet.*
- Every self-inflating bag has an *oxygen inlet*, which is a small nipple or projection to which oxygen tubing is attached.
- The *patient outlet* is where gas exits from the bag to the baby and where the mask or endotracheal tube attaches.
- When the bag is squeezed during ventilation, the valve opens, releasing oxygen/air to the patient. When the bag reinflates the valve is closed. This prevents the patient's exhaled air from entering the bag and being re-breathed.
- Most self-inflating bags have a *pressure-release valve* (*pop-off valve*) which is generally set to 30 to 40 cm H_2O. If pressure greater than this is generated, the valve closes.
- Concentration of oxygen actually received by the patient without reservoir is 40%. High concentrations of oxygen can be achieved by using an *oxygen reservoir*. The concentration of oxygen achieved with a self-inflating bag with an oxygen reservoir attached will be between 90% and 100%.
- Current recommendations are that a baby who requires resuscitation should be given a high concentration of oxygen (90 to 100%).

FACE MASK (FIG. 1.4)

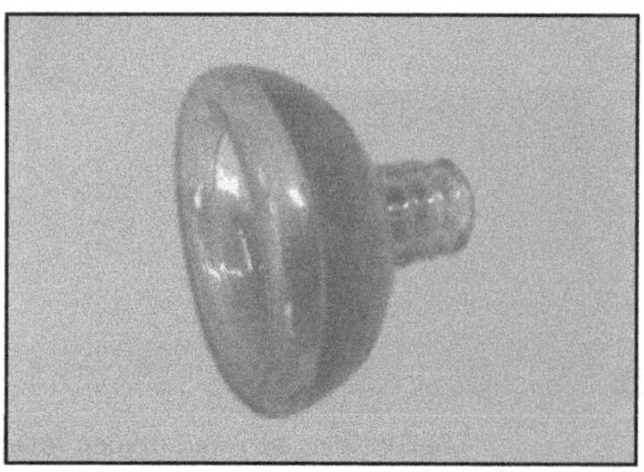

Fig. 1.4: Face mask *(For color version, see Plate 1)*

- Resuscitation masks have thin rims that are either cushioned or noncushioned.
- The rim on a cushioned mask makes it easier to form a seal. It requires less pressure on newborns face to obtain a seal. There is less chance of damaging the newborn's eyes.
- A mask with noncushioned rim, makes more difficult to obtain a seal, can damage the eyes, and can bruise the newborn's face.
- Two shapes are available—Round and Anatomically shaped.
- For the mask to be of *correct size*, the rim will cover the tip of the chin, the mouth, and the nose but not the eyes. Too large may cause possible eye damage. Too small will not cover the mouth and nose and may occlude the nose.

OXYGEN MASK (FIG. 1.5)

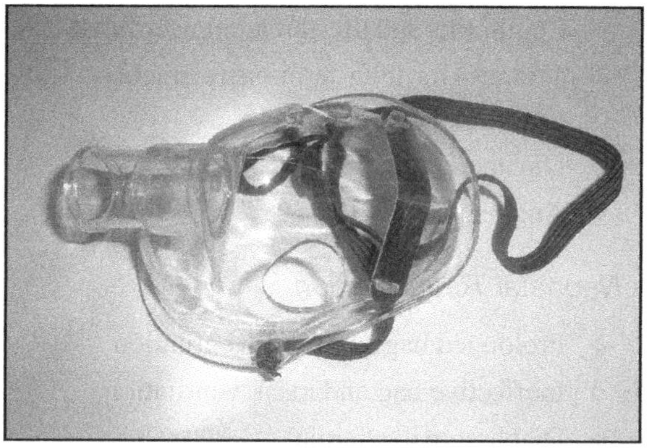

Fig. 1.5: Oxygen mask
(For color version, see Plate 1)

- It has elongated design for visual patient assessment (cyanosis, regurgitation) with adjustable nose clip and elastic head strip which helps in proper positioning of mask on mouth and nasal area.
- It also has exhalation ports in the side and between mask and face.
- Lumen tube is provided to ensure continuous flow of oxygen.

- Proximal end of tube is fitted with soft funnel shaped connector for easy connection to oxygen source.
- It should have low under mask volume (dead space) which will decrease the chances of rebreathing of exhaled gases.

Uses

- ❖ Administration of oxygen (with gas flow rate of 6-18 L/min, it provides 30-60% of oxygen)
- ❖ Nebulization
- ❖ Provide supplemental oxygen for shorter period of time like transportation.

DISADVANTAGES

- Interference with feeding and suction procedures
- If oxygen flow rate is less than 6 L/min, rebreathing of exhaled CO_2.
- Tightly fitted mask is not accepted by children and poorly fitted mask provide only 30-40 percent oxygen.
- Variable FiO_2 delivery.

NASAL OXYGEN CATHETER (FIGS 1.6A AND B)

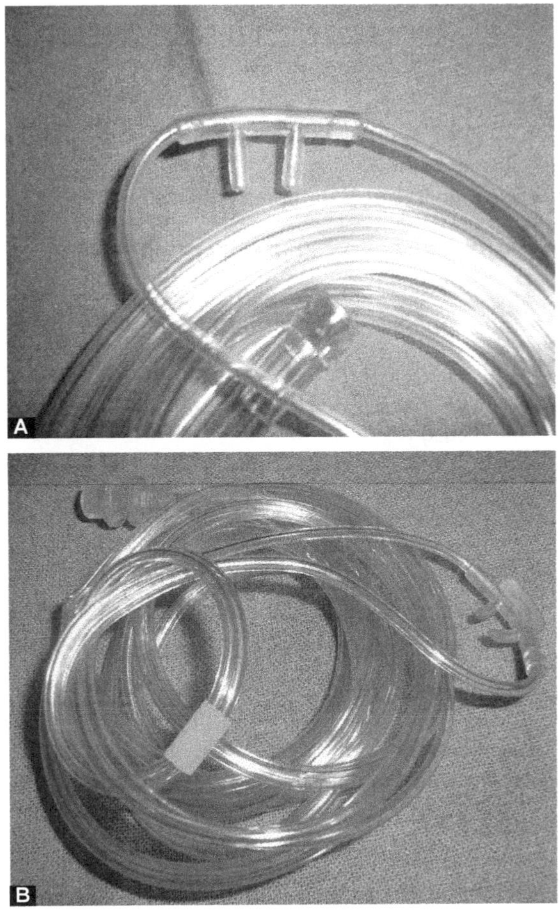

Figs 1.6A and B: Nasal oxygen catheter
(For color version, see Plate 2)

- It contains soft twin prong nasal tips to ensure equal volume of oxygen to both air passages and has star lumen main tube to avoid accidental blockage.
- Prongs are inserted into anterior nares and oxygen is delivered into nasopharynx.
- Sizes available: Adult and paediatric.

Use

Administration of oxygen (with gas flow rate of 2-4 L/ min, it provides 30-40% of oxygen).

ADVANTAGES

- CPAP
- Leaves mouth free for nutritional purpose.

DISADVANTAGES

- Does not provide humidified oxygen
- Frequent displacement of prongs
- Nasal mucosa injury.
- Contraindicated in chonal atresia, deviated nasal septum, nasal polyp.

OTHER OXYGEN DELIVERY DEVICES

- Oxygen mask
- Oxygen hood
- Nasal cannula
- Nasopharyngeal catheter.

MONITORING OXYGEN THERAPY

- Clinical assessment by color.
- Pulse oximetry:
  - Recommended levels of oxygen saturation- 89-95%.
  - Pulse oximetry is based on measurement of the proportion of light transmitted by oxy-genated forms of hemoglobin; a sensor is placed over a finger, toe, earlobe, or the bridge of the nose, and a numerical output is produced.
  - Pulse oximetry is generally accurate only for oxygen saturations greater than 80%; therefore, arterial blood gas analysis is recommended for oxygen saturations less than 80%.
- PaO_2 estimation by arterial blood gas analysis
- Transcutaneous oxygen measurement for SpO_2 monitoring
- Estimation of tissue oxygenation by estimation of serial lactate.

Strategies to Improve Oxygenation

- Noninvasive
  - Prone position
  - Relief of pain
  - Correction of anemia and shock
- Invasive
  - Hyperbaric oxygen
  - Conventional mechanical ventilation
  - High frequency ventilation
  - Nitric oxide therapy
  - Extracorporeal membrane oxygenation.

ACRYLIC OXYGEN HOOD (FIG. 1.7)

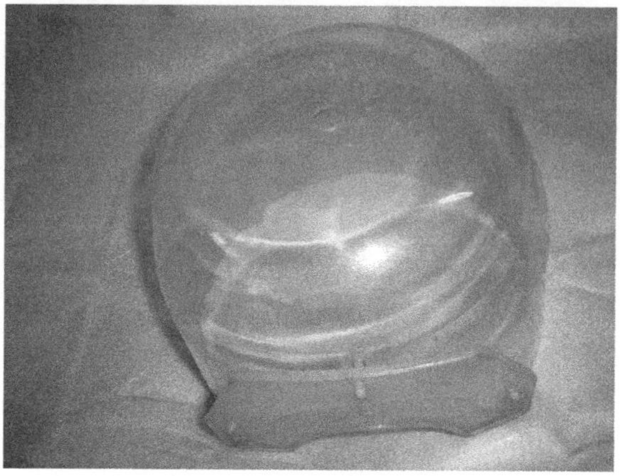

Fig. 1.7: Acrylic oxygen hood
(For color version, see Plate 2)

It is clear transparent acrylic shell that encompasses the infant's head with oxygen inlet nozzle and port hole for easy access. With gas flow rate of 10-12 L/ min it provides 80-90% of oxygen. A minimum gas flow of 4L/min is necessary to avoid rebreathing of O_2.

Uses

- Hypoxemia
- Oxygen administration

ADVANTAGES

- Humidification decreases the size of oxygen molecule, therefore, reaches alveoli easily.
- Humidification prevents drying of secretions as dried secretions may block the airway.
- Well tolerated by infant.
- Allows easy access to rest of body.
- No risk of airway obstruction and gastric dilatation.

DISADVANTAGES

- Prolonged exposure to humidified oxygen increases the risk of cutaneous fungal infections.

- Low temperature within enclosure system may result in cold stress injury.
- Inadequate oxygen flow rate, may result in hypoxia or hypercapnia.
- Any opening in the enclosure may result in decrease in the concentration of oxygen.
- Difficulty in feeding and suction procedures.
- Carbon dioxide build up can occur.

Sterilization: Autoclaving

INFANT FEEDING TUBE (FIG.1.8)

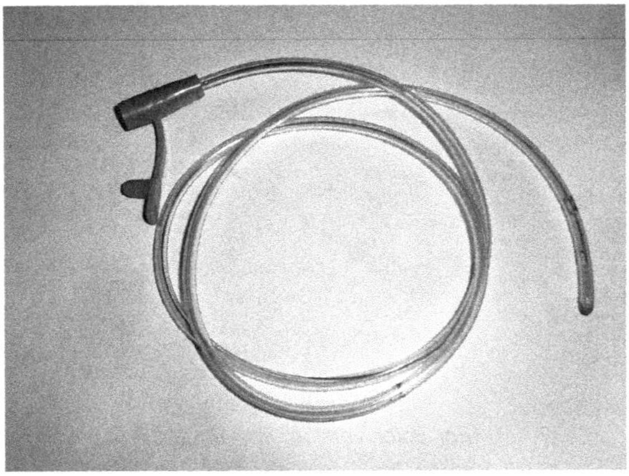

Fig. 1.8: Infant feeding tube
(For color version, see Plate 2)

- It has closed distal end with two lateral eyes and soft and rounded tip to prevent trauma during application.
- Length is 52 cm and is marked at 25 cm from the tip for accurate placement.
- Radiopaque line is provided throughout the length for X-ray visualization.
- Proximal end is fitted with mount for easy connection to feeding funnel or syringe.
- Color coding is done for size identification.

HOW TO INSERT

- Always measure the length of the tube. The length of the inserted tube should be equal to the distance from the *Bridge* of the nose to the tragus and from the tragus to the *Xiphoid Process* (the lower tip of the sternum).
- Insert the tube through the mouth rather than the nose. The nose should be left open for ventilation. Ventilation can be resumed as soon as the tube has been placed.
- Once the tube is inserted the desired distance, attach a syringe and gently remove the gastric contents.
- Remove the syringe from the tube and leave the end of the tube open to provide a vent for air entering the stomach.
- A large tube may cause difficulty in making a seal. A smaller tube can be occluded by secretions.

Uses

- Feeding
  - Gavage feeding in infants < 34 weeks of gestation
  - Feeding of child with respiratory distress, bulbar palsy, polio, unconscious child and palatopharyngeal insufficiency
  - Forced feeding in protein energy malnutrition
- Aspiration
  - Gastric aspirate for shake test, acid-fast bacilli, macrophages, polymorphs, fungus, poisoning.
  - To decompress stomach in intestinal obstruction
  - In unconscious child
- Bag and mask ventilation (prolonged) to avoid gastric distention
- Injecting drugs per rectal, enema
- Gastric lavage
- Catheterization
- Umbilical catheterization for ABG, blood sampling, exchange transfusion

- Detect congenital anomalies:
  - Choanal atresia
  - Anal atresia
  - Tracheo-esophageal fistula
  - Meatal Stenosis:
    - Infant (inability to insert FG 5)
    - 4 years (inability to insert FG 8)
    - 10 years (inability to insert FG 10)

SUCTION CATHETER (FIGS 1.9A AND B)

- Atraumatic, soft and rounded open tip with two lateral eyes
- For removal of secretion from oropharynx and trachea
- Length: 52 cm.

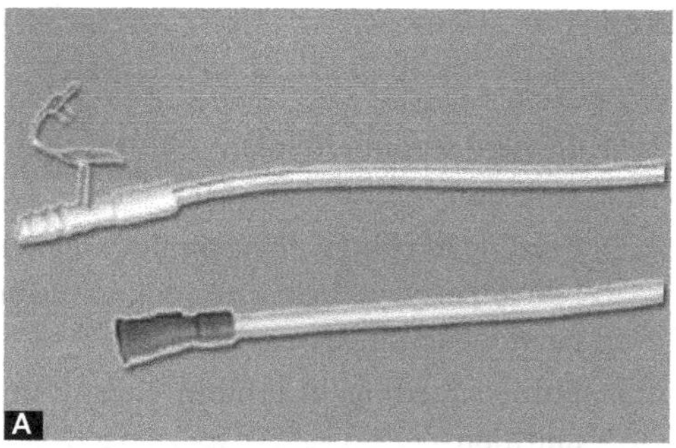

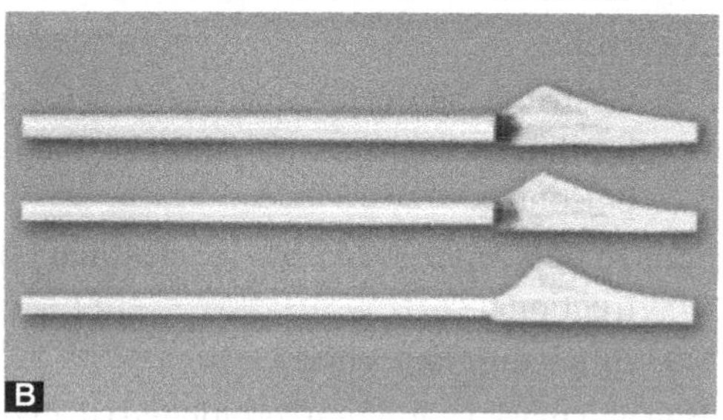

Figs 1.9A and B: Suction catheter
(For color version, see Plate 2)

UMBILICAL CATHETER (FIG. 1.10)

- Designed for intermittent or continual access to the umbilical artery or vein of the newly born or premature baby
- Tube with radiopaque line, marked at every cm from 5 to 25 cm from the open distal tip for accurate placement:
  - 1st marking: Under surface of liver
  - 2nd marking: Hepatic vein
  - 3rd marking: Inferior venae cava
- Open distal end without lateral eyes eliminates the chance of clot formation in the blind spaces

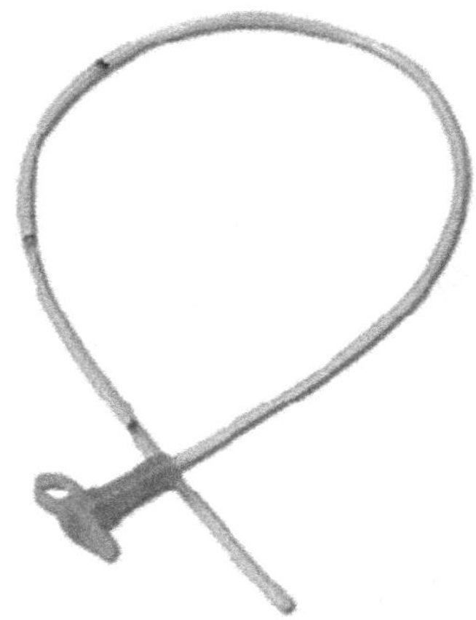

Fig. 1.10: Umbilical catheter
(For color version, see Plate 3)

- Has female flexible mount and luer lock
- Color coded funnel end connector for easy identification of size
- *Length* : 40 cm
- *Sizes available* : FG 4, 5, 6, 8
- *Optimal length for umbilical vein catheterization*: 20 percent of crown heel length or 50 percent of shoulder umbilicus length.

Uses

Can be used with venous or arterial routes for
- Infusion
- Transfusion
- Administration of medication
- Blood sampling
- CVP monitoring.

COMPLICATIONS

Immediate

- Bleeding
- Thromboembolism
- Infection.

Late

- Portal hypertension (extrahepatic)

DILEYS MUCUS EXTRACTOR (FIG. 1.11)

- It has atraumatic, soft and rounded, open tip with two lateral eyes and clear transparent container permiting visual examination of aspirate.
- Spare screw top lid is provided to seal the container for safe transportation of specimen to the laboratory or aseptic disposal of container
- Suction tube lengths available: 40 cm, 50 cm
- Capacity: 25 ml.
- Pressure: 100 mm Hg.

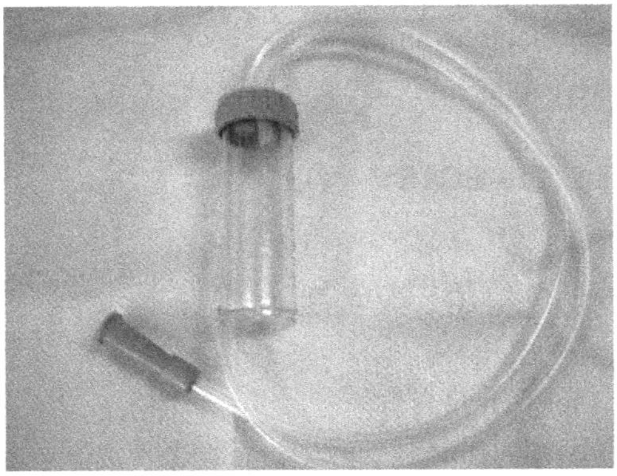

Fig. 1.11: Dileys mucus extractor
(For color version, see Plate 3)

Uses

- Obtaining mucus specimen for microbiological examination
- Aspiration of secretion from oropharynx of newborn babies to ensure free respiration.

TONGUE DEPRESSOR (FIG. 1.12)

Uses

- To see the gag reflex
- To examine the pharynx, oral cavity and tonsils
- To examine the movements of the palate and the uvula
- *Spatula test* – To test for the spasm of the masseter muscle in a suspected tetanus case by trying to insert the tongue depressor in between the teeth.

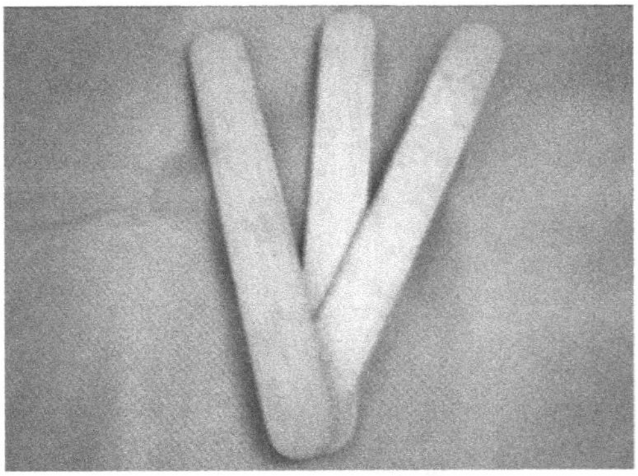

Fig. 1.12: Tongue depressor
(For color version, see Plate 3)

TUBERCULIN SYRINGE (FIG. 1.13)

It is a 1 cc syringe with a white piston (plastic syringes) or metal piston (glass syringes).

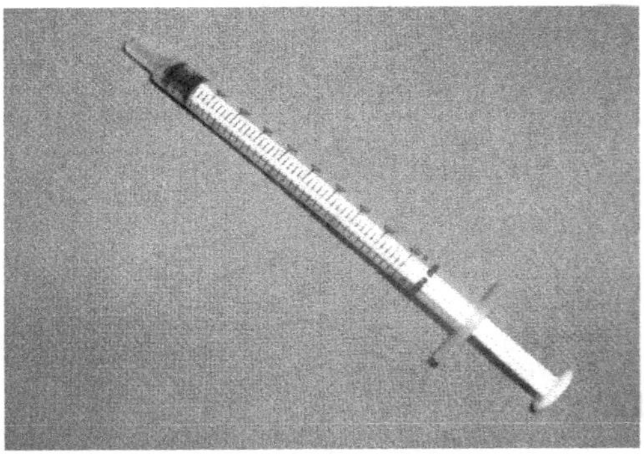

Fig. 1.13: Tuberculin syringe
(For color version, see Plate 3)

Uses

- To administer PPD for Mantoux test
- To administer BCG vaccine
- To administer test doses of drugs such as Penicillin
- Provocative testing – To test for allergens in bronchial asthma, atopy
- Insulin injection in diabetes mellitus. (1cc is graduated to 40, 80 or 100 units)
- Giving small doses of drugs e.g. Digoxin.

INHALERS (FIGS 1.14A AND B)

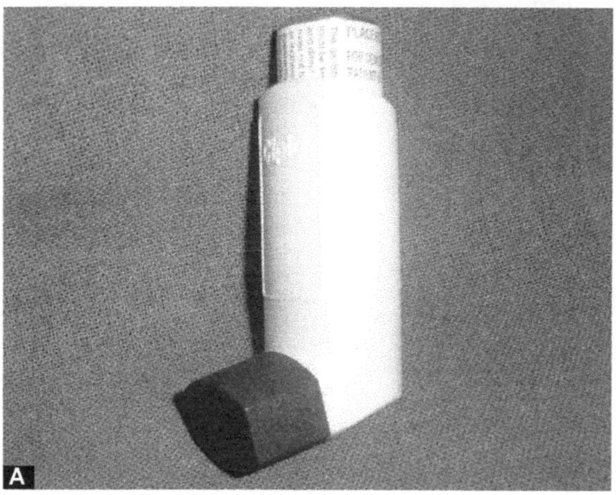

A

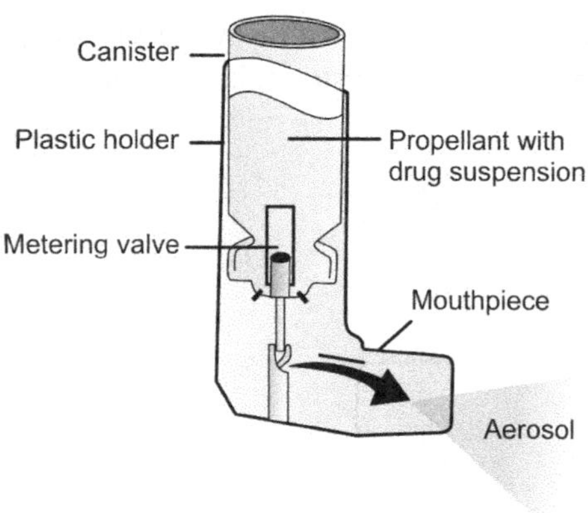

B

Figs 1.14A and B: Metered dose inhaler
(For color version of Figure 1.14A, see Plate 3)

METERED DOSE INHALER

- Most commonly used device
- Cannister with drug (1%), surfactant, preservatives and propellent (80%) (CFC/HFA)
- Metered dose chamber (finite volume released)
- A metering valve that dispenses a constant volume of a solution or suspension of the drug in the propellant.

DRUGS DELIVERED THROUGH MDI

- β_2 agonist
- Ipratropium bromide
- Inhaled steroids—beclamethasone, budesonide, fluticasone
- Mast cell stabilizers—cromolyn sodium, nedocromolyn.

Uses

- Bronchial asthma (acute episode and symptomatic asthma)
- Hyperkalemia

SIDE EFFECTS

- Tremors
- Oral thrush
- Ankle edema
- Tachycardia
- Hypokalemia.

ADVANTAGES

- Portable
- Quick delivery
- Precise and constant dose
- Light, compact, resistant to moisture
- No drug preparation
- No contamination of contents.

DISADVANTAGES

- Needs hand breath coordination
- *Cold Freon effect* (inability to breath when propellent is released in mouth)
- Contains CFC
- Used with spacer (increases cost)
- Time consuming to teach
- Oropharyngeal deposition

How to Use Metered Dose Inhaler

- Remove cap and shake inhaler in vertical direction
- Breathe out gently
- Put mouthpiece in mouth and at start of inspiration which should be slow and deep, press canister down and continue to inhale deeply
- Hold breath for seconds or as long as possible then breathe out slowly
- Wait for few seconds before repeating above steps.

How to Use Metered Dose Inhaler with Spacer Device

- Remove cap, shake inhaler and insert into spacer device
- Place mouthpiece of spacer in mouth
- Start breathing in and out gently and observe movements of valve
- Once breathing pattern is established press canister and continue to breath 5-10 times (tidal breathing)
- Remove the device from mouth and wait for 3 minutes before repeating above steps

How to Use MDI + Spacer + Baby Mask

- Attach baby mask to the mouth end of spacer
- Shake MDI and insert it in the MDI end of spacer device
- Cover baby's mouth and nose with baby mask
- Press canister and encourage the child to take tidal breathing with mouth open (if possible) 5-10 times
- Remove baby mask and wait for 30-60 seconds before repeating above steps.

WHY YOU MUST SHAKE MDI

You must shake MDI before each actuation to give correct mix of propellent and medication as one is heavier than the other.

FLOAT TEST (FIG. 1.15)

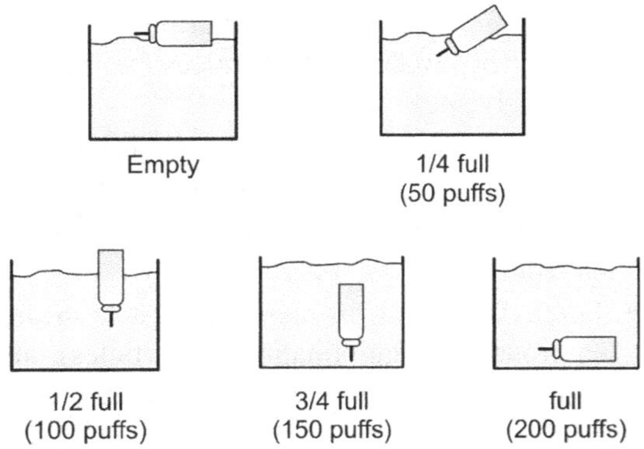

Fig. 1.15: Float test

HOW TO PRIME MDIS

- If a new inhaler OR if you have not used the MDI for one week spray two doses into the air before use to mix properly and check it working.

Aerosol Delivery Systems

- MDI: Metered dose inhalers
- DPI: Dry powder inhalers
- Nebulizers

Selection of Device

- < 3 years : Metered dose inhaler + Spacer + mask
- 3-6 years : Metered dose inhaler +Spacer
- > 6 years : Metered dose inhaler + Spacer OR Dry powder inhaler

PARTICLE SIZE

MMAD	:Mass median aerodynamic diameter
MMAD <1µm	:Exhaled out
MMAD 1~5µm	:Target particle that reaches lung
MMAD >5µm	:Deposited in oropharynx

DRY POWDER INHALER (DPI) (FIG. 1.16)

- Rotahaler is used in children above 4-5 years of age
- Contains mouthpiece and reservior
- *Drugs administered*: Salbutamol, Beclomethasone, Budesonide, Fluticasone, Sodium cromoglycate
- They have the advantage of being portable and eliminate the need to co-ordinate actuation with breathing environmental friendly, as they do not contain CFC
- There may be a problem in high humidity environment (agglutination of particles), and high oropharyngeal deposition of drugs.

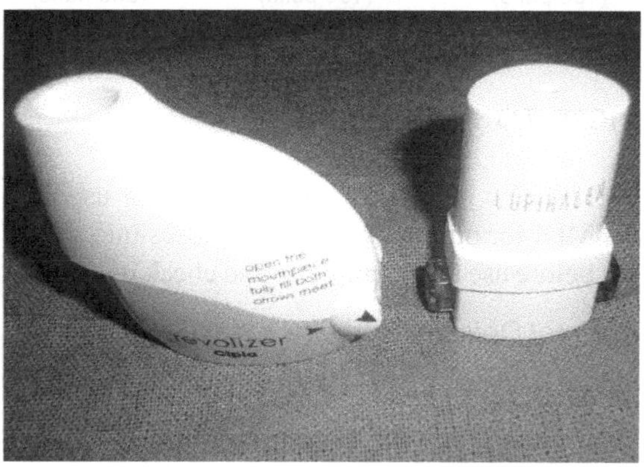

Fig. 1.16: Dry powder inhaler (DPI)
(For color version, see Plate 3)

Comparison between Metered Dose Inhaler and Dry Powder Inhaler

MDI

- Contains CFC
- High velocity aerosols
- Requires hand breath co ordination
- Delivery of medicines independent of external factors
- Time consuming to teach
- Requires deep and slow breathing only.

DPI

- No CFC
- Aerosol velocity depends on inspiratory flow rate
- No hand breath coordination needed
- Delivery of medication largely dependent on external factors
- Easy to teach
- Requires high inspiratory flow >28 L/min.

NEBULIZER CHAMBER (FIG. 1.17)

- Nebulizers are used for delivering nebulized β-agonist in acute severe asthma.
- Dose of salbutamol used in nebulizers is 0.15 mg/kg/dose at 0, 20 min and 40 min and then depending on the response of patient 2 hourly or 4 hourly.

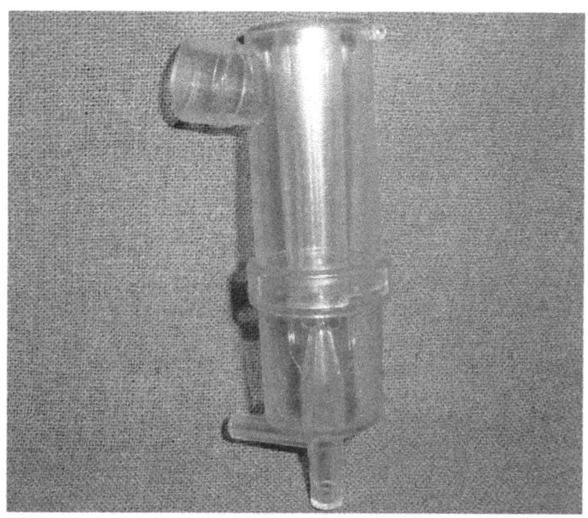

Fig. 1.17: Nebulizer chamber
(For color version, see Plate 4)

STEPS TO USE NEBULIZER

1. Calculate the dose of medicine (0.15 mg/kg/dose; minimum dose: 1.25 mg)
2. Add saline to make a fill volume of 3-5 ml.
3. Switch on the compressor and give aerosol for 8-10 minutes.
4. As many patients are hypoxic, oxygen from central supply or a oxygen cylinder should be given, at a flow rate of 6-8 L/minute in place of compressed air.
5. Nebulization is given over 8-10 minutes, till you hear a spluttering sound.

Can we combine two drugs:
- Avoid combining steroids with other medications
- Can combine salbutamol and ipratropium

What is the optimal total volume:
- 3-5 ml

What should be time for nebulization:
- 8-10 minutes.

The following measures can improve the amount of drug delivered to the lung by nebulizer.
- The total fill volume should be about 3-5 mL
- Tapping the sides
- The optimal flow rate is 6-12 L/min, 30-50% of aerosol are in the respirable range of 1-5 µm
- Slow deep inhalations and breath holding can improve delivery:

Drug Delivery

Device	Drug delivery
• MDI + Spacer	10-15 %
• MDI	5-10 %
• DPI	5-10 %
• Nebulizer	1-5 %

SPACER (FIG. 1.18)

- Holding chamber/resevoir types:
  - Small volume/large volume
  - With/without valve
  - Polyamide/polycarbonate.

Home made: water bottle

Usually of 140–750 mL capacity. Incorporates one way valve that permits aerosol to be drawn from chamber during inhalation only, diverting exhaled gas to atmosphere & not disturbing remaining aerosol suspended in the chamber. Combines the benefits of spacer with advantage of protecting the patient from loss of dose due to poor hand breath coordination.

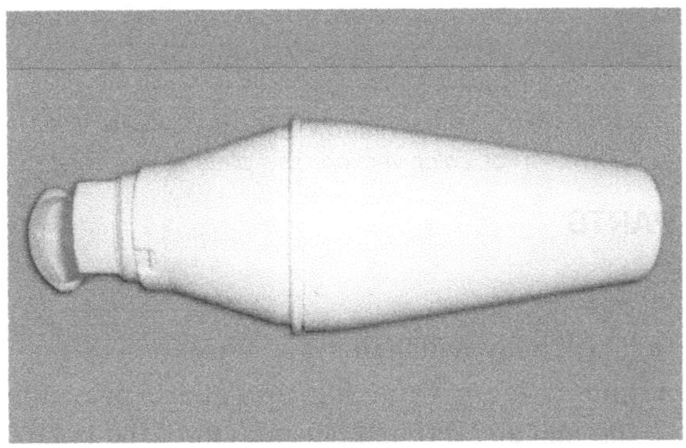

Fig. 1.18: Volume spacer
(For color version, see Plate 4)

ADVANTAGES

- No need to actuate with inspiration
- Increased drug deposition in lungs
- Less deposition in mouth
- *Eliminates Cold Freon effect:* (inability to breath when propellent is released in mouth)
- Decreased chance of oral thrush
- As effective as nebulizer.

DISADVANTAGES

- Initiation can be more complex
- More expensive than MDI alone
- Less portable than MDI alone
- Can reduce dose if not correctly given.

BONE MARROW ASPIRATION NEEDLE (FIG. 1.19)

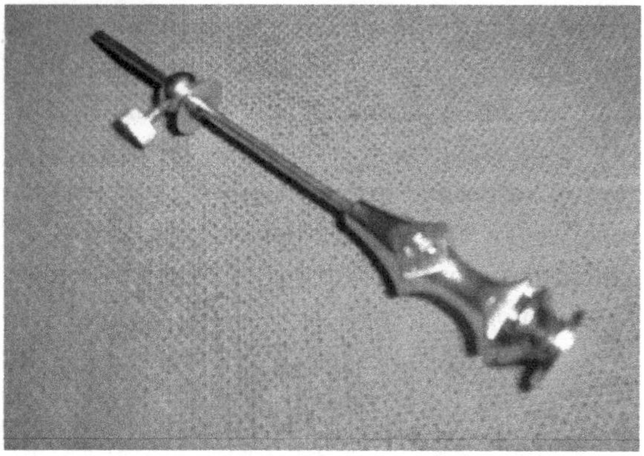

Fig. 1.19: Bone marrow aspiration needle
(For color version, see plate 4)

PARTS

- Stillete
- Thick body with nail
- Guard 2 cm from the tip (guard prevents through and through penetration of the bone).

USES

Bone marrow aspiration.

SITE

1. Posterior iliac crest (both aspiration and biopsy)
2. Sternum (aspiration only in adults)
3. Anterior iliac crest (both aspiration and biopsy).

Indications

Diagnostic

- Idiopathic thrombocytopenic purpura
- Aplastic anemia
- Leukemia
- Megaloblastic anemia
- Storage disorders, e.g. Gaucher's disease
- Infection, e.g. kala azar
- Pyrexia of unknown origin
- Myelofibrosis.

Therapeutic

- Bone marrow transplantation

CONTRAINDICATIONS

- Coagulation disorders like hemophilia
- Infection at biopsy area.

COMPLICATIONS

- Infection
- Bleeding
- Cardiac injury (if deep penetration occurs in sternal aspiration).

BONE TREPHINE BIOPSY (FIG. 1.20)

The Jamshidi needle is the most popular needle for this procedure. The needle is tapered at the distal end to help retain the specimen. Currently, disposable needles are used.

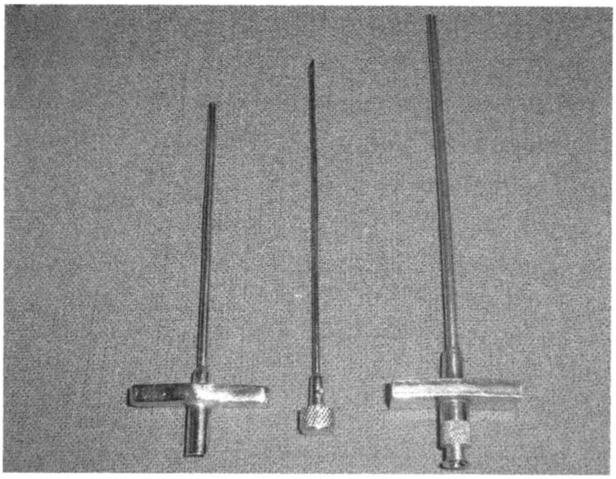

Fig. 1.20: Bone trephine biopsy
(For color version, see Plate 4)

Indications

- Macrocytic anemias in which blood changes are minimal
- Microcytic hypochromic anemias to help distinguish iron deficiency from anemia of chronic disease and sideroblastic anemia

- Normocytic normochromic anemia to detect degree of ineffective erythropoiesis, pure red cell aplasia or aplastic anemia
- Myelofibrosis (dry tap)
- Evaluation of a "dry tap" aspirate
- Acute leukemias
- Lipid storage diseases

LUMBAR PUNCTURE NEEDLE (FIG. 1.21)

It is 10-12 cm in length and stilette of the needle has pin which fits into the slot of the head of the needle. Spinal needle provides exceptional control when penetrating the dura mater.

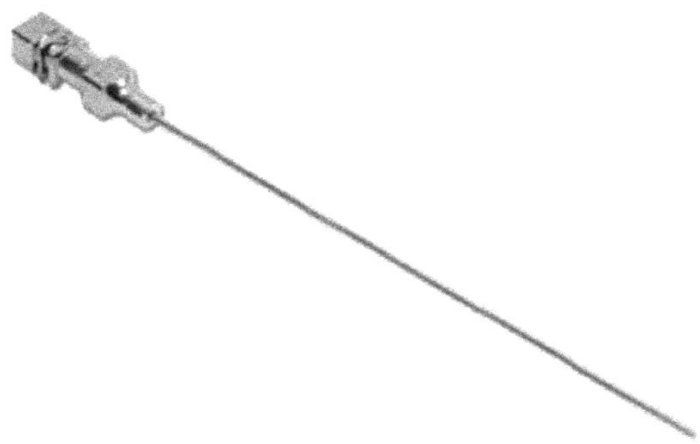

Fig. 1.21: Lumbar puncture needle

Uses

- Lumbar puncture
- Cisternal puncture
- Carotid angiography
- Splenoportogram
- For tapping fluids from the cavity, e.g. ascites or pleural fluids

Note

- In children, ordinary needle is often used for lumbar puncture.
- The advantage with the lumbar puncture needle is that the stilette helps to keep the lumen of the needle patent.

VIM-SILVERMAN'S NEEDLE (FIG. 1.22)

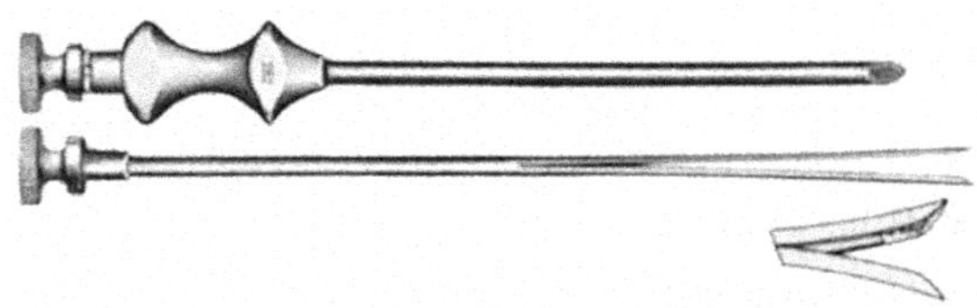

Fig. 1.22: Vim-Silverman's needle

PARTS

- Trocar
- Cannula
- Bifid needle.

ADVANTAGES

Large tissue is obtained and failure rate is low.

DISADVANTAGES

Complications are more compared to trucut needle.

TRUCUT BIOPSY NEEDLE (FIG. 1.23)

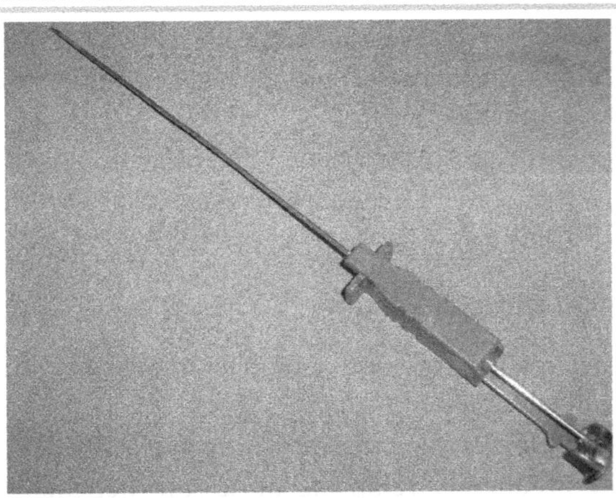

Fig. 1.23: Trucut biopsy needle
(For color version, see Plate 4)

Uses of Biopsy Needle

- Liver biopsy
- Kidney biopsy
- Lung biopsy – rarely

INDICATIONS OF LIVER BIOPSY

Neonate

- Neonatal hepatitis
- Biliary atresia
- Galactosemia.

Children

- Chronic hepatitis
- Cirrhosis
- Metabolic: Wilson's disease, Tyrosinosis, Hemochromatosis
- Malignancy Staging: Wilms' tumor, Hodgkin's lymphoma, Neuroblastoma
- Diagnosis of malignancy: Hepatoma, hepatoblastoma.

INDICATIONS FOR KIDNEY BIOPSY IN NEPHROTIC SYNDROME

At Onset

- Age <1 year or > 8 years
- Persistent microscopic or gross hematuria, low serum C3
- Sustained hypertension (>3 weeks)
- Suspected secondary causes of nephrotic syndrome.

After Initial Treatment

- Proteinuria persisting despite 4 weeks of daily corticosteroid therapy
- Before starting treatment with cyclosporine A
- Frequently relapsing or steroid dependant nephrotic syndrome (discretion of the pediatric nephrologist).

INDICATION FOR KIDNEY BIOPSY IN ACUTE GLOMERULONEPHRITIS

- Systemic features: Fever, rash, joint pain, heart disease.
- Absence of serologic evidence of streptococcal infection; normal levels of C3.
- Mixed picture of AGN and nephrotic syndrome
- Severe anemia, very high levels of blood urea or anuria requiring dialysis.
- Delayed resolution.
  - Oliguria, hypertension and/or azotemia persisting past 2 weeks.
  - Gross hematuria persisting past 3-4 weeks.
  - Low C3 levels beyond 6-8 weeks.
  - Persistent hematuria or proteinuria beyond 6 to 12 months.

THREE WAY (FIG. 1.24)

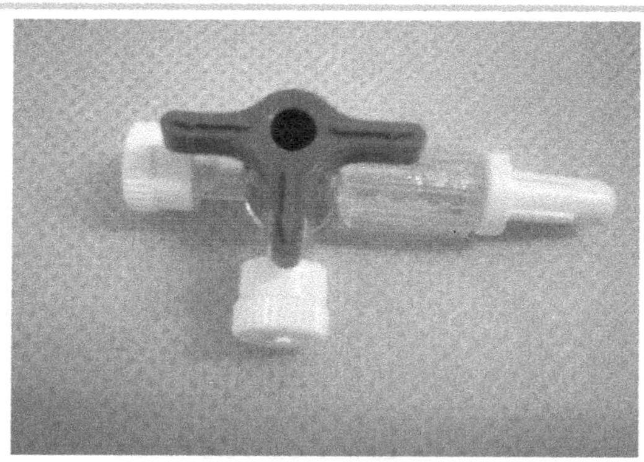

Fig. 1.24: Three way
(For color version, see Plate 4)

- Three way is a T-shaped instrument with two inlets and one outlet. By a screw, either of the inlets can be connected to the outlet.
- Transparent polycarbonate main body facilitates observation of flow. Arrow on the handle indicates the direction of flow.
- Minimum priming volume required for accurate drug administration.

Uses

- It is commonly connected to an intravenous set where through one inlet IV fluids pass and through the other inlet, medications can be given or CVP can be monitored.

- ❖ Aspirating fluid from the body cavities, e.g. pleural tap. Through one inlet fluid is withdrawn from the body cavity and by changing the direction of the screw the fluid from the syringe is pushed into the kidney tray.
- ❖ Exchange transfusion
- ❖ Total parental nutrition
- ❖ Dialysis

MICRODRIP SET (FIG. 1.25)

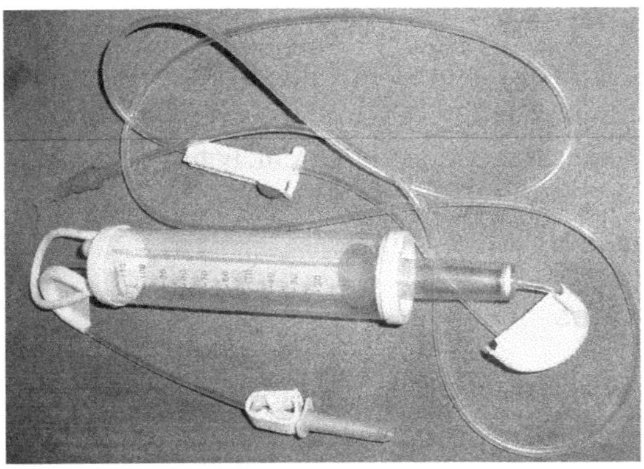

Fig. 1.25: Microdrip set
(For color version, see Plate 5)

- Clear, soft, cylindrical and calibrated measured volume chamber with bold graduation.
- Chamber injection port allows medication to be injected into burette chamber for medication mixture.
- Chamber vent allows air to enter chamber through hydrophobic membrane to prevent solution contamination.
- Burette sizes available: 110 ml, 150 ml.
- 1 ml of it contains 64 drops.
- It contains *Murphy chamber* through which it is possible to regulate the number of drops falling per minute. A fluid level must be maintained in the Murphy's chamber. If the chamber gets full, it has to be reset.
- If you want to give 40 ml/hr fluid through microdrip set, adjust it to set at just 40 drops/min.

Uses

- ❖ Intravenous fluid administration
- ❖ Drug administration
- ❖ Parental nutrition

BLOOD SET (FIG. 1.26)

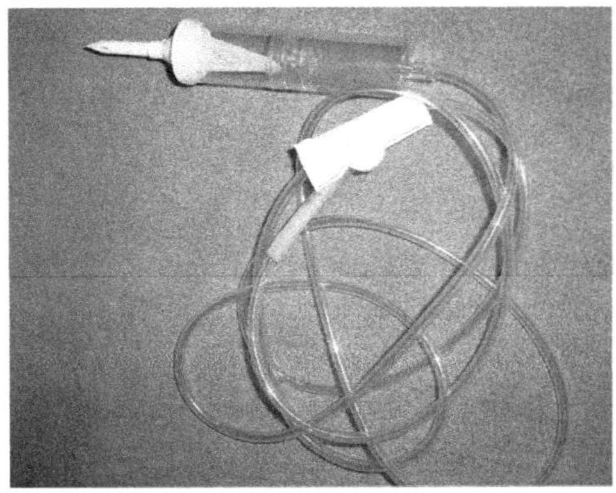

Fig. 1.26: Blood set
(For color version, see Plate 5)

This is similar to intravenous set except that there is a filter in Murphy's chamber that filters out clots. Hence, it is useful when blood has to be transfused.

GUEDEL AIRWAY (FIG. 1.27)

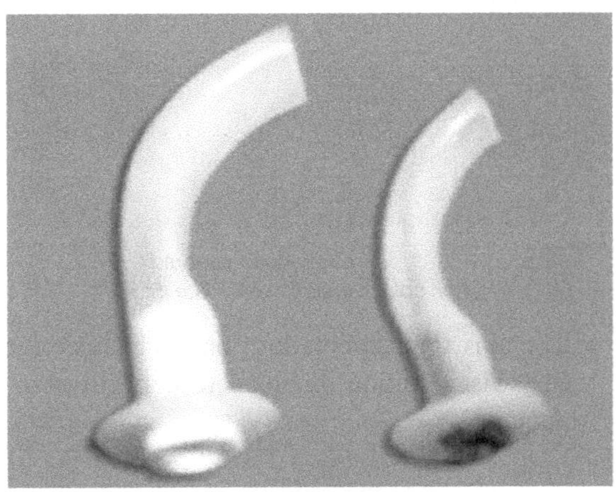

Fig. 1.27: Guedel airway
(For color version, see Plate 5)

- Suitable for maintaining an unobstructed oropharyngeal airway during general anesthesia and in unconscious patients. It has rounded atraumatic edges with smooth airway path for easy cleaning
- *Length* of Guedel airway used is 2/3rd of distance between angle of mouth and temporo-mandibular joint.

Uses

- ❖ Macroglossia
- ❖ Retrognathia
- ❖ Choanal atresia
- ❖ Neonatal resuscitation
- ❖ Seizuring child
- ❖ Unconscious child
- ❖ Pierre Robin syndrome

INTRAVENOUS CANNULA (FIG. 1.28)

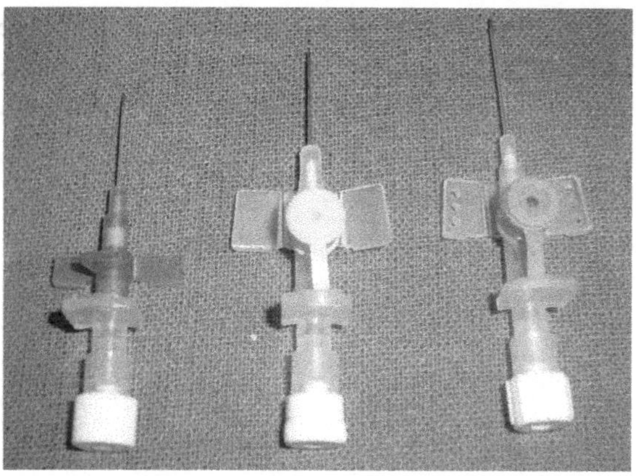

Fig. 1.28: Intravenous cannula
(For color version, see Plate 5)

- Contains transparent flash back chamber for easy visualization of blood to confirm veni-puncture.

Uses

- ❖ Venipuncture

SPHYGMOMANOMETER (BP APPARATUS)

Various phases are:

- Phase I : First appearance of clear, tapping sound. It represents the systolic blood pressure
- Phase II : Tapping sounds are replaced by soft murmurs
- Phase III : Murmurs become louder
- Phase IV : Muffling of sounds
- Phase V : Disappearance of sounds

Diastolic pressure closely corresponds to phase V. However, in aortic regurgitation, the disappearance point is extremely low, sometimes 0 mm Hg and so phase IV is taken as diastolic BP in adults as well as children.

Uses

- ❖ To measure the blood pressure (principal use of the instrument)
- ❖ Hess' capillary fragility test
- ❖ Latent tetany – When the pressure is raised above the systolic BP for 2-3 minutes, typical carpal spasm appears and is known as Trousseau's sign
- ❖ To assess the respiratory reserve – Blow the mercury column (by placing the mouth to the inlet tube) upto 40-50 mm of Hg and try to hold it at this level
- ❖ Diagnosis from recording of BP of lower limb: Lower limb systolic BP > upper limb systolic BP and if crosses 20 mm of Hg, it is known as *Hill's sign*, which is diagnostic of Aortic regurgitation. Again, Lower limb BP < upper limb BP occurs in coarctation of aorta
- ❖ To draw venous blood
- ❖ To draw blood during blood donation

PULSES CONFIRMED BY SPHYGMOMANOMETER

Pulsus paradoxus: Systolic BP is always more in expiration than in inspiration by > 10 mm of Hg.

Water-hammer pulse: Pulse pressure is usually greater than at least 50 mm of Hg.

Pulsus alternans: When the strong beats are heard during measurement of systolic BP (initial part of measurement), the pulse rate remains half of the actual rate (as weak beats do not reach the radial artery). With gradual lowering of the mercury column, the weak beats are also heard and thus, the pulse rate doubles, i.e. returns to the actual pulse rate.

CONDOM CATHETER (FIG. 1.29)

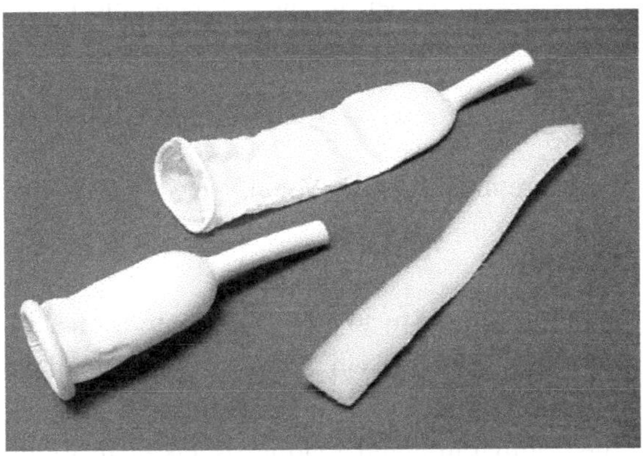

Fig. 1.29: Condom catheter
(For color version, see Plate 5)

- It has penile sheath/External catheter
- Male catheter is specially designed for urine incontinence for day and night use in male patient
- Proximal end is designed for easy connection to urine bag, making it simple to use
- Provided with self-adhesive coated strip for proper fixing on to the penis

CORD CLAMP (FIG. 1.30)

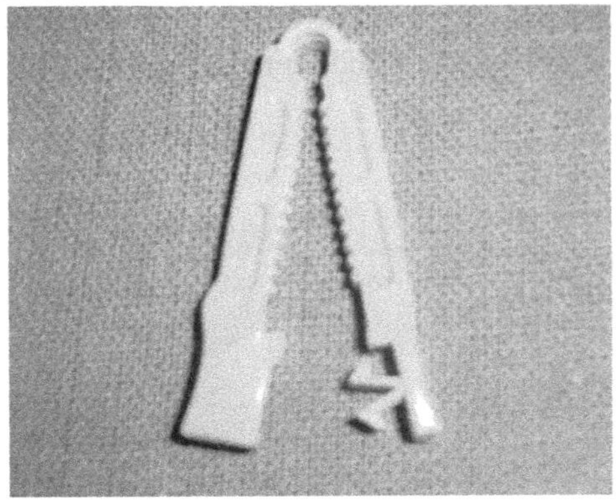

Fig. 1.30: Cord clamp
(For color version, see Plate 5)

- Provided with finger grip for safe and convenient handling
- Security lock to prevent accidental opening after clamping
- Grooved clamping area to prevent slipping of umbilical cord.

Uses

- Clamping the umbilical cord of newborn baby immediately after the birth

RESPIRATORY EXERCISER (FIG. 1.31)

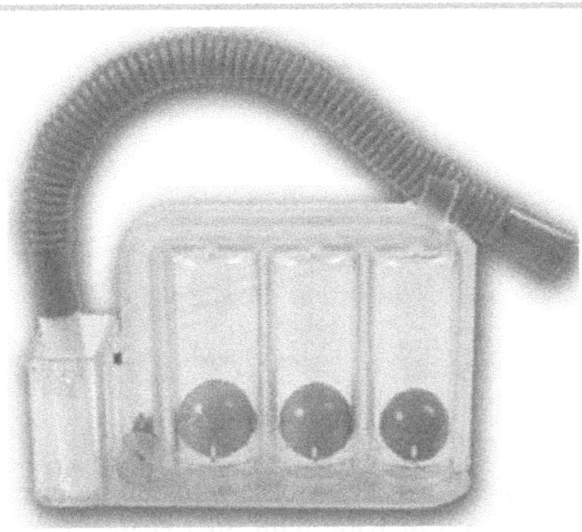

Fig. 1.31: Respiratory exerciser
(For color version, see Plate 6)

- It consists of three balls
- It helps the patient to recover normal respiration after a chest or abdominal surgery

URINE COLLECTION BAG (FIG. 1.32)

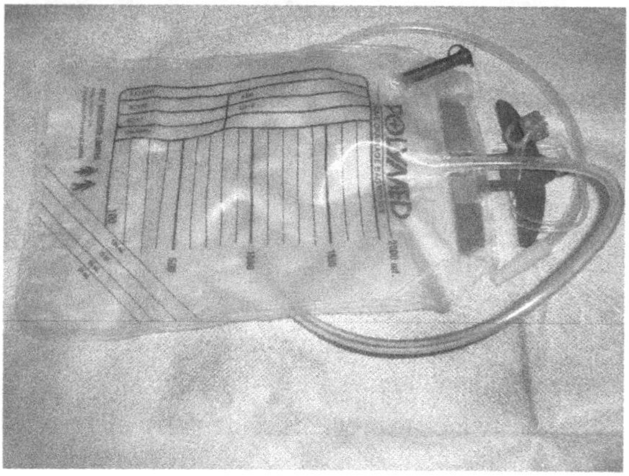

Fig. 1.32: Urine collecting bag
(For color version, see Plate 6)

- Bag graduated in ml to measure urine output
- Contains non-return valve
- Conical inlet connector with cap

INFANTOMETER (FIG. 1.33)

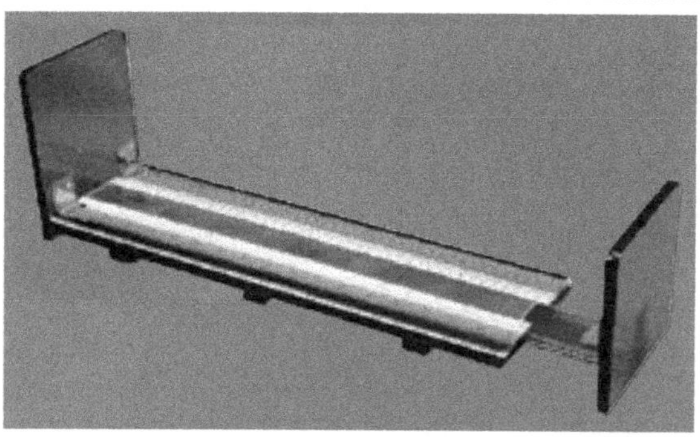

Fig. 1.33: Infantometer
(For color version, see Plate 6)

It has a broad acrylic base with one sliding side as per length of baby with dual scale for direct reading in cm from 0 to 45 and 45 to 90 cm. It has folding sides for easy storage.

Uses

Recording length/height of baby.

SAHLI'S HEMOGLOBINOMETER (FIG. 1.34)

INSTRUMENT

i. *Comparator:* It contains Sahli tube. Comparator has brown tinted glass pieces on either side for color matching an opaque white glass is present at back to provide proper illumination.
ii. *Sahli tube:* Calibrated in gram% hemoglobin (2 to 24) on one side and in percentage (20 to 140) on other side. 100 percent being equivalent to Hb 17.3 g/dl blood.
iii. *Sahli pipette* Graduated to .02 ml (20 mm3) mark with rubber tubing and mouthpiece.
iv. Glass rod stirrer

Uses

Measurement of hemoglobin.

Principle

Blood is diluted in an acid solution, to form acid hematin. The brown color so developed is matched against standard brown tinted glass in the comparator and reading is taken in gram percent.

PROCEDURE

- Fill the Sahli tube to the 20 mark (3 g%) with N/10 HCl
- Draw blood to the 0.02 ml mark of Sahli pipette
- Wipe out any blood stick to the pipette from outside with cotton
- Blow the blood from pipette into Sahli tube containing N/10 HCl

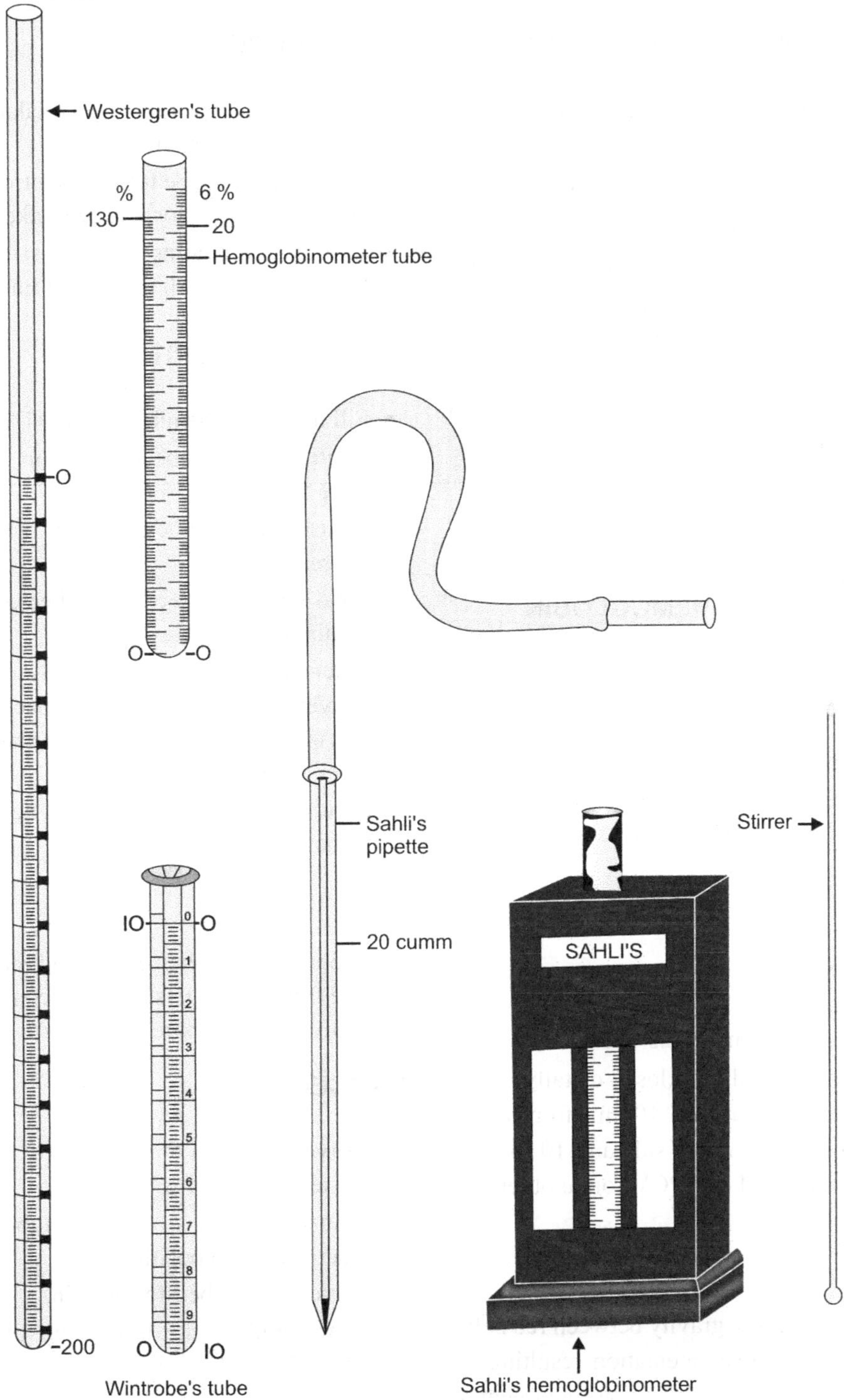

Fig. 1.34: Sahli's hemoglobinometer

- Mix the content quickly by gently shaking the tube
- Keep the Sahli tube back into comparator for 10 min
- Acid reacts with hemoglobin and converts it into acid hematin (brown color)
- Compare it with color of standard com parator
- If the color of blood is darker than that of standard continue to dilute by adding distilled water drop by drop and stir it after adding each drop of distilled water till the color of solution matches with standard.
- Note the reading in gram percent. It gives reading with error of 10%.

OTHER METHODS FOR MEASUREMENT OF HEMOGLOBIN

- Cyanmethemoglobin method—Best method
- Alkaline haematin method
- Oxyhemoglobin method
- Carboxyhemoglobin method
- Copper sulfate specific gravity method.

WINTROBE'S TUBE

INSTRUMENT

- Length 11 cm, diameter 2.5 cm
- It is open at top end and closed distally

It is calibrated from 0 to 10 cm, from above downward (for ESR) on one side and 10 to 0 cm from above downward (for PCV) on another side of tube.

Principle of ESR

Differences in specific gravity between red cells and plasma leads to sedimentation resulting in red cells to form roulex, which are aggregates of large volume but have small surface area.

PROCEDURE

- Fill the Wintrobe tube from oxalate blood with pipette up to zero mark.
- Keep the Wintrobe tube in Wintrobe stand in a vertical position for 1 hr and take the reading.
- Express the reading in mm 1st hour. Normal ESR value: 1 to 10 mm in 1st hour.

PCV (HEMATOCRIT)

- Fill the Wintrobe tube with EDTA blood.
- Centrifuge the tube for 20 min at 2500 rpm. Take the reading in percent.
- Centrifuge the tube again for 5 min and note the reading.
- Final reading is recorded when 3 consecutive readings are identical.
- After centrifugation blood is separated into 3 layers, tall bottom layer of packed red cells, thin middle layer of WBCs and platelets and top layer of clear plasma.
- Percentage of height of red cell volume is hematocrit (PCV).

WESTERGREN TUBE

The recommended Westergren sedimentation tube is made from either glass or plastic, has a length of about 30 cm and a bore of 2.5 mm.

PROCEDURE

- Draw the EDTA sample into clean dry Westergren tube.
- Adjust the rack so that the tube rests in an exactly vertical position.
- Leave undisturbed for 60 min.
- At the end of the hour read the height of clear plasma above the upper margin of the column of sedimenting cells to the nearest millimetre.

- A poor delineation of the upper layer of red cells, so-called 'stratified' sedimentation, has been attributed to the presence of many reticulocytes.
- Report this measurement as the ESR (Westergren) in units of mm in 1 hour.

NEUBAUER'S CHAMBER

See Figures 1.35 and 1.36.

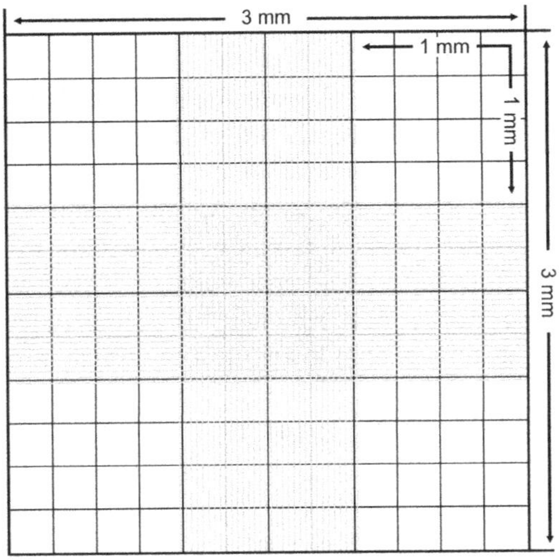

Fig. 1.35: Neubauer's chamber

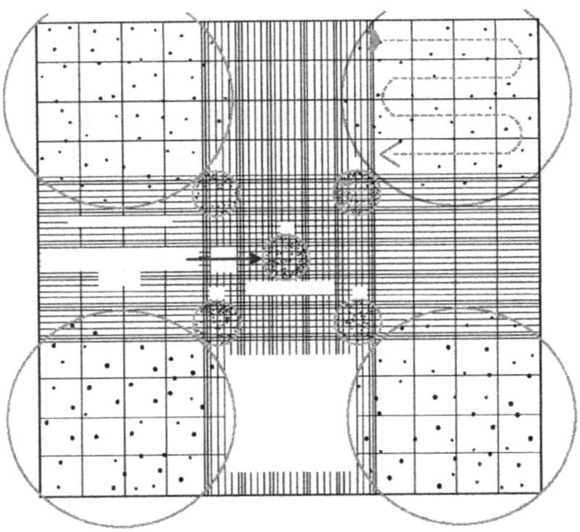

Fig. 1.36: Method of counting cells in Neubauer chamber

RBC PIPETTE (FIG. 1.37)

INSTRUMENT

- Glass stem has 3 marking 0.5,1 and 101 (volume)
- Glass capillary tube opens into wide bulb containing red glass bead
- Red bead helps in mixing the contents of bulb.

USES

Total RBC count.

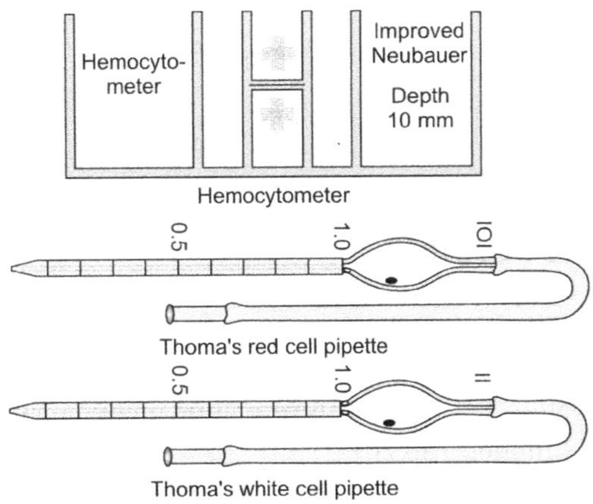

Fig. 1.37: RBC and WBC pipette

PROCEDURE

- Fill the RBC pipette exactly upto 0.5 mark with blood
- Now fill RBC diluting fluid (formal citrate solution) up to mark 101 (dilution 1 in 200)
- Mix the content thoroughly for 2 minutes. Discard first 2-3 drops of diluted blood
- Adjust the chamber and put coverslip in such a manner that both the ruled platforms are evenly covered by it
- Now charge the chamber (improved Neubauer chamber)

- Wait for 2 min for settling of cells and then count
- In erythrocyte count central double-ruled square is used. Red cells lying in 80 very small squares have to be counted.

No of RBC/mm^3 of Blood

Number of cells counted in 5 squares (4 from corner and 1 from central) × 10,000.

WBC PIPETTE (FIG. 1.37)

- Glass stem has 3 marking 0.5,1 and 11 (volume)
- Glass capillary tube opens into wide bulb containing white bead
- White bead helps in mixing the contents of blood

USE

Total leukocyte count.

PROCEDURE

- Fill the WBC pipette exactly up to 0.5 mark with blood.
- Now fill WBC diluting fluid upto mark 11 (dilution 1 in 20).
- Mix the content of pipette thoroughly for 2 minutes.
- Expel first 3 drops of diluted blood.
- Adjust the chamber under microscope.
- Wait for 2 minutes for settling of cells.
- Cells lying in 4 large corner squares are counted.

Total Number of WBC per mm^3 of Blood

Number of cells counted in 4 squares × 50.

GROWTH CHART (FIGS 1.38A AND B)

REFERENCE CURVES

- For purposes of comparison, growth charts are provided with reference curves. The WHO reference curves are based on extensive cross sectional data of well nourished healthy children, assembled by the National Centre for Health Statistics which are considered the best available for international use.
- 50th percentile of NCHS weight for age chart normally corresponds to the reference median. It gives the value of the 50th child of a group of 100 when they are arranged in ascending or descending order and where equal number of children will have measurements smaller or larger than the 50th value.
- When we say 3rd percentile it means that only 3 percent (3 in each 100) of children weighed had values which fall below that line. The 3rd percentile corresponds approximately to 2 standard deviations below the median of the weight for age reference value (2 SD below 50 percentile of NCHS chart). It is considered as the conventional lower limit of normal range.

WHO GROWTH CHART

- The WHO growth chart has 2 reference curves. The upper reference curve is the median (50th percentile NCHS) for boys (slightly higher than that for girls), and the lower reference curve is the 3rd percentile for girls (slightly lower than that for boys)
- The space between the two growth curves has been called the "road to health", i.e. road to normality.

Space is also provided on the growth chart for recording and presenting information on the following:

- Identification and registration
- Birth date and weight
- Chronological age
- History of sibling health
- Immunization
- Introduction of supplementary foods
- Episodes of sickness
- Child spacing and reasons for special care.

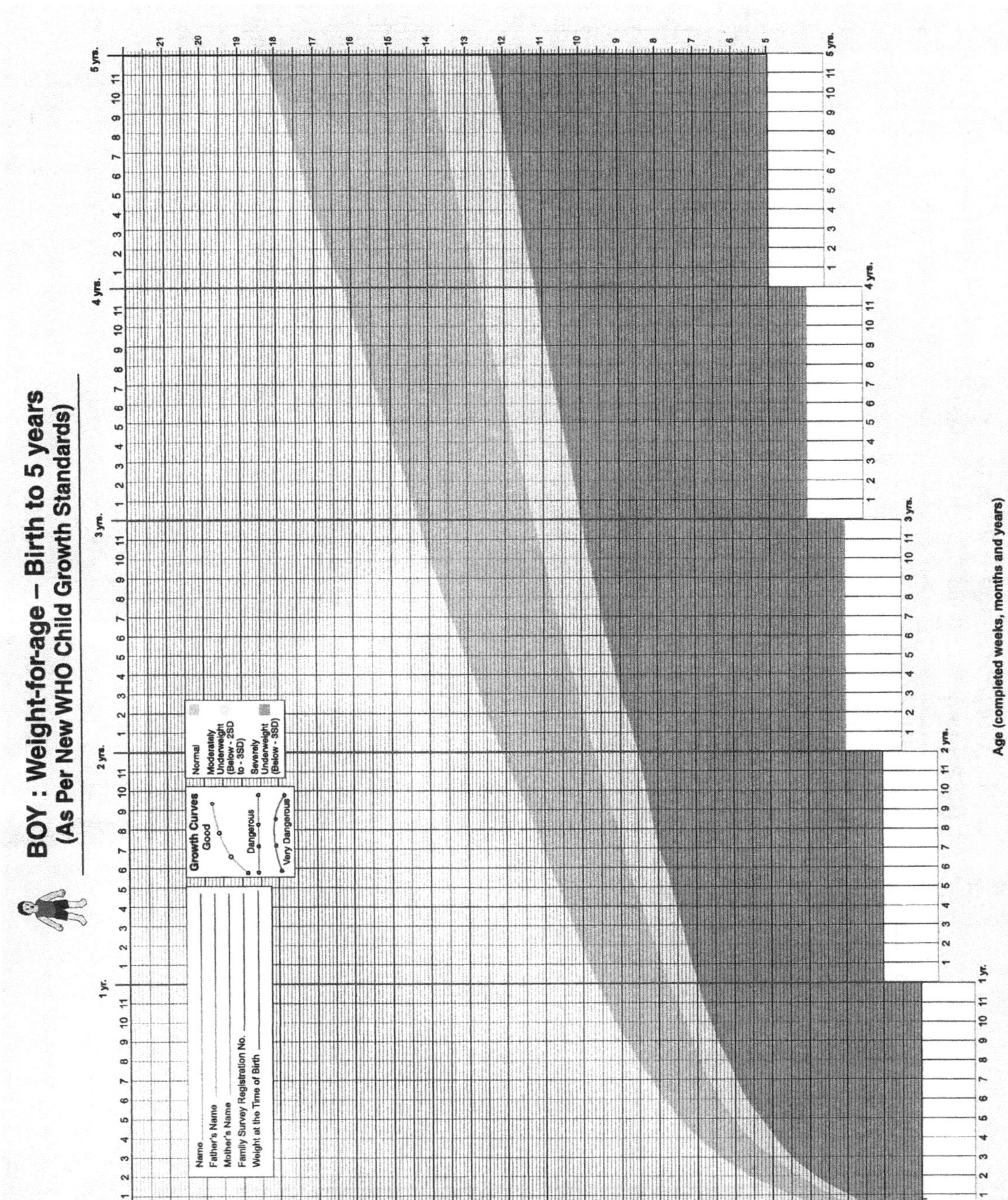
BOY : Weight-for-age – Birth to 5 years
(As Per New WHO Child Growth Standards)
Name
Father's Name
Mother's Name
Family Survey Registration No.
Weight at the Time of Birth
Growth Curves
Good
Dangerous
Very Dangerous
Normal
Moderately Underweight (Below - 2SD to - 3SD)
Severely Underweight (Below - 3SD)
Weight (kg)
Age (completed weeks, months and years)

Fig. 1.38A

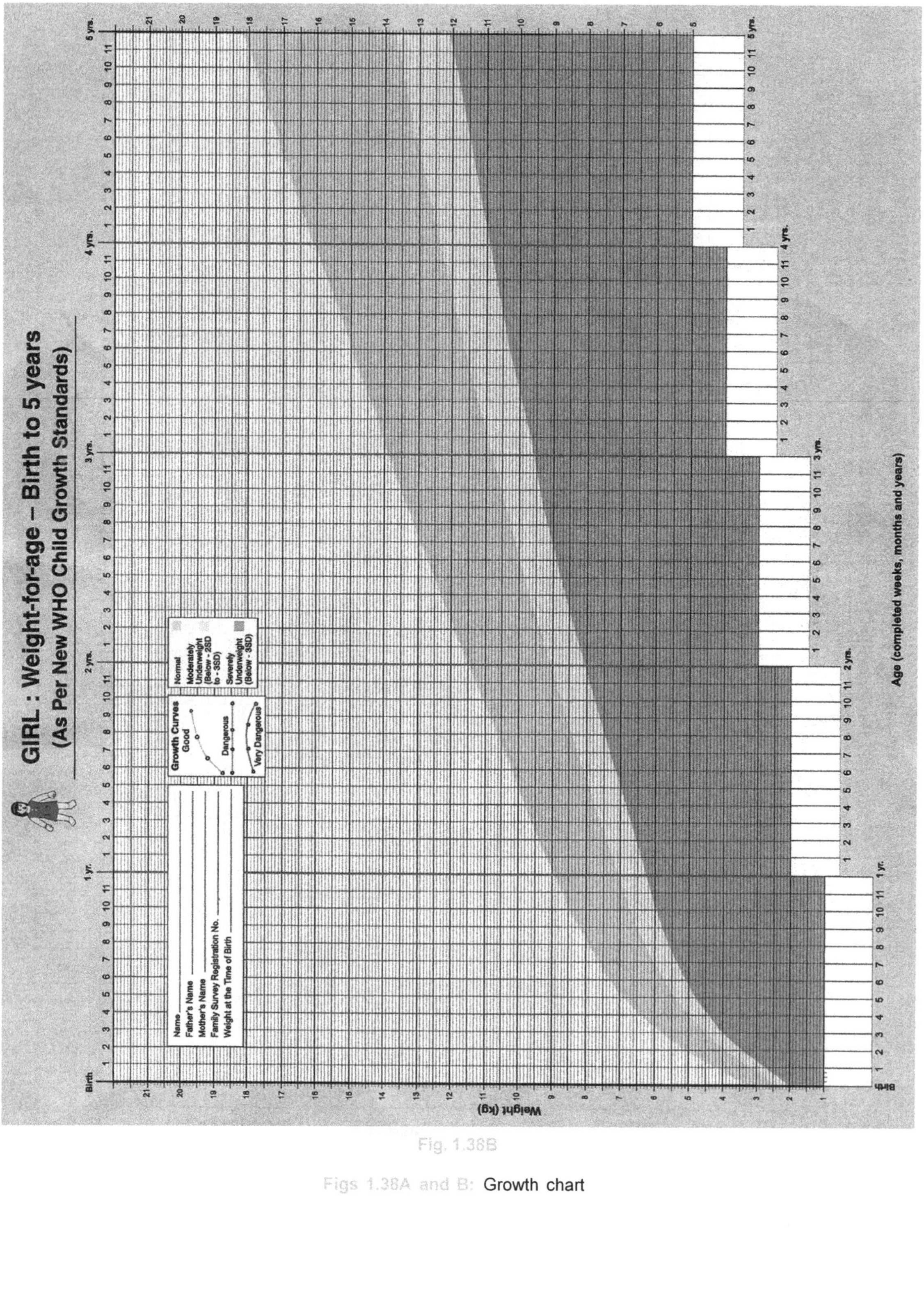

Fig. 1.38B

Figs 1.38A and B: Growth chart

GROWTH CHARTS USED IN INDIA

- There are 49 different types of growth charts in use in India.
- Growth chart recommended by the government of India has four reference curves.
- Topmost curve corresponds to the median (50th percentile of WHO reference standard) which represents the level of optimum growth.
- Second line represents 80 percent of the median weight (3rd percentile) which is approximately equivalent to 2 SD below the median which is the conventional lower. limit of normal range.
- 3rd and 4th line represents 70 and 60 percent of the median weight.
- *1st degree malnutrition*: Weight is between 80 and 70 percent line
- *IInd degree malnutrition*: Weight is between 70 and 60 percent
- *IIIrd degree malnutrition*: Weight is below 60 percent line
- *IVth degree malnutrition*: Weight below 50 percent.

Any weight between the top two lines is considered satisfactory. The growth charts used in ICDS contain 3 reference lines in addition to the standard (median), representing 80, 60 and 50 percent.

IAP CARD

Based on NCHS standards. It has additional information regarding immunization, developmental assessment using Trivandrum developmental scale and other informations.

INTERPRETATION OF GROWTH CURVES

- There are 3 patterns of curves
- Direction of the growth curve is more important than the position of the dots on the line at any time
- If child is growing normally, growth line will be above the 3rd percentile and run parallel to the road to health curves.
- Flattening of the weight curve shows persistent failure to gain weight. It is the earliest sign of malnutrition.
- Falling of the weight curve shows definite malnutrition.
- When there is increase in the rate of weight gain after a flattening or a falling curve that is the earliest evidence of recovery (catch up growth)
- Weight chart can be misleading in Kwashiorkor. The weight increases due to edema and the weight can go above 50th percentile also.

Uses of Growth Chart

- To make growth a tangible visible attribute.
- For growth monitoring and promotion.
- Diagnostic tool for identifying "high risk" children, before signs and symptoms of malnutrition become apparent.
- Educational tool for the mother. Because of its visual character the mother can be educated and motivated in the care of her own child.
- Planning and policy making: By grading malnutrition it provides an objective basis for planning and policy.
- Tool for action: It helps the health worker on the type of intervention that is needed and helps to make referrals easier.
- Evaluation: Helps to evaluate the effectiveness of corrective measures and the impact of a program or of special interventions for improving child growth and development.

CHAPTER 2

DRUGS

ORS (ORAL REHYDRATION SOLUTION)

Table 2.1: Composition of reduced osmolarity ORS

Reduced osmolarity ORS	*grams/litre*	*Reduced osmolarity ORS*	*mmol/ litre*
NaCl	2.6	Sodium	75
Glucose, anhydrous	13.5	Chloride	65
KCl	1.5	Glucose anhydrous	75
Trisodium citrate, dihydrate	2.9	Potassium	20
		Citrate	10
		Total osmolarity	245

Table 2.2: Composition of standard and reduced osmolarity ORS solutions

	Standard ORS (mEq or mmol/L)	*Reduced osmolarity ORS (mEq or mmol/L)*
Glucose	111	75
Sodium	90	75
Chloride	80	65
Potassium	20	20
Citrate	10	10
Osmolarity	311	245

Indications

For prevention and treatment of dehydration, potassium depletion and base deficit due to diarrhea.

Mechanism of Action

Glucose in ORS helps in transporting sodium and water across the intestinal membrane during diarrhea.

How to Prepare

Mix full packet of ORS in 1 liter of clean household drinking water.

Precaution Guidelines for Administration

ORS should be used within 24 hours of preparation.

- *Infant*: 1 tsf every 1 to 2 min.
- *Child*: Sips with cup of glass.
- If child vomits then wait for 10 minutes, then give ORS more slowly.

Side Effects

Puffness of face, hypernatremia.

Reduced Osmolarity ORS

The *classical full-strength WHO-ORS* contains Na 90 mmol/L.

Reduced osmolarity solution, which is the current WHO-ORS, contains Na 75mmol/L.

Hypotonic osmolarity solution, not recommended by WHO, but recommended by European society for pediatric gastroenterology and nutrition, contains Na 60 mmol/L.

Reduced or hypotonic osmolarity ORS should be used as first line therapy for the management of children with acute gastroenteritis (AGE).

Role of Improved ORS in Diarrhea

Improved ORS was made by:

- Reducing the osmolarity of WHO-ORS
- Reducing glucose and salt concentration in the solution or by replacing glucose with a complex carbohydrate or amino acids
- Preserving the 1:1 molar ratio of sodium to glucose that is critical for efficient co-transport of sodium and water.

Reduced Osmolarity ORS associated with

- Less frequent use of unscheduled intravenous fluid
- Less vomiting
- Less stool output
- No significant difference in the incidence of hyponatremia and total duration of diarrheal episode.

Racecadotril (Acetorphan)

Racecadotril is an antisecretory drug that exerts its antidiarrheal effects by inhibiting intestinal enkephalinase; this prevents the breakdown of endogenous opioids (enkephalins) in the gastrointestinal tract and reduces the secretion of water and electrolytes into the gut without interfering with motility.

Racecadotril is effective in reducing the volume and frequency of stool output and in reducing the duration of diarrhea (particularly in children with rotavirus).

Rice Based ORS

Rice based ORS can be used as an alternative therapy to standard ORS in children with cholera diarrhea.

Rice based ORS is not recommended for children with noncholera diarrhea, because it does not result in any additional benefit compared with standard ORS.

Super ORS

Substrates and substances other than rice or cereals have been added to ORS to enhance clinical efficacy.

Aims and Rationales

- Reduces osmolality while providing increased calories (this has been done with rice as well as glucose polymers);
- Contains peptides and amino acids that enhance fluid uptake by coupled transport
- Contains amylase resistant starch that release shortchain fatty acids, that increase salt and water colonic absorption.
- Include therapeutic agents like probiotic Lactobacillus GG and with diosmectite, a clay that reduces the duration of symptoms of acute gastroenteritis (AGE).

ORS + Probiotics

ORS with Lactobacillus GG may be of benefit in children with acute gastroenteritis (AGE), but there is insufficient evidence to recommend its routine use

Zinc Fortified ORS

While zinc-ORS is superior to ORS alone, it is less efficacious in reducing duration of the episode than zinc supplements given separately from the ORS solution. However, evidence is insufficient to recommend in favor or against the universal addition of zinc to ORS.

Adsorbents

Smectite is a natural hydrated aluminomagnesium silicate that binds to digestive mucus and has the ability to bind endo and exotoxins, bacteria, and rotavirus.

Probiotics

Probiotics have beneficial effect on rotavirus diarrhea which was present in >75% of cases in studies from the west. Rotavirus constitutes about 25% of diarrhea in hospitalized children and 15% in outpatient practice in India.

The following probiotics showed benefit in meta-analyses of Randomised controlled trials: *Lactobacillus GG* and *Saccharomyces boulardii.*

Prebiotics

Prebiotics should be used with caution in the management of children with AGE. However, only a few prebiotics have been studied.

Role of Zinc

- 30-50% children in developing countries are zinc deficient
- High prevalence of zinc deficiency is due to
  - Malnutrition
  - Low intake of animal source food
  - Low levels in breast milk
  - High consumption of cereals and legumes rich in phytates
  - Low level in soil and crops.

Zinc Deficiency Causes

- Reduced brush border enzyme activity
- Disrupts intestinal mucosa
- Increased mucosal permeability and intestinal secretion
- Making the diarrheal episode more severe and prolonged.

Zinc Supplementation Causes

- Early regeneration of intestinal mucosa thus improving intestinal permeability
- Restoration of intestinal brush border enzymatic function, overall causing reduction in intestinal secretion and regulation of water and electrolyte transport
- Maintains the integrity of the gut mucosa and reduces and prevents the fluid losses
- It is essential mineral for cell growth, differentiation and DNA synthesis
- Improves water and electrolyte absorption.

Role of Zinc Supplementation in Diarrhea

- Reduction in the incidence (11-15%) and prevalence (18-30%) of diarrhea in children less than 5 years
- 15 -26% faster recovery
- 9-43% reduction in episodes lasting more than 7 days and 16-24% reduction in the mean duration of diarrhea
- 9-23% reduction in stool frequency.

Recommendations

- WHO and UNICEF recommendation in acute diarrhea:
  - Children > 6 months: 20 mg zinc daily for 10–14 days.
  - Children < 6 months: 10 mg per day for 10-14 days.

Additional Information for Diarrhea

- *Persistent diarrhea*: Diarrhea starts acutely which lasts 14 days or longer. It is usually infective and occurs in a previously normal child. The main danger is malnutrition and serious non-intestinal infection; dehydration may also occur.

- *Chronic diarrhea*: Diarrhea starts gradually and last beyond 14 days, in children who have some basic defect either in the GI tract, immune system or other organs. Therefore, chronic diarrhea need not be infective, often only controllable, unlike persistent diarrhea which is potentially curable. Diarrhea due to inflammatory bowel diseases, immunodeficiency, malabsorptions, etc. would be classified as chronic. The main dangers are severe systemic infection, malnutrition, vitamin and mineral deficiency. Dehydration is unusual.

Bacterial Versus Viral Etiology of Diarrhea

High fever (>40^{0}C), overt fecal blood, abdominal pain, and central nervous system (CNS) involvement each suggests a bacterial pathogen. Vomiting and respiratory symptoms are associated with a viral etiology.

Clinical severity, vomiting, and dehydration are worse in rotavirus infections. Children with Adenovirus infections have less severe general symptoms. Vomiting is less prominent in astrovirus infections than in rotavirus infections.

Role of Investigations in Diarrhea

Stool cultures and stool routine/microscopy should be considered in cases of persistent diarrhea when antimicrobial treatment is started (in case of immunocompromised host or dysentery), when intestinal infection must be excluded to verify another etiology such as inflammatory bowel disease, and in case of an outbreak.

Role of Electrolytes in Dehydration

In moderately dehydrated children whose history and physical examination findings are inconsistent with a straight diarrheal disease, and in all severely dehydrated children.

In all children starting intravenous (IV) therapy, and during therapy, because hyper-or hyponatremia will alter the rate at which IV rehydration fluids will be given.

Recommendations for Hospital Admission

- Shock
- Severe dehydration (>9% of body weight)
- Neurological abnormalities (lethargy, seizures, etc)
- Intractable or bilious vomiting
- ORS treatment failure
- Caregivers cannot provide adequate care at home
- Suspected surgical condition.

Indications for Discharge in Gastroenteritis

Sufficient rehydration is achieved as indicated by clinical status:

- Intravenous fluids are not required
- Oral intake of fluids equals or exceeds losses
- Adequate management by parents is ensured
- Medical follow-up is available (Table 2.3).

Table 2.3: The amount of ORS

Age	*Amount of ORS after each liquid stool*
6 months	Quarter glass (50 ml)
7 months -2 years	Quarter to half glass (50-100 ml)
2 years -5 years	Half to one glass (100-200 ml)

Empiric Antibiotic Therapy

Severe invasive diarrhea: The common causes are Shigella, Campylobacter, and Salmonella.

Bloody diarrhea with low or no fever, which is typical of Shiga toxin–producing *E coli,* but can be mild shigellosis or salmonellosis.

Watery diarrhea. Antibiotic therapy is not recommended unless the patient has traveled recently or may have been exposed to cholera.

SODIUM BICARBONATE

AVAILABLE STRENGTHS

- 7.5% and 8.4% (8.4% strength sodium bicarbonate is very unstable and hence only 7.5% strength solution is routinely used)
- 1 mL (7.5%) = 0.9 mEq
- 1 ampoule = 10 mL
- Route: Intravenous/Oral. Never via endotracheal tube.
- Diluent: Distill water.
- Sodium bicarbonate when used IV is to be diluted 6 times in distilled water.
- However, in labor room, for neonatal resuscitation, it is given as 1:1 dilution at rate of 2 mEq/kg through umbilical vein.

Mode of Action

- Acts by increasing pH of blood
- Causes volume expansion since it is hypertonic
- Increases tissue perfusion
- Increases vascular volume.

Uses

Neonates

- Birth asphyxia with documented metabolic acidosis (ensure adequate ventilation)
- During neonatal resuscitation
- Respiratory distress syndrome
- Metabolic acidosis.

Older Children

- Metabolic acidosis which may occur during.
  - Gastroenteritis
  - Diabetic ketoacidosis
  - Cardiac arrest
  - Status asthmaticus
  - Salicylate or barbiturate poisoning
  - Renal tubular acidosis
- Cyanotic spells
- Hyperkalemia
- Alkalinization of urine
- Dissolve ear wax
- Bladder washes.

Side Effects

- Tissue necrosis if extravasation occurs
- Hypernatremia (in hypernatremia THAM, i.e. tris hydroxy methyl methane is used. 2 mL of THAM = 1 mL of 7.5% $NaHCO_3$)
- Intraventricular hemorrhage in premature children (if given fast)
- Tetany (increases binding of calcium to tissue proteins thus decreasing ionized calcium)
- Hypokalemia (shifts potassium intracellularly)
- Metabolic alkalosis
- Paradoxical acidosis (Intracellular) $NaHCO_3 \rightarrow Na + HCO_3 \rightarrow H_2O + CO_2 \rightarrow CO_2$ diffuses into brain and forms H_2CO_3 which causes acidosis.

Interaction

Forms precipitate on interaction with calcium.

RINGER LACTATE

Composition in 1 Liter

Na	– 131 mEq/L
Cl	– 111 mEq/L
K	– 5 mEq/L
Ca	– 2 mEq/L
Lactate	– 29 mEq/L

Uses

- In dehydration – In shock as a plasma expander
- After hemorrhage – As an initial replacing solution and if blood is not available urgently
- Differentiate between oliguria of prerenal and renal origin
- Therapeutic effect – In case of prerenal oliguria

Side Effects

- Worsens lactic acidosis in case of shock–due to slow conversion of lactate to bicarbonate in poor peripheral circulation
- It cannot be used in case of liver dysfunction

Table 2.4: Choice of IVF in various conditions

Dehydration	Ringer lactate
Maintinence fluid	Isolyte P (N/6 + 5% Dextrose + 20 mEq/L Potassium)
Shock	Normal saline
Hypernatremic dehydration	N/5 in 2.5% Dextrose (2.5% Dextrose due to risk of hyperglycemia)
ARF	5% Dextrose
Nasogastric replacement	N/2 with added Potassium
Post ileostomy losses	Normal saline or Ringer lactate with added Potassium
Acute liver failure	N/5 in 10% Dextrose

25% GLUCOSE

- Each 100 mL supplies 25 gm of dextrose/L
- 1 ampoule = 25 mL

DOSE

2-4 mL/kg.

Uses

- Hypoglycemia
- Total parenteral nutrition
- Acute intermittent porphyria
- To make 5%, 10% 12.5%, 15% Dextrose drips Formula is (5c–25) where c is concentration of drip wanted

  e.g.: To make D 7.5 % drip: c = 7.5

  5 (7.5) – 25 = 37.5 – 25 mL = 12.5

  Thus, add 12.5 mL of 25% Dextrose to 87.5 mL of 5% Dextrose. This will give 100 mL of 7.5% Dextrose

Side Effects

- Rebound hypoglycemia
- Necrosis if extravasation occurs
- Thrombophlebitis
- Intraventricular hemorrhage (in premature and newborns) due to hyperosmolar solution
- Hyperglycemia.

TAble 2.5: Composition of intravenous solutions (mEq per liter)

Fluid	*Na+*	*Cl–*	*K+*	*Ca^{2+}*	*Glucose (g)*	*Others*
Normal saline (0.95% NaCl)	154	154				
N/2 (0.45% NaCl)	77	77				
Ringer Lactate	131	111	5	3		29 (Lactate)
5% Dextrose					50	
10% Dextrose					100	
Isolyte P	25	20	20	50		Acetate 23 Phosphate 3 Magnesium 3

Precaution

Concentration of glucose through peripheral vein should not be more than 12.5%.

MANNITOL (20% SOLUTION)

DOSAGE

5-8 mL/kg/dose 8 hourly given fast over 20 minutes.

Uses

- Cerebral edema
- Forced alkaline diuresis.

Contraindications

- Congestive heart failure
- Dehydration
- Subdural hemorrhage
- Renal failure

CALCIUM GLUCONATE

PREPARATIONS

Calcium gluconate contains 9% Calcium, preferred injectable calcium

Calcium lactate: 13% Calcium, given orally

Calcium chloride: 27.2% Calcium, not preferred due to highly irritating tissue necrosis

- 1 mL = 1 mEq of Calcium
- 1 mL = 9.3 mg of Elemental Calcium
- Ampoule of 10 mL

Uses

- Hypocalcemia due to any cause
- Cardiopulmonary resuscitation
- Hyperkalemia
- Antidote to verapamil
- Parental nutrition (30 mg/dL of elemental Ca)
- Prophylaxis of hypocalcemia in extremely premature babies, severe birth asphyxia and severe IUGR.
- Septic shock

Side Effects

- Necrosis occurs if extravasation occurs in the subcutaneous tissue
- Bradycardia and cardiac arrest (calcium should be given very slowly IV, in a diluted form, under heart – rate – monitoring)
- Hypercalcemia.

Drug Interaction

Incompatible with sodium bicarbonate. Forms calcium carbonate precipitate.

Precaution

Severe bradycardia if patient is on digoxin (cardiac asystole).

Dosage

- *Deficiency*: 75-100 mg/kg/day of elemental calcium in divided doses.
- *Prophylactic dose*: 50 mg/kg/day of elemental calcium in divided doses.
- *Premature infants*: May require 120-150 mg/kg/day of elemental calcium.

Withhold the drug if there is bradycardia.

POTASSIUM CHLORIDE (KCl)

PREPARATIONS

- *Oral:*
  - Syrup Potchlor: 15 mL = 20 mEq of Potassium
  - Syrup Kesol: 1 tsp = 13 mEq of Potassium.

- *Injection:*
  - 10 mL of 15% solution of KCI
  - 1 mL = 2 mEq of Potassium
  - 1 Ampoule = 10 mL.

Daily Requirement of Potassium

- 2-3 mEq/kg/day
- Maximum concentration in Intravenous fluid should be 40 mEq/L.

Route

Intravenous infusion.

Uses

- Hypokalemia
  - Persistent vomiting
  - Acute gastroenteritis
  - Prolonged intravenous fluids
  - Protein energy malnutrition
  - Diuretic therapy (especially with furosemide)
  - Renal tubular acidosis, paralytic ileus.
- Digitalis toxicity
- Diabetic ketoacidosis
- Glucose – insulin – potassium drip
- Bartter's syndrome
- Hypokalemic periodic paralysis.

Side Effects

- Hyperkalemia
- Cardiac arrest (if given as bolus)
- Respiratory paralysis
- Hypotension.

Monitoring

- ECG
- Serum potassium level.

AMINOPHYLLINE

PREPARATION

10 mL ampoule contains 250 mg of aminophylline.

Uses

1. *Neonatal apnea (Apnea of prematurity)*: *Mechanism of action:*
   - Direct stimulation of respiratory center
   - Makes respiratory center more sensitive to increased CO_2 concentration in blood
   - Improves contractility of diaphragm.
2. *Bronchial asthma*: As a bronchodilator *Mechanism of action:*
   - Phosphodiesterase inhibition: Increased cAMP concentration causes bronchodilatation
   - Effect on Calcium flux across cell membrane
   - Prostaglandin antagonism
   - Improved contractility of diaphragm.
3. *Left ventricular failure:* Acts as a cardiotonic and diuretic.
4. *Drug induced Apnea.*

Dosages

- *Bronchial asthma*: 5 mg/kg/dose oral or Intravenous (dilute in 5% Dextrose)
- Apnea of prematurity: *Loading dose*: 5 mg/kg/dose.
  Maintenance dose: 2 mg/kg/dose 8 hourly.

Serum Concentration

5-15 μg/mL

Side Effects

- Gastrointestinal disturbance—Nausea, vomi-ting, hematemesis, cramping

- Tachyarrhythmias
- Shock, hypotension
- Convulsions
- Hyperglycemia, glycosuria
- Hypokalemia and hallucinations.

ADRENALINE

PREPARATION

1 mL ampoule (1: 1000 dilution).

Dose

- 0.01 mL/kg/dose of 1: 1000 dilution subcutaneous (for anaphylaxis).
- 0.1 mL/kg/dose of 1:10,000 intravenous (for resuscitation).
- *Higher dosage*: 0.1 mL/kg/dose (1:1000 dilution) can be used in cardiac arrest when given via endotracheal tube. Then flush endotracheal tube with saline.
- *Intravenous infusion:* 0.6 × Body weight. Dissolve in 100 mL fluid. Then give 1 mL/hour which gives 1 μg/kg/min.

Route

- Intravenous, Endotracheal, Subcutaneous, Local.
- Never Intramuscular.

Uses

- Cardiac arrest
- Neonatal resuscitation
- Anaphylaxis
- Bronchial asthma
- Hypoglycemia
- Local bleeding (epistaxis and gastointestinal bleeding)
- Septic shock
- Along with local anesthetics to prolong duration and decrease systemic toxicity.

Side Effects

- Pallor, palpitation, arrhythmias
- Tremor, headache
- Hypertension.

Contraindications

- Congestive cardiac failure
- Diabetes mellitus
- Hypertension.

Drug Interaction

Inactivation with sodium bicarbonate.

DOPAMINE

PREPARATION

1 mL = 40 mg
1 ampoule = 5 mL

Indications

Persistent hypotension not related to hypovolemia.

Action

- *2 to 5 μg/kg/min:* Increases renal blood flow by acting on dopaminergic receptors (useful in ARF).
- *5 to 10 μg/kg/min:* Cardiotonic beta agonist with some dopaminergic action (in congestive cardiac failure).
- *10-15 μg/kg/min*: Vasoconstrictor action useful in septic shock, shock following removal of pheochromocytoma.
- *20 μg/kg/min:* As a vasoconstrictor by acting on alpha agonist (causes side effects).

Side Effects

- Hypovolemia
- Arrhythmia
- Extravasation causes subcutaneous necrosis.

Interaction

Inactivation with sodium bicarbonate.

DOBUTAMINE

Preparation

Injection: 25 mg/mL or 12.5 mg/mL (10 or 20 mL vial)

Dose

2 to 20 μg/kg/min (dilute in 5% dextrose).

Route

Slow intravenous infusion.

Action

- Catecholamine
- Inotropic (β_1 agonist)
- Decreases pulmonary capillary pressure and systemic vascular resistance.

Uses

- Refractory CCF
- Normotensive cardiogenic shock.

Precautions

- Should not be mixed in alkaline solution as it inactivates dobutamine
- Should not be used in hypovolemia.

Side Effects

- Nausea, vomiting
- Palpitation, hypertension, arrhythmias
- Extravasation leads to subcutaneous necrosis.

Contraindications

Idiopathic hypertrophic subaortic stenosis.

ATROPINE

Preparation

0.6 mg/mL.

Dosage

- 0.01 mg/kg/dose
- Minimum dose 0.1 mg (dose less than 0.1 mg can cause paradoxical bradycardia)
- Maximum dose 0.5 mg for child and 1 mg for adolescents
- Repeat after 5 min.

Uses

Neonates

- Resuscitation

Older Children

- Pre-anesthetic medication to inhibit secretions (blocks action of acetylcholine and antagonizes histamine and serotonin)
- Organophosphorus poisoning every 10-20 min till atropine effect (mydriasis, tachycardia, fever)
- Bradycardia and heart block
- Snake bite (antimuscarinic effect)
- Myasthenia gravis (antimuscarinic effect)

Side Effects

- Dryness of mouth
- Constipation

- Retention of urine
- Palpitation
- Hyperpyrexia
- Blurring of vision (due to mydriasis)
- Atropine psychosis.

FUROSEMIDE

PREPARATIONS

- *Injection:*
  - 10 mg/mL ampoule.
  - 40 mg/mL ampoule.
- *Tablet:*
  - 40 mg/tablet.

Dosage

- *Oral*: 2 mg/kg/dose
- *Injection*:1mg/kg/dose (maximum 6 mg/kg/day).

Uses

- Acute renal failure
- Nephrotic syndrome/Acute glomerulonephritis
- Bronchopulmonary dysplasia
- Congestive cardiac failure and left ventricular failure with pulmonary edema
- Hypertension
- Hyperkalemia
- Raised intracranial tension
- Forced alkaline diuresis.

Precaution

To be used cautiously in patients of hypoproteinemia (Nephrotic syndrome, PEM).

DIGOXIN

PREPARATIONS

- Injection: 0.25 mg/mL
- Tablet: 0.25 mg
- Syrup Digoxin Elixir: 0.25 mg/5 mL (0.05 mg/mL; dropper contains 5 markings for 1 mL thus each marking corresponds to 0.01 mg).

Ideal Blood Levels

- 1-2 ng/mL

Actions

- Decreases conduction via AV node
- Increases myocardial contraction
- Decreases myocardial oxygen consumption
- Increased automaticity.

Mechanism of Action

It inhibits the Na^+K^+ATPase pump, thus causing faster entry of sodium into cells, which promotes calcium influx with increased intracellular calcium and thus improved contractility.

Uses

- Congestive heart failure
- Atrial flutter and fibrillation
- Paroxysmal supraventricular tachycardia
- Left ventricular failure and pulmonary edema.

Side Effects

- GI side effects: Gastritis, nausea, vomiting
- Arrhythmias: Ventricular tachycardia, extrasystoles and fibrillation
- CNS side effects: Headache, Vertigo

- Allergic rashes
- Gynecomastia.

Digitalization

Oral

- Calculate the total digitalizing dose for 24 hours:
  - Neonates – 0.04 mg/kg
  - Infants and older children – 0.05 mg/kg.
- Half the dose calculated should be given stat
- 1/4th of the dose after 8 hours
- 1/4th of the dose after 16 hours
- No dose for next 8 hours and then maintenance dose ¼ dose to be divided twice daily.

Intravenous

- 75% of per oral dose.

ECG Response

Shortening of QTc interval followed by sagging ST segment and decreased T amplitude followed by slowing of heart rate.

Contraindications

- AV Block
- Hypertrophic cardiomyopathy
- Diastolic dysfunction
- WPW syndrome with atrial fibrillation.

Antidote

Digitalis specific FAB fragment.

Precautions

- Hypokalemia
- Hypercalcemia
- Hypomagnesemia.

VITAMIN D

Preparation

Cholecalciferol

- Injection 1 mL = 6 Lac IU.
- Sachet 60,000 i.u.
- Vitamin D_2 is ergocalciferol, and Vitamin D_3 is cholecalciferol.
- 1 μg vitamin D = 40 IU.

Daily Requirement

- 400 IU/day: older children
- 1000 IU/day: premature babies.

Actions

- Increased absorption of calcium and phosphorus from the gut
- Decreased excretion of calcium and increased excretion of phosphorus from urinary tract
- Causes bone mineralization.

Dosage

- Six lacs units, oral or intramuscular
- In patients with rickets who respond to this therapy, are further put on oral calcium for approximately 3 months.

Uses

- Rickets
- Hypoparathyroidism
- Total parenteral nutrition
- Malabsorption
- Biliary atresia.

Side Effects

- Gastrointestinal upset—Nausea, vomiting, constipation

- CNS irritability—Pseudotumor cerebri, hydrocephalus
- Nephrocalcinosis and hypertension
- Hypokalemia.

Contraindications

- Hypercalcemia
- Vitamin A toxicity.

Antidote

Sodium sulphate orally as 0.5% solution in milk. Increase it to 1% till diarrhea occurs.

VITAMIN A

PREPARATION

- Syrup 1 mL = 1 Lakh units
- Injection 1 mL = 40,000 units
- Each ampoule = 2.5 mL.

Dosage

Vitamin A Deficiency

- Day 1: 2 Lacs IU oral or 1 Lac IU Intramuscular.
- *Day 2*: 2 Lacs IU oral or 1 Lac IU Intramuscular
- *Day 14 or at discharge*: 2 Lac IU oral or 1 Lacs IU Intramuscular.

Measles or Severe PEM

- 2 doses of vitamin A on 2 consecutive days

Persistent diarrhea or prolonged febrile illness:

- One dose in each episode, keeping at least 1 month interval between 2 doses.

Prophylaxis

Age	*Dose*
< 6 months	50,000 IU
6 months -1 year	1 Lac IU
> 1 year	2 Lac IU

Every infant should be administered one dose of 1 Lac units of vitamin A along with measles vaccine at 9 months to be followed by four more doses of 1 lakh IU at 18, 24, 30 and 36 months.

In national program, vitamin A is supplied in drug kit to female multipurpose worker. Each kit supplied every 6 months contains 5 bottles of 100 mL each.

Recommended Daily Allowance

Newborn	:	1000 IU
Infant	:	2500 IU
Child	:	5000 IU

Uses

- Vitamin A deficiency
- Biliary atresia
- Total parental nutrition
- Acute respiratory tract infection
- Pregnant women
- Familial hyperkeratosis
- Malabsorption states
- Renal calculi
- Topical disease – Icthyosis, Psoriasis
- Measles (vitamin A is known to decrease mortality and morbidity in measles).

Side Effects

- Gastrointestinal upset
- Pseudotumor cerebri
- Hypervitaminosis A

- Neural tube defects in baby (vitamin A toxicity in pregnant mother)

VITAMIN K

PREPARATION

1 mL = 10 mg
Vit K_1 (derived from plants): Phytonadione
Vit K_2 (derived from bacteria): Phytoquinone
Vit K_3 (synthetic): Menadione

Action

Required for synthesis of clotting factors II, VII, IX, X.

Route

Intramuscular, Intravenous (Dilute in 5% dextrose).

Uses

- Prevention of hemorrhagic disease of newborn dose:
  - Weight > 1.5 kg - 1 mg Intramuscular
  - Weight < 1.5 kg - 0.5 mg Intramuscular
- Treatment of hemorrhagic disease of newborn dose:
  - 2-5 mg Intravenous
- Cholestasis
- Hypoprothombinemia (drug induced, anti-coagulant)

Side Effects

- Hemolytic anemia
- Anaphylaxis
- Hyperbilirubinemia.

Monitoring

PT/PTTK

DIAZEPAM

PREPARATION

- Injection: 5 mg/mL
- Tablet: 2 mg and 10 mg tablets
- Syrup: 2 mg/5 mL

Dose

- 0.2 - 0.3 mg/kg/dose

Uses

- Acute convulsive episode
- Tetanus
- As a muscle relaxant in tuberculous meningitis, spasticity
- Febrile convulsion prophylaxis
- Sedation
- Preanesthetic medication

Side Effects

- Drowsiness
- Hypotension
- Respiration depression.

Contraindications

- Jaundice (displaces bilirubin from albumin-bilirubin complex)
- CNS depression
- Myasthenia gravis

Antidote

Flumazenil

PHENOBARBITONE

PREPARATIONS

- Tablet: 15 mg, 60 mg
- Injection: 1 mL = 200 mg
- Syrup: 5 mL = 20 mg.

Dosage

- Loading dose: 15-20 mg/kg with infusion rate 1 mg/kg/min
- Maintenance dose: 5-8 mg/kg/day.

Therapeutic Level

15-40 μg/mL.

Mechanism of Action

- Inhibits GABA reductase, thus it increases the concentration of GABA
- Decreases Post-tetanic potentiation
- Inhibits reticular activating system.

Uses

Neonates

- Convulsions
- Status epilepticus
- Hypoxic – ischemic – encephalopathy (to stabilize neuronal membrane)
- Neonatal hyperbilirubinemia
- Crigler-Najjar syndrome Type II
- Cholestasis (facilitates excretion of conjugated bilirubin from hepatocyte).

Older Children

- Epilepsy
- Status epilepticus
- Prophylaxis to prevent convulsions:
  - Febrile convulsions
  - Tubercular meningitis
  - Encephalitis.
- Rheumatic chorea
- Raised intracranial tension (decreases brain metabolism thus decreasing cerebral blood flow).

Side Effects

CNS	: Drowsiness—irritability, hyperkinetic syndrome, disturbance in cognitive function (prolonged use)
Skin	: Rash, Stevens–Johnson's syndrome, porphyria
Metabolic	: Osteomalacia, anemia, ataxia
Hematologic	: Megaloblastic anemia.

Contraindication

Porphyria

PHENYTOIN

Preparation

- Tablet: 50 mg, 100 mg
- Syrup Dilantin: 125 mg/5 mL
- Syrup Eptoin: 30 mg/5 mL
- Injection: 50 mg/mL (should be diluted in normal saline, forms precipitate in glucose)

Dosage

- Loading dose: 10-15 mg/kg/day at 1 mg/kg/min with heart rate monitoring
- Maintenance dose: 5-8 mg/kg/day
- Always flush Intravenous line with normal saline after giving phenytoin because it is highly irritant to vein due to its high pH (12).

Therapeutic Levels

- 10-12 μg/mL—Therapeutic
- >35 μg/mL—CNS depression, coma

Mechanism of Action

Decreases post tetanic potentiation and prevents seizure spread.

Uses

- Seizure - Grand mal epilepsy/Focal epilepsy
- Digitalis toxicity (as antiarrhythmic)
- Epidermolysis bullosa
- Trigeminal neuralgia
- Myotonia congentia
- Head injury

Side Effects

Dose Related

- Nystagmus (20 mg/kg)
- Ataxia (30 mg/kg).

Drug Related

- Megaloblastic anemia
- Hirsutism
- Rickets
- Stevens-Johnson syndrome and allergic rashes.

Contraindications

- Heart block
- Sinus bradycardia

PHOSPHENYTOIN

Phosphenytoin is a parenterally administered prodrug of phenytoin, used in the treatment of patients with seizures.

PREPARATIONS

- 10 mL per vial: Each vial contains Phosphenytoin sodium 750 mg equivalent (PE) to 500mg of phenytoin sodium
- 2 mL per vial: Each vial contains Phosphenytoin sodium 150 mg equivalent to 100mg of phenytoin sodium.

Dosage

- Loading dose is 10-20 mg PE/kg given intravenous or intramuscular. The rate of administration for IV administration should be no greater than 150 mg PE/min.
- The initial daily maintenance dose is 4-6 mg PE/kg/day.

Advantages over Phenytoin

- More rapid intravenous administration than phenytoin
- No need for an in line filter
- May be administered by intramuscular injection
- Lower potential for local tissue and cardiac toxicity than phenytoin
- Associated with less pain and phlebitis at the injection site, fewer reductions in infusion rate and fewer changes of administration site because of injection site complications than phenytoin.
- The rapid achievement of effective concentrations permits the use of Phosphenytoin in emergency situations, such as status epilepticus.

Disadvantages

- Approximately 10-fold higher acquisition cost as compared to phenytoin.

MIDAZOLAM

Available Strengths

- Midazolam Hydrochloride Injection contains 5mg midazolam/mL OR
- Midazolam Hydrochloride Injection contains 1 mg midazolam/mL
- Routes of Administration: Intravenous, Intranasal, Sublingual.

Dose

To initiate sedation, an intravenous loading dose of 0.05 to 0.2 mg/kg administered over at least 2 to 3 minutes. The initial dose of midazolam should be administered over 2 to 3 minutes to avoid hypotension.

This loading dose is followed by continuous intravenous infusions of midazolam at a rate of 0.05 to 0.12 mg/kg/hour (1 to 2 μg/kg/min).

The rate of infusion can be increased or decreased (generally by 25% of the initial or subsequent infusion rate) as required.

Uses

- As an anticonvulsant when seizures are not controlled by phenytoin and phenobarbitone.
- Preoperative sedation/anxiolysis/amnesia.
- Sedation prior to or during diagnostic, therapeutic or endoscopic procedures, such as bronchoscopy, bone marrow aspiration/biopsy, oncology procedures, radiologic procedures, suture of lacerations.
- Induction of general anesthesia, before administration of other anesthetic agents.

Side Effects

- Respiratory depression, airway obstruction, oxygen desaturation, apnea
- Hypotension (more frequently in patients premedicated with narcotics and in neonates)
- Reactions such as agitation, involuntary movements, hyperactivity and combativeness.

PENICILLIN

Crystalline Penicillin (Penicillin G Aqueous)

Preparation

Ampoule: 5 Lac Units, 10 Lac Units.

Uses

Neonates:

- Congenital syphilis: 50,000 units/kg/day
- Tetanus neonatorum
- Septicemia: due to Group B streptococci
- Skin infection – Cellulitis, pustules, impetigo, Staphylococcal scalded skin syndrome.

Older children:

- Pneumonia especially due to Streptococci, Pneumococci, H. influenza- 1 lakh units/kg/day
- Meningitis/Infective endocarditis- 3 lakhs/kg/day
- Meningococcal meningitis and meningococcemia
- Diphtheria
- Tetanus
- Pyoderma.

Procaine Penicillin

Preparation

PPF (Procaine Penicillin Fortified): 1 ampoule = 4 Lac U (3 Lac U Procaine penicillin + 1 Lac U crystalline Penicillin).

Route

Deep Intramuscular (Intravenous use can cause ischemic necrosis).

Uses

- Acute rheumatic fever
- Acute glomerulonephritis
- Congenital syphilis
- Osteomyelitis
- Septicemia.

Benzathine Penicillin

Preparation

Vials of 6 lac Units/1.2 million Units/2.4 million Units.

Uses

- Rheumatic fever prophylaxis (Secondary Prevention)
  - Weight < 28 kg: 6 lac units 3 weekly
  - Weight > 28 kg: 12 lac units 3 weekly
- Streptococcal sore throat infection (Primary Prevention of Rheumatic fever)
  - Weight < 28 kg: 6 lac units, single dose
  - Weight > 28 kg: 12 lac units, single dose
- Syphilis (Asymptomatic) 50,000 units/kg, single dose
- Treatment of gonorrhea

Side Effects of Penicillin

- Anaphylaxis – Can give rise to all types of hypersensitivity reactions. Hence test dose of penicillin should always be given before starting therapy. Test dose: 0.1 cc of 1: 10,000 dilution, injected intradermally. Wheal + Urticaria within 15-30 minutes and Erythema > 5 mm are taken as a positive reaction.
- Thrombophlebitis.
- Jarisch – herxheimer reaction.
- Hemolytic anemia.

ACTH

PREPARATION

40 IU/mL in 5 mL ampoule.

Uses

- Infantile myoclonic spasms
- Subacute sclerosing panencephlitis
- ACTH suppression test.

Side Effects

- Hirsutism
- Acne
- Hypertension
- Cushingoid facies.

METHYL PREDNISOLONE

Methylprednisolone is a synthetic (man-made) corticosteroid. Corticosteroids are naturally-occurring chemicals produced by the adrenal glands located adjacent to the kidneys.

AVAILABLE STRENGTHS

- Injection: 20, 40, and 80 mg/mL
- Tablets: 2, 4, 8, 16, 24, and 32 mg.

Dose

Dosage requirements vary depending upon the disease being treated.

Uses

- *Inflammatory conditions*: rheumatoid arthritis, systemic lupus erythematosus, acute gouty arthritis, psoriatic arthritis, ulcerative colitis, and Crohn's disease.
- *Severe allergic conditions*: bronchial asthma, allergic rhinitis, drug-induced dermatitis, and contact and atopic dermatitis.
- *Chronic skin conditions:* dermatitis herpetiformis, pemphigus, severe psoriasis and severe seborrheic dermatitis.
- *Hematological conditions:* idiopathic thrombo-cytopenic purpura, Aplastic anemia.

Side Effects

- Fluid retention, weight gain, high blood pressure, potassium loss, headache, muscle weakness, puffiness of the face, hair growth on the face, thinning and easy bruising of the skin, glaucoma, cataracts, peptic ulceration, worsening of diabetes, irregular menses, growth retardation in children.
- Psychic disturbances: depression, euphoria, insomnia, mood swings, personality changes, and even psychotic behavior.
- Osteoporosis and an increased risk of bone fractures. Supplemental calcium and vitamin D are encouraged to slow this process of bone thinning.
- Prolonged use can depress the ability of the body's adrenal glands to produce corticosteroids. Abruptly stopping can cause symptoms of corticosteroid insufficiency, with accompanying nausea, vomiting, and even shock.
- This product contains benzyl alcohol which is potentially toxic when administered locally to neural tissue. Exposure to excessive amounts of benzyl alcohol has been associated with toxicity (hypotension, metabolic acidosis), particularly in neonates, and an increased incidence of kernicterus, particularly in small preterm infants.

DIFFERENCE BETWEEN PREDNISOLONE AND METHYL PREDNISOLONE

- Compared with prednisone, methylprednisolone has higher antiinflammatory potency.
- Methylprednisolone tends to cause less salt retention, but on the downside it is more likely to raise blood sugars, even in people without diabetes.
- Prednisone is available only as an oral medicine while methylprednisolone can be given by oral or injection.
- Methylprednisolone has slightly greater glucocorticoid and less mineralocorticoid activity than Prednisolone.

CHAPTER 3

NEONATAL RESUSCITATION

INTRODUCTION

- Birth asphyxia accounts for about 19% of the 5 million neonatal deaths that occur each year worldwide.
- American Academy of Pediatrics (AAP) and American Heart Association (AHA) developed a neonatal resuscitation program which has shown to protect and prevent harmful effects on the vital organs of the body due to perinatal asphyxia and ischemia (Fig. 3.1).

BASICS OF ASPHYXIA

APNEA

- The asphyxiated infant passes through following series of events:
  - Rapid breathing and fall in heart rate
  - Primary apnea
  - Irregular gasping respiration, further fall in heart rate and drop in blood pressure
  - Secondary apnea
- Most infants in primary apnea will resume breathing, when stimulated. Once in secondary apnea, infants are unresponsive to stimulation.
- Apnea at birth should be treated as secondary apnea of unknown duration and resuscitation should begin at once.

CLEARING ALVEOLAR FLUID

- The first few breaths of a normal infant are usually adequate to expand the lungs and clear the alveolar lung fluid.
- The pressure required to open the alveoli for the first time may be two to three times that for normal breaths.
- Problems in lung fluid clearance occur with:
  - Apnea at birth
  - Weak initial respiratory effort caused by:
    - prematurity
    - depression by asphyxia, maternal drugs, or anesthesia.

PULMONARY CIRCULATION

- At birth, pulmonary blood flow increases as the lung arterioles open up and blood is no longer diverted through the ductus arteriosus.
- With asphyxia, hypoxemia and acidosis cause further pulmonary vasoconstriction and maintain the fetal pattern of circulation.

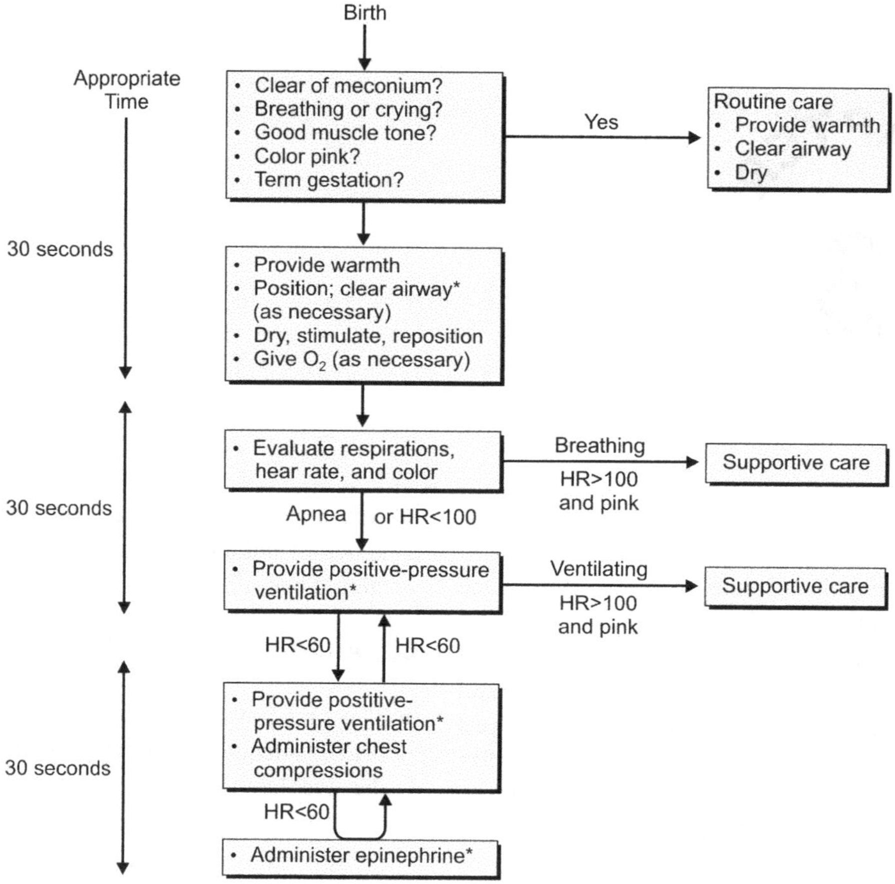

Fig. 3.1: Flow chart of neonatal resuscitation

SYSTEMIC CIRCULATION

- Early in asphyxia, vasoconstriction in the gut, kidneys, muscles and skin redistributes blood flow to the heart and brain as an attempt to preserve function.
- With progressive hypoxemia and acidosis, myocardial function deteriorates and cardiac output declines.

HISTORY REVIEW

- Age of the mother
- Any antenatal/perinatal complications:
  - Pregnancy induced hypertension
  - Diabetes
  - Drug therapy
  - Any cardiac/renal dysfunction.
- Blood group of mother
- Past obstetric history.

CHECK FUNCTIONING OF EQUIPMENT

- Warmer
- Linen – prewarmed
- Suction apparatus
- Oxygen supply
- Self-inflating bag:
  - Air inlet and attachment for oxygen reservoir
  - Oxygen inlet

- Patient outlet
- Valve assembly
- Oxygen reservoir
- Pressure release valve.

Bags used for newborns should have a volume of 200-750 ml. Term newborn require 15-25 ml with each ventilation.

- Mask—should cover chin, mouth and nose but not eyes
- Laryngoscope
- Endotracheal tube.

RESPONSE TO BIRTH

- Baby is received in prewarmed towel
- Quick assessment:
  - Clear of meconium
  - Crying or breathing
  - Good muscle tone
  - Term gestation
  - Color-pink.

INITIAL STEPS OF RESUSCITATION

- Child to be placed under radiant warmer with neck slightly extended in sniffing position. A folded towel (approximately 2.5 cm thick) can be placed under the infant's shoulders to maintain this position. This will bring posterior pharynx, larynx and trachea in line.
- *Suction mouth and then nose*. If the nose were cleared first the infant may gasp and aspirate secretions in the pharynx. Limit suctioning to 5 seconds at a time and monitor heart rate for bradycardia which may be associated with deep oropharyngeal stimulation.
- Immediately dry the baby.
- If drying and suctioning do not induce effective breathing, additional safe methods include:
  - flicking the soles of the feet
  - rubbing the back gently.
- Do not waste time continuing tactile stimulation if there is no response after 10-15 seconds.

EVALUATION (FIG. 3.2)

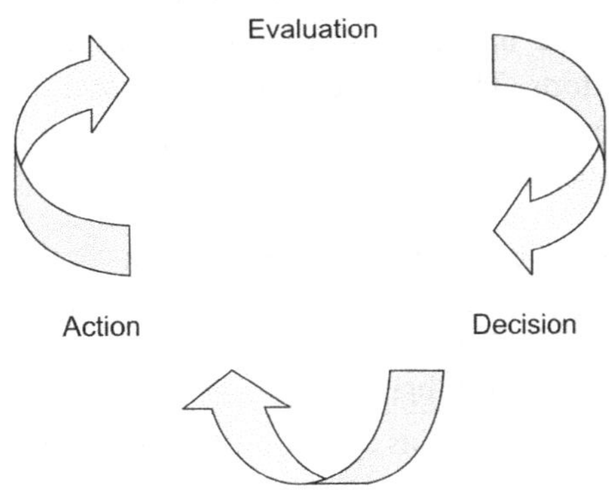

Fig. 3.2: Decision action cycle

- *Respirations*:

  Infants who are apneic or gasping despite brief stimulation attempts should receive positive pressure ventilation. If there is adequate spontaneous breathing, go to next step.
- *Heart Rate*:

  Monitor either by auscultating the apical beat or by palpating the base of the umbilical cord. Do not count heart rate for 1 full minute; count for 6 seconds and multiply it by 10. If the heart rate is below 100 bpm, begin positive-pressure ventilation, even if the infant is making some respiratory efforts. If the heart rate is above 100 bpm, go to the next step.
- *Color*:

  The presence of central cyanosis indicates that although there is enough oxygen passing through the lungs to maintain the heart rate, the infant is still not well oxygenated. Free-flow 100% oxygen using a mask held closely to the infant's face should be administered until the infant becomes pink, when the oxygen should be gradually withdrawn.

BAG AND MASK VENTILATION

- Most babies do not require more than this and child may be covered and swaddled and handed over to mother for breastfeeding.
- Some babies require further resuscitative efforts. This baby did not have good cry and require Intermittent positive pressure ventilation.

Indications for Bag and Mask

- Not breathing/gasping
- HR < 100 bpm
- Color remains cyanotic after 100% free flow Oxygen.

VENTILATING PROCEDURE

- Mask should be placed so that it covers the nose and mouth and tip of chin and not the eyes.
- Mask is held on the face with thumb, index and middle finger encircling much of the rim of the mask, while ring and fifth fingers bring the chin forward to maintain patent airway.
- Squeeze the bag to generate required pressure.
- *Rate*:
  40-60 breaths per minute.
- *Pressure*:
  Initial lung inflation may require a pressure as high as 30-40 cm H_2O but subse-quent breaths should be in the 15-20 cm H_2O range.
- *Method*:
  Speak 'SQUEEZE-TWO-THREE' while ventilating. Bag should be squeezed when you mention 'SQUEEZE' and relaxed when you mention 'TWO-THREE'.
  - Squeeze-Two-Three
  (Inspiration) (Expiration which is longer)
- Adequate ventilation is assessed by observing chest wall motion and hearing breath sounds bilaterally. If chest expansion is inadequate, the following steps should be followed in sequence:
  - Reapply the face mask to rule out a poor seal
  - Reposition the head - extend the head a bit further - reposition the shoulder towel
  - Check for secretions - suction if necessary
  - Try ventilating with the infant's mouth slightly open - perhaps with an oral airway
  - Increase pressure to 20-40 cm H_2O
  - Abandon bag and mask - intubate trachea
- After 30 seconds of effective ventilation, the heart rate of the neonate should be evaluated. To save valuable time, the heart rate over a 6 second period is counted and multiplied by 10 to give an approximation of the 1-minute heart rate. (e.g. 9 beat in 6 seconds = 90 bpm).

CHECK HR

If HR > 60: Bag and mask ventilation
↓ after 30 sec.
If HR > 60: Continue bag and mask ventilation
↓ after 30 sec.
If HR< 60: Start Chest compression.

CHEST COMPRESSIONS

Indication of Chest Compression

- HR< 60/min after 30 sec of bag and mask ventilation.

RATIONALE

- Babies who have HR < 60 bpm probably have low oxygen levels. As a result myocardium is depressed and unable to contract strongly enough to pump blood to lungs. Therefore, we need to mechanically pump the heart.

- Chest compressions must always be accompanied by ventilation with 100% oxygen.
- Pressing on the sternum compresses the heart and increases the intrathoracic pressure, causing blood to be pumped into the arterial circulation. Release of the sternal pressure will increase venous blood to return to the heart.

TECHNIQUES

- *Positioning of thumb/finger:*
  Run your fingers along the lower edge of ribs until you locate the xiphoid. Place your finger/ thumb 1 cm above the xiphoid.
- *Thumb technique*
  Thumbs can be placed side by side or in small baby one above another. Thumb should be flexed at the first joint and pressure applied vertically to press the heart between sternum and spine.
- *Two finger technique*
  Position fingers perpendicular to the chest and press the fingertips. Second hand should be used to support the newborns back so that heart is more effectively compressed between sternum and spine.
- Depress sternum—1/3rd of A-P diameter
  - Duration of downward stroke < duration of release
  - Thumb and fingers should remain in contact with chest all the time.
- *Method*:
  While performing chest compression; speak loudly 'ONE AND TWO AND THREE AND BREATH AND.

  When you speak 'ONE, TWO and THREE'- do chest compression and when you speak 'BREATH'—other person delivers breath by compressing self inflating bag. 'AND' signifies relaxation.

ONE AND TWO AND THREE AND BREATH AND
↓ ↓ ↓ ↓

- At any stage, endotracheal intubation can be performed
- A 3:1 ratio of chest compressions to ventilation is recommended. The three compressions are followed by a pause to interpose an effective breath. The combined rate of compressions with ventilation should be 120 per minute - resulting in 90 compressions and 30 ventilations each minute.
- Although bag and mask ventilation can be performed effectively over a prolonged period of time, ventilation is much easier if the infant is intubated.

ENDOTRACHEAL INTUBATION

Indications of Endotracheal Intubation

- Meconium stained liquor
- Prolonged bag and mask ventilation/ ineffective bag and mask ventilation
- Diaphragmatic hernia
- Extreme prematurity

INSTRUMENTS

- *Laryngoscope:*
  Turn on the laryngoscope light and hold the laryngoscope in your left hand, between your thumb and first two or three fingers, with the blade pointing away from you. One or two fingers should be left free to rest on baby's face to provide stability.

  Laryngoscope is designed to be held in left hand by both right and left handed persons. If held in right hand, the closed covered part of blade will block your view of glottis, as well as make insertion of ET tube impossible.
- *Blade:*
  The laryngoscope blade must be straight. The straight blade is preferred for infants since it provides better visualization of glottis.

- *Endotracheal tube:*
  Endotracheal tube should be sterile, disposable and constructed of translucent polyvinyl chloride with a radiopaque vocal cord guide.

Endotracheal tube of uniform internal diameter is preferable to a tapered tube (Table 3.1).

A standerd 15 mm adapter is firmly fixed to proximal end for attachment to ventilating device.

Table 3.1: Size of ET tube

Tube size (mm)	*Weight (gms)*	*Gestation age (weeks)*
2.5	<1000	Below 28
3.0	1,000-2,000	28-34
3.5	2,000-3,000	34-38
3.5-4.0	Above 3,000	Above 38

$$\text{Age} > 2 \text{ yrs} = \frac{\text{Age in years}}{4} + 4$$

PREPARATION FOR INTUBATION

- Before ET is attempted ventilation is provided with a bag and mask device using 100% oxygen.
- Monitoring of heart rate and oxygen saturation by pulse oximetry should be performed during the procedure.
- Intubation attempts should be brief, since those lasting more than 20 seconds, may produce profound hypoxemia.
- Laryngoscope and suction equipment should be checked before laryngoscopy to ensure they are in working order.
- A variety of blades should be available for proper blade size.
- A blade is attached to a handle by inserting a U shaped indentation onto the small bar at the end of the handle.
- After the intubation is aligned with bar, the blade is pressed forward, clipped onto bar, and elevated until, it snaps into position perpendicular to the handle.
- If the light is dim, flickers or does not illuminate blade may be improperly seated on the handle or bulb or batteries may be faulty.

PROCEDURE

- The correct position of newborn for intubation is on a flat surface with the head in midline position and the neck slightly extended with a roll placed under the baby's shoulder
- Do not hyperextend the neck, because this will raise the glottis above your line of sight and narrow the trachea.
- If there is too much flexion towards the chest, you will be viewing the posterior pharynx and may not be able to directly visualize the glottis.
- First stabilize the baby's head with your right hand; it may be helpful to have a second person hold the head in the desired "sniffing" position.
- Free flow oxygen should be delivered throughout the procedure.
- Slide the laryngoscope blade over the right side of the tongue, pushing the tongue to the left side of the mouth and advance the blade until the tip lies in the vallecula, just beyond the base of the tongue.
- Lift the blade slightly, thus lifting the tongue out of the way to expose the pharyngeal area. When lifting the blade raise the entire blade by pulling up in the direction the handle is pointing.
- Application of cricoid pressure by an assistant may facilitate visualization of the glottis opening.
- Holding the tube in your right hand introduce it into the right side of the baby's mouth.
- Keep the glottis in view and when the vocal cords are apart insert the tip of the endotracheal tube until the vocal cord guide is at the level of the cords.
- If the cords are together, wait for them to open. Do not touch the closed cords with the tip of

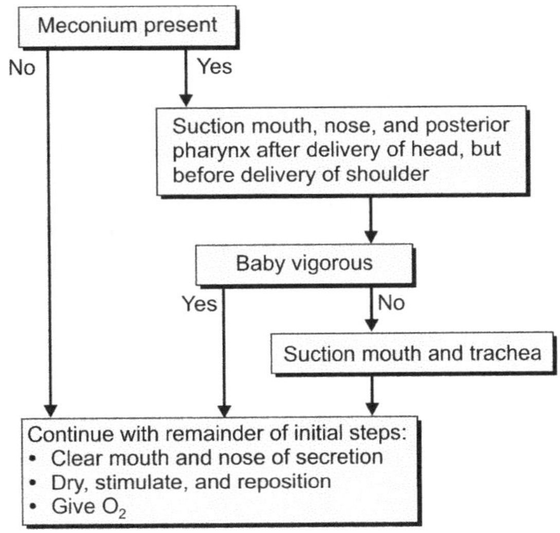

Fig. 3.3: Diagram outlining suctioning of newborns with meconium

the tube because it may cause spasm of the cords. If the cords do not open within 20 sec, stop and ventilate with a bag and mask.

- After the heart rate and colour have improved, you can try again.
- With right hand held against the face, hold the tube firmly at the lips and/or use a finger to hold the tube against the baby's hard palate. Use you left hand to carefully remove the laryngoscope without displacing the tube.
- Fix the endotracheal tube.

Confirmation of Placement of Endotracheal Tube

- Clinical: On IPPV symmetrical chest movements on right and left side and minimal abdominal movements.
- Auscultation of equal breath sounds over left and right chest just lateral to nipples.
- Documentation of absent breath sounds over the stomach.
- Noninvasive measurement of end tidal CO_2 levels.
- Chest X-ray in the NICU.

IF TUBE WAS INSERTED TO SUCTION MECONIUM (FIG. 3.3)

- If there is meconium in the amniotic fluid and the baby has depressed muscle tone, depressed respiration and heart rate less than 100 beats/min trachea should be intubated and suctioned.
- Connect the ET to a meconium aspirator connected to suction source.
- Occlude the suction control part on the aspirator to apply suction to the endotracheal tube, and gradually withdraw the tube as you continue suctioning any meconium that may be in trachea.

- Repeat intubations and suction as necessary until little additional meconium is recovered or until baby's heart indicates that positive pressure ventilation is needed.

"*Vigorous*" is defined as strong respiratory efforts, good muscle tone and heart rate greater than 100 bpm.

Precaution

- Do not apply suction to the ET longer that 3-5 sec as you withdraw the tube.
- If no meconium is recovered don't repeat the procedure.
- If you recover meconium with the first suction check the heart rate.
- If baby does not have significant bradycardia, reintubate and suction again.

IF TUBE INSERTED FOR VENTILATION

- If the purpose was to ventilate the baby, then you should quickly attach a ventilation bag to the tube, take steps to be certain that the tube is in the trachea and resume IPPV with 100% oxygen.

Table 3.2: Neonatal resuscitation guidelines 2005

AAP/AHA 2000 guidelines	*AAP/AHA 2005 guidelines*
INITIAL STEPS	
❖ *Ask 5 questions* Full term Clear of meconium Breathing or crying Good muscle tone Color	❖ *Ask 4 questions(No mention of Color)* Full term Clear of meconium and no evidence of infection Breathing or crying Good muscle tone
❖ *Temperature control:* Need of more assistance for maintaining normal temperature *in preterms recognized*	❖ *Temperature control:* *Additional warming techniques* like plastic wrapping and monitoring for development of hypothermia should be used *in VLBW neonates*
❖ *Give supplemental oxygen if needed.*	❖ Giving supplemental oxygen is highlighted as a *separate next step* (Fig. 3.4). It is not a part of initial steps. Give positive pressure ventilation if cyanosis persists despite free flow oxygen
MECONIUM STAINED LIQUOR	
❖ In case of meconium stained liquor, before delivery of shoulders *routine intrapartum oropharyngeal and nasopharyngeal suctioning* should be done	❖ *No longer advisable*
OXYGEN	
❖ Use of 100% oxygen is recommended when baby is cyanotic or when positive pressure ventilation is required during neonatal resuscitation.	**For term babies** In addition to these 2 points: ❖ One *may begin with less than 100% oxygen* or room air.
❖ In situations where 100% oxygen is not available positive pressure ventilation should be started with room air	❖ Use supplementary oxygen if there is no appreciable improvement within 90 seconds after birth ❖ Use of *pulse oximetry* may help to achieve normoxia more quickly

Contd...

Contd...

AAP/AHA 2000 guidelines	*AAP/AHA 2005 guidelines*
	For very preterm babies (< 32 weeks) ❖ Begin PPV with oxygen concentration between room air and 100% oxygen ❖ Keep oxygen saturation between 90 and 95% by increasing or decreasing oxygen concentration ❖ Use an oxygen blender and pulse oximeter during resuscitation ❖ Correct ventilation problem and use 100% oxygen if heart rate does not increase rapidly to > 100 per minute. If no facility of blender use 100% oxygen
POSITIVE PRESSURE VENTILATION (PPV) **Devices** ❖ Use self-inflating bag or flow Inflating bag to provide PPV during resuscitation	❖ Flow controlled pressure limited mechanical devices,e.g. *T-piece resuscitator* (for preterm babies) and *Laryngeal Mask Airway* (term and Near term babies) can also be used.
Checking Effectiveness of PPV ❖ Improvement indicated by three signs: *increasing heart rate; improving color and spontaneous breathing.*	❖ Primary measure of improvement is *increasing heart rate.* ❖ If heart rate not improving assess chest movements and check breath sounds.
MEDICATIONS ❖ Epinephrine or naloxone can be given through *endotracheal (ET) route.*	❖ Epinephrine or Naloxone should be given preferably by *intravenous route* only
ENDOTRACHEAL INTUBATION ❖ Tube position may be confirmed by capnography.	❖ Capnography (exhaled CO_2) is recommended method of confirming tube placement. This may have no role in brief period of intubation for clearing meconium from trachea.
DISCONTINUATION OF RESUSCITATION ❖ *After 15 minutes* of complete and adequate efforts	❖ If there are no signs of life discontinue *after 10 minutes.*
WITHHOLDING RESUSCITATION ❖ Non-initiation of resuscitation in: ❐ Confirmed gestation less than 23 weeks or birth weight < 400 g ❐ Anencephaly ❐ Confirmed trisomy 13 or 18	❖ Non-initiation of resuscitation in: ❐ Confirmed gestation less than 23 weeks or birth weight < 400 g or Anencephaly ❐ Babies with confirmed trisomy 13 ❖ Resuscitation always indicated with gestation of 25 weeks or more ❖ In conditions with uncertain prognosis in which survival is borderline take into account parental desires.

PRECAUTIONS DURING INTUBATION

- ET intubation is an invasive procedure, and exaggerates hypoxia, so oxygenate the baby appropriately with bag and mask before beginning intubation and between repeated intubation attempts.
- Hold 100% free flow oxygen by the baby's face.
- Do not try to intubate for longer than approx 20 sec.
- If intubation is not possible in 2 attempts, ask your colleague to do the intubation.

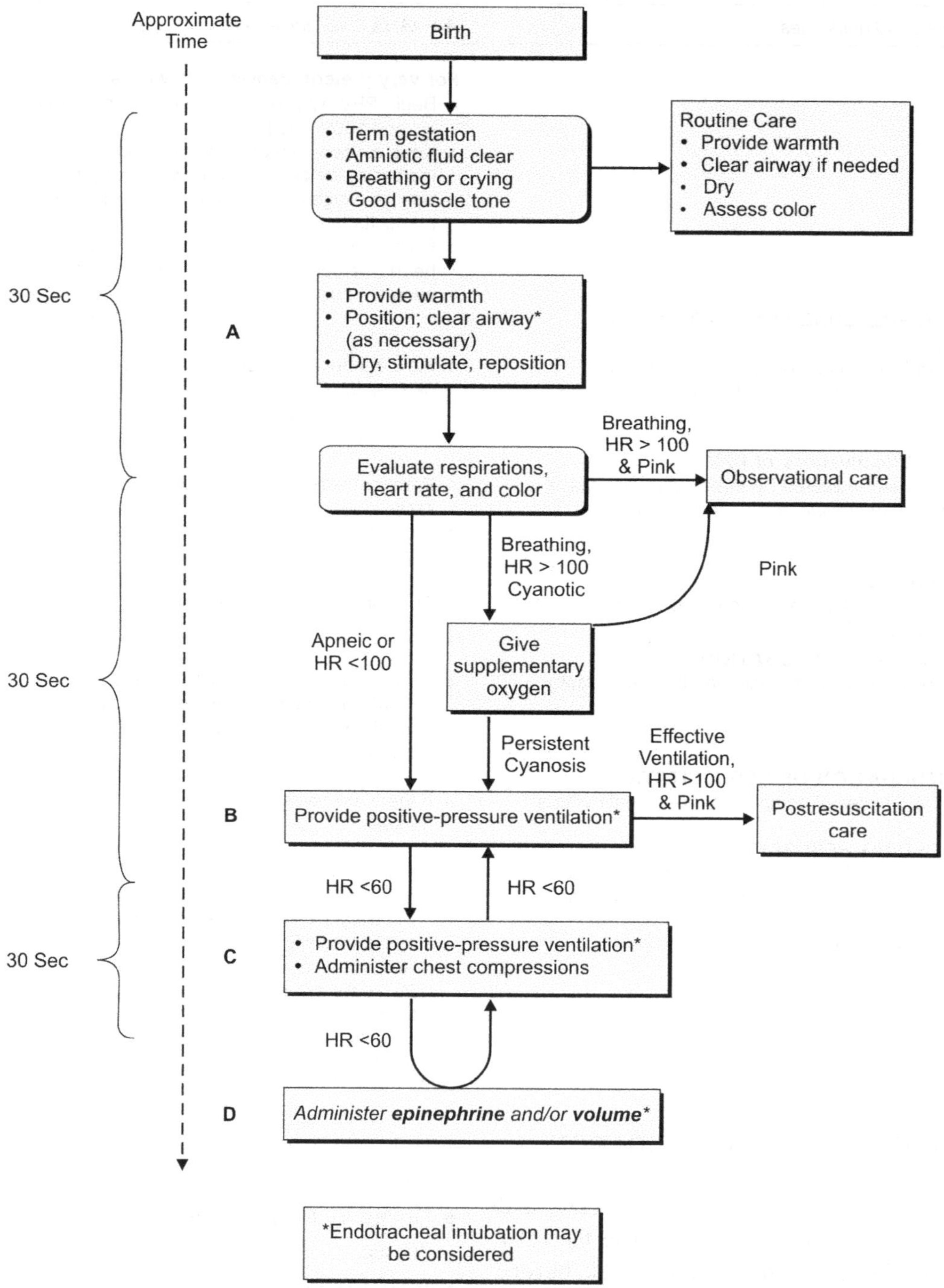

Fig. 3.4: Neonatal resuscitation flow chart, AAP 2005 guidelines

- Do not hyperextend the neck or cause too much flexion of the head as this will remove glottis from your line of sight.
- Do not elevate the tip of the blade by using a rocking motion and pulling the handle toward you. Raise the entire blade by pulling up in the direction the handle is pointing.
- Record cm marking of the endotracheal tube.
- Use of stylette is generally not preferred. If used do not take beyond tip of the endotracheal tube.

MEDICATIONS

Indications

- HR < 60 bpm after 30 sec of chest compressions.

EPINEPHRINE

- Recommended concentration – 1:10,000
- Recommended route – Endotracheal tube/ Intravenous
- Recommended dose – 0.1-0.3 ml/kg of 1:10,000 solution
- Recommended rate – as quickly as possible.

CRYSTALLOIDS

- Normal saline, Ringer lactate
- Dose – 10 ml/kg
- Route – Umbilical vein
- Rate – over 5-10 minute.

SODA BICARBONATE

- Dose – 2 mEq/kg
- Route – Umbilical vein
- Preparation – 0.5 mEq/ml (4.2%)
- Rate – 1 mEq/kg/min.

POSTRESUSCITATION CARE

- Resuscitated (Table 3.2 and Fig. 3.4) newborns will require close monitoring in a neonatal intensive care unit.
- Postresuscitation care may include:
  - Arterial pH and blood gas determinations
  - Correction of documented metabolic acidosis
  - Appropriate fluid therapy
  - Treatment of seizures
  - Screening for hypoglycemia and hypocalcemia
  - Chest X-rays for diagnostic purposes
- Complete documentation of all observations and actions should be entered in the infant's chart. This should include recording the APGAR scores calculated at one and five minutes. If the 5-minute APGAR score is less than 7, then additional scores should be obtained every 5 minutes for up to 20 minutes or until two successive scores are 8 or greater. Although the APGAR score is not used as a decision-making tool, it has been of value in assessing the progress of the resuscitation.

CHAPTER 4

IMMUNIZATION

Immunization History

Take Immunization history specifying following points:

- Immunization history, regarding administration of BCG, Polio, DPT, Measles, Boosters (depending on the age of the child)
- Look for the BCG Scar on the deltoid of the left arm to confirm the history regarding BCG administration
- OPV doses received through Pulse Polio immunization
- Reason for missing immunization. Usual reasons are lack of faith, side effects to previous immunization, lack of availability or awareness, illness at time of vaccination
- Any optional vaccines taken
- Any complications due to vaccination.

History of Immunization

- **Expanded program on Immunization (EPI)**
  - Started in 1974
  - Target population – Children < 5 yrs and Pregnant women
  - Vaccine included – BCG, DPT, OPV, Measles and TT
  - India adopted EPI in 1978 with typhoid vaccine replacing measles vaccine
- **Universal Immunization Program (UIP)**
  - Introduced in India in 1985
  - Concentration on target population < 1 year
  - Under UIP the earlier target of 85% coverage of EPI was removed, so that every infant was targeted for immunization (Table 4.1)
- ***Global alliance for vaccine and immunization (GAVI):*** started in 1999 which aims at immunization of all children using all vaccines with major contribution from Bill Gates Foundation
- In India, UIP became a component of child survival and safe motherhood programme (CSSM) in 1992 and then part of RCH in 1997

National Immunization Schedule

Birth	BCG, OPV-0
6 weeks	DPT 1, OPV 1
10 weeks	DPT 2, OPV 2
14 weeks	DPT 3, OPV 3

9 months	Measles
16-18 months	DPT booster, OPV 4
5 years	DT
10 years	TT
16 years	TT
Pregnant women	TT (2 doses at 4 weeks interval)

IAP Immunization Schedule

Vaccine	*Age Recommended*
BCG	Birth to 2 weeks
OPV	Birth, 6, 10, 14 weeks, 16-18 months, 5 years
DPT	6 weeks, 10 weeks, 14 weeks, 16-18 months, 5 years
Hepatitis B	Birth, 6 weeks, 14 weeks OR 6 weeks, 10 weeks, 14 weeks
Hib Conjugate	6 weeks, 10 weeks, 14 weeks, 16-18 months
Measles	9 months plus
MMR	15 months plus
Typhoid	2 years
TT/Td	10, 16 years
2 doses of TT	Pregnant women
Newer Vaccines	
Varicella	Above 1 year
Hepatitis A	Above 1 year

Table 4.1: Vaccination schedule of an unimmunized child

Age	*Less than 5 years*	*More than 5 years*
First visit	BCG, OPV, DPT, Hep.B	TT/Td, Hep. B
2nd visit (1 month later)	OPV, DPT, Hep.B	TT/Td, Hep.B
3rd visit (1 month later)	OPV, DPT, MMR/Measles Typhoid	MMR, Typhoid
1 Yr later	OPV, DPT, Hep.B	Hep.B
Every 3 years	Typhoid booster	Typhoid booster

No other vaccine should be administered within 4 weeks interval after the administration of Measles/ MMR vaccine.

Types of Vaccines

Live bacteria, attenuated	BCG, Ty21a
Live virus, attenuated	OPV, MMR, Varicella
Killed bacteria	Pertussis
Killed virus	IPV, Rabies, HAV
	Toxoid DT, TT
Capsular polysaccharide	Typhoid Vi, Hib Meningococcal, Pneumococcal
Viral subunit	HbsAg
Bacterial subunit	Acellular Pertussis

WHAT IS ROUTINE IMMUNIZATION

- Essentially covers national schedule of government of India
- Includes vaccines against six major diseases
- These are – Tuberculosis, Polio, Diphtheria, Pertussis, Tetanus and Measles
- All the vaccines are available free of cost.

NEWER (ADDITIONAL) VACCINES

- Vaccines yet to be considered for universal immunization on routine basis
- May be offered on one to one basis as per need
- Vaccines – Varicella vaccine, Hepatitis A vaccine and Pneumococcal Vaccine

Immunization Coverage (NFHS 3)

BCG	78%
Oral polio drops (3 doses)	78%
Measles	59%
DPT (3 doses)	55%

(NFHS 3) DATA ON IMMUNIZATION

- Nationwide, only 44 percent of children aged 12-23 months are fully vaccinated. This represents only a very slight change from 42 percent in NFHS-2, but a more substantial improvement from NFHS-1 when only 35 percent of children were fully vaccinated.
- Children who received BCG, measles, and three doses each of DPT and polio (excluding Polio 0) are considered to be *fully vaccinated.*
- 5 percent have not received any vaccinations.
- Coverage for BCG, DPT, and polio (except Polio 0) vaccinations is much higher than for 'all vaccinations'. BCG, the first dose of DPT, and all three doses of polio vaccine have each been received by at least 76 percent of children. Fifty-five percent of children have received three doses of DPT.
- Although DPT and polio vaccinations are given at the same time as part of the routine immunization programme, the coverage rates are higher for polio than for DPT (for all three doses), undoubtedly because of the Pulse Polio campaigns. The difference between the percentages of children receiving the first and third doses is 21 percentage points for DPT and 15 percentage points for polio.
- Fifty-nine percent of children age12-23 months have been vaccinated against measles.
- The relatively low percentages of children vaccinated with the third dose of DPT and measles are mainly responsible for the low proportion of children fully vaccinated.
- The 12-23 month age group was chosen for analysis because both international and government of India guidelines specifies that children should be fully vaccinated by the time they complete their first year of life.

BCG VACCINE

- BCG induces cell mediated immunity.
- Protection maximum against the hematogenous spread of *M. tuberculosis*, which results in miliary TB or TB meningitis.
- Preparation:
  - Supplied as a lyophilized *(freeze dried)* preparation in a vacuum sealed multidose dark coloured ampoule or 2 ml vials.
  - To be reconstituted with sterile normal saline.
  - Once reconstituted, should be *used within 4-6 hours* since it contains no antibacterial substance and organism is temperature sensitive.
  - Long necked BCG ampoule should be cut carefully by gradual filing at the junction of its neck and body, as sudden gush of air in the vacuum sealed ampoule may lead to spillage of contents.
- *Administration*:
  - *Intradermal* using 26 Gauze needle and tuberculin syringe.
  - Subcutaneous administration is associated with increased incidence of BCG adenitis.
- *Site*:
  - Convex aspect of the left shoulder so that inspection for BCG scar may be made easy.
  - A wheal of 5 mm at the injection site indicates successful administration of vaccine.
  - The selected site may be swabbed clean using sterile saline and local antiseptics should be avoided.
  - Sequence of events after BCG administration

♦ No skin reaction visible:	2-3 weeks
♦ Papule appears:	3-4 weeks
♦ Papule increases in size of 4-8 mm:	5-6 weeks
♦ Scar formation:	6-12 weeks

- *Dose*:
  - 0.1 ml irrespective of age and weight of baby.

- *Storage*
  - 2-8°C
- *Side effects*
  - Ipsilateral axillary/cervical lymphade nopathy: Spontaneous regression occurs and antitubercular therapy is not recommended.
  - Abscess formation: Surgical removal of nodes or repeated fine needle aspiration is treatment of choice.

Existing Coverage

According to recent countrywide National Family Health survey (NFHS-3), about 78% of children aged 12-23 months had received BCG vaccine. This figure is about 6% higher than NFHS-2 survey in 1998.

BCG Vaccine Controversies

Efficacy

BCG has an efficacy of 50-80% for prevention of miliary and meningeal form of the disease. Protective efficacy for pulmonary tuberculosis is around 50%.

BCG may be given with all vaccines on the same day or at any interval with the exception of Measles and MMR where a gap of 4 weeks between the two vaccines is recommended.

No BCG Scar After 90 Days of Inoculation

If no scar is seen after 90 days of BCG, it is assumed as failed BCG vaccination but it does not necessarily mean that it had failed to induce immune response. Since it is clinically impossible to distinguish between failed vaccination and failure to develop scar in spite of immune response, the better clinical option is to inoculate BCG a second time.

Success Rate of BCG 'Take up'

A success (of 'take' with scar formation) rate of BCG inoculation is 90%, provided the vaccine is satisfactory and the inoculation technique is good.

BCG and Tuberculin Testing

The interpretation of tuberculin test results in BCG recipients is the same as for people who have not received BCG vaccine. Positive test result (≥ 10 mm) should not be attributed to BCG vaccine.

BCG Vaccine and HIV Infection

BCG vaccine is not recommended for HIV infected children in areas of low prevalence of tuberculosis. However, in developing countries with high prevalence of tuberculosis, WHO recommends that BCG vaccine be given to all infants at birth if they are asymptomatic, regardless of maternal HIV infection. However, BGG should not be given to symptomatic immunosuppressed patients because of the risk of disseminated BCG infection.

BCG Vaccine and Anti-Tubercular Therapy

Children who are on or have received antitubercular therapy (ATT) for tuberculosis have been exposed to natural infection so BCG vaccine is not useful for them. INH resistant BCG vaccine should be used for children receiving ATT for reasons such as chemoprophylaxis, but it is not available in most countries. In such circumstances, it is better to wait till completion of INH therapy. Other option of giving regular BCG with INH chemoprophylaxis is also acceptable as there is hardly any evidence that INH renders regular BCG vaccine ineffective.

Newer Vaccines for Tuberculosis

Major antigens of *M. tuberculosis*, including the 6 kDa early secreted antigen target (ESAT6) and its peptide (aa51-70) protects mice challenged with *M. tuberculosis*. The protective efficacy of immunization further improves when ESAT6 is recombinantly fused with *M. tuberculosis* antigen 85B. In addition, ESAT6 delivered as DNA vaccine is also protective in mice.

ORAL POLIO VACCINE

- Suspension of over 1 million particles of poliovirus types 1, 2 and 3 together.
- *Contains* stabilizing agent, magnesium chloride
- The vaccine viruses establish infection in GIT (+ vaccine virus take) before an immune response occurs.
- Multidoses of OPV are necessary because
  - 'Take rate' is low in our children
  - Vaccinated children do not participate in the chain of transmission of wild polio viruses by a high level of gut immunity
- *Polio eradication* is defined as no case of paralytic poliomyelitis by wild polio virus in last three calendar years along with absence of wild polio virus in the community, where excellent clinical and virological surveillance exists and the coverage of routine OPV is more than 80 percent.
- *Polio elimination* is defined as Zero cases of paralytic poliomyelitis by the wild polio virus in one calendar year with other criteria same as in eradication
- When any poliovirus is detected it should be examined by genomic analysis to identify it as wild poliovirus and to distinguish from vaccine strain of poliovirus, to facilitate recording the incidence of *Vaccine associated Paralytic Poliomyelitis (VAPP)*. VAPP may occur in vaccine recipient within 4-40 days of receiving OPV or in contact of vaccine recipient. The risk of VAPP in India is estimated to be 1 per 4.1 to 4.6 million doses distributed. Half of all VAPP cases are associated with Type 2 OPV strain.
- *Vaccine Derived Polio Viruses (VDPV)*: Mutants that re-acquire wild virus like properties and have been associated with outbreaks of paralytic polio. VDPV usually arise in communities with low population immunity.

Storage

- 20°C at state and district level
- In freezer at clinic level
- Must reach outreach facility at 2 to 8°C in vaccine carriers with ice packs.

EXISTING COVERAGE

According to recent countrywide National Family Health survey (NFHS-3), about 78% of children aged 12-23 months had received 3 doses of oral polio vaccine. This figure is about 16% higher than NFHS-2 survey in 1998.

INJECTABLE POLIO VACCINE (IPV)

- Formaldehyde killed poliovirus grown in monkey kidney cell/human diploid cell
- Contains 40, 8 and 32 D antigen units of types 1, 2 and 3 polioviruses respectively.
- Seroconversion rates are 90 to 95% after two doses and 99% after three doses
- It produces excellent humoral immunity as well as local pharyngeal and, possible intestinal immunity
- The vaccine is very safe but not easily available at present in the Indian market
- IPV can be used in combination with DPT and Hib vaccines without compromising seroconversion and increasing side effects

- Ideal age to give first dose of IPV is 8 weeks and the interval between two doses should also be 8 weeks
- As the number of wild poliovirus cases in the country decreases, it is inevitable that one would have to gradually shift from OPV to IPV in the next few years. *The government should, therefore, consider incorporating IPV gradually in the national immunization schedule in a phased manner, starting from the states where polio has been eliminated.*
- IPV is also the vaccine of choice in patients with immunodeficiencies and the preferred vaccine in children with HIV infection
- *Adverse reactions*
  The vaccine is very safe. As IPV contains trace amounts of streptomycin, neomycin and polymyxin B, allergic reactions may be seen in individuals with hypersensitivity to these antimicrobials.

Advantages of IPV over OPV

- Relatively heat stable
- No risk of VAPP, VDPV
- Safe for immunocompromised
  - *OPV:* Major weapon for polio eradication, onset of action of OPV is faster as compared to IPV and thus OPV is vaccine of choice for outbreak control.
  - *IPV:* Also important for current and further polio control.

Monovalent Versus Trivalent Vaccine

- The live vaccine containing the 3 types of viruses is called trivalent OPV (tOPV); if it contains individual types, it is called mono-valent OPV (mOPV).
- Monovalent OPV is 3 times more efficacious than trivalent OPV as competition between different polio viruses is eliminated.
- The benefit of decline in P1 cases has been partially offset by resurgence of P3. Pulse immunization with monovalent P3 and bivalent OPV (bOPV containing P1 and P3) are strategies to offset this risk.

Polio Vaccine Controversies

Polio Eradication

India will have to achieve polio eradication in 2 stages, first interrupt wild viruses using OPV and later eliminate vaccine viruses using IPV.

Endemic wild polio virus transmission, with periodic outbreaks, is now restricted to Uttar Pradesh (UP) and Bihar. When the number of Vaccine associated paralytic poliomyelitis cases exceeds wild polio virus cases, the continued use of OPV will become unacceptable. This situation has already become real for type 2 virus in all states and types 1 and 3 in all but Uttar Pradesh and Bihar. Thus, the Government of India will have to stop using OPV sooner than later. Gradual withdrawal of OPV is highly risky since it creates a milieu conducive for the emergence of vaccine derived wild like (VDWL) viruses. Similar risks exist with abrupt stopping of OPV also. The safest approach is to use IPV, achieve high (>85%) coverage, and then only withdraw OPV. Thus, IAP recommended Government of India to include IPV in the routine schedule, and plan to stop OPV when IPV coverage reaches over 85%.

Reason for Variable 'Take' Rates of OPV

- Infection with other enteroviruses and competition between three polioviruses
- Poor efficacy in Uttar Pradesh and Bihar is attributed to high population densities, mal-nutrition, poor sanitation that increases the risk of infection with other enteroviruses and NOT due to poor vaccine potency.

Effect of Pulse polio?

- Routine immunization coverage fell after start of pulse polio program

- More publicity to pulse polio on the cost of routine immunization
- Community mistook it as if this covers all immunizations
- Health staff very busy in pulse polio for almost one month in each round
- Too many rounds - It is perceived that some kind of fatigue has also crept in.

DT_wP VACCINE

- Combination of diphtheria toxoid (20 to 30 Lf), whole cell killed pertussis vaccine and tetanus toxoid (5 to 25 Lf), popularly known as the triple antigen.
- While the two toxoids are highly immunogenic and antibodies to them are almost completely protective, the pertussis vaccine, given in 3 doses, has a protective efficacy of about 70 to 80% only.
- Life long immunity is necessary for tetanus. Therefore, at least 5 doses are recommended during the preschool age followed by boosters at 10 and 16 years of ages.
- Regarding Diphtheria, 5 doses are important with no boosters.
- The UIP recommends 4 doses of pertussis vaccine – 3 during infancy and fourth during the second year of life. Hence, while UIP recommends DT vaccine at 5 years, IAP recommends DPT vaccine for continued protection against whooping cough.
- Route: Intramuscular.
- *Site*: Anterolateral aspect of the thigh. The gluteal region is avoided because:
  - May injure the sciatic nerve
  - Deposits in the fat pad so immune response is less
  - This phenomenon has been shown to be important in the case of Hepatitis.B and Rabies vaccine; although not shown directly with DPT, it is better to adhere to the principle of no Intramuscular injection gluteally.
- *Precautions*:
  If any of the following events occurs the risks and benefits of administering subsequent doses of Pertussis containing vaccine should be evaluated:
  - Collapse or shock-like state (hypotonic hyporesponsive episode) within 48 hours.
  - Persistent crying lasting greater than 3 hours, occurring within 48 hours.
  - Temperature of greater than or equal to 105° F within 48 hours, not attributable to another identifiable cause.
  - Convulsions with or without fever, occurring within 7 days.

  In circumstances in which the benefits of further pertussis vaccination outweigh the possible risks (e.g., during an outbreak of pertussis), DTaP should be administered for the subsequent doses.
- *Efficacy*:
  The immunogenicity (protective titer for diphtheria > 0.1 IU/ml and for tetanus > 0.01 IU/ml) and effectiveness against diphtheria/tetanus of three doses of the vaccine exceeds 95%.

  Immunogenicity against all three components wanes over next 6-12 years and thus regular boosting is required.

  DTwP is not recommended in children aged 7 years and older due to increased risk of side effects.

Existing Coverage

According to recent countrywide National Family Health survey (NFHS-3), only 55% of children have received all three doses of DPT vaccine by one year of age.

History of Confirmed Disease

Vaccination against diphtheria, tetanus and pertussis should be given even if the child has suffered from a confirmed disease as these diseases usually do not confer complete protection.

DTaP VACCINE (ACELLULAR PERTUSSIS VACCINE)

The components of pertussis bacilli used for preparation of the acellular vaccines include pertussis toxin (PT) as the essential component with or without filamentous hemagglutinin (FHA), pertactin (PRN) and fimbrial hemagglutinins 1,2 and 3 (FIM).

The efficacy and duration of protection with DTaP vaccines against diphtheria / tetanus and pertussis is similar to that afforded by the whole cell vaccines.

The DTaP vaccines have advantage over the whole cell vaccines in both minor and major adverse effects, is reduced by two thirds with the acellular vaccines.

The absolute contraindications to DTaP vaccines are same as those for whole cell vaccines and include history of anaphylaxis/ encephalopathy following past pertussis vaccination.

DTaP vaccines are not more efficacious than DTwP vaccines, they have fewer adverse effects.

DTaP Vaccine Controversies

Should DTaP replace DPT in national Immunization schedule?

The cost benefit analysis does not favor DPT replacement by acellular pertussis in national schedule.

Can different acellular pertussis vaccines be used in same Individual?

As pertussis components are different in different types of acellular vaccines, they cannot be used interchangeably (unlike Hemophilus influenzae vaccine).

DT VACCINE

This vaccine comprises of diphtheria and tetanus toxoid in similar amount as in DTwP/DTaP, should be stored at 2 to 8°C and dose is 0.5 ml intramuscularly.

It is recommended in children below 7 years of age where pertussis vaccination is contraindicated.

The DT vaccine is also recommended by the Government of India in EPI as the second childhood booster at the age of 5 years instead of DTP vaccine due to fear of side effects with the pertussis component of DTwP.

However, studies with DTwP in school aged children have shown no serious adverse events attributable to the vaccine. Additionally boosting of pertussis immunity is important to protect against childhood pertussis.

TETANUS TOXOID (TABLE 4.2)

- After completing the full course of 7 doses, there is no need for additional doses during pregnancy, at least for the next 10 years. Thereafter a single booster would be sufficient to extend immunity for another 10 years.
- For previously unimmunized pregnant women give 2 doses of TT at 4 weeks interval; second dose at least 2 weeks before delivery. A single dose would suffice for pregnancies that occur in next 5 years; thereafter, 2 doses of TT would again be necessary.

Table 4.2: Guide to tetanus prophylaxis in routine wound management

H/o prior TT doses	*Clean, minor wounds*		*All other wounds*	
	TT	TIG*	TT	TIG
Unknown or < 3	Yes	Yes	Yes	Yes
3 or > 3	No**	No	No***	No

* TIG (Tetanus immunoglobulin) 250 IU I.M.

** Yes if more than 10 years since last dose

*** Yes if more than 5 years, DPT is given and above 7 years TT or Td (if available). More frequent boosters are not needed and can accentuate adverse effects

TETANUS IMMUNOGLOBULIN (TIG) (TABLE 4.2)

- Liquid or freeze dried preparation containing immunoglobulins, mainly IgG.
- *Adverse effects*:
  - Pain, fever, chills
- *Dosage*:
  - Prophylaxis- 250-500 IU Intramuscular
  - Therapeutic- 500-1000 IU Intramuscular
- *Indications*:
  - Burns, injuries, open and compound fractures
  - Unimmunized or inadequately immunized mothers.

TD VACCINE (TETANUS, DIPHTHERIA TOXOID)

- DTwP, DTaP, DT cannot be used in children aged 7 years and above to increased reactogenicity.
- Td which contains usual dose of tetanus toxoid and only 2 units of diphtheria toxoid
- Given at 10 years and 16 years and then every 10 years thereafter in doses of 0.5 ml intramuscularly.

Tdap VACCINE

In India the currently available Tdap vaccine is Boostrix.

It contains tetanus toxoid 5 Lf, diphtheria toxoid 2 Lf and the three acellular pertussis components namely, pertussis toxoid 8 mg, filamentous hemagglutinin 8 mg, and pertactin 2.5 mg. It contains aluminium hydroxide as adjuvant and no pre-servative.

The dose is 0.5 ml intramuscularly. Vaccine efficacy against clinical disease exceeds 90%.

Commonest side effect with Tdap is pain at the local injection site followed by redness and swelling.

The contraindications are serious allergic reaction to any component of the vaccine or history of encephalopathy not attributable to an underlying cause within 7 days of administration of a vaccine with pertussis component.

Recommendations:

- In those children who have received all five doses of DTwP/DTaP vaccine, Tdap vaccine is recommended at age of 10-12 years.
- It is also acceptable to use Tdap as a replacement for TT/Td in would management of children aged 10 and above if they have not received Tdap in the past, and at least 5 years have elapsed since receipt of Td/TT vaccine.
- The single booster dose of Tdap may be followed by Td boosters every 10 years.

MEASLES VACCINE

- Contains live attenuated measles virus
- The original virus strain was isolated from a child by the name Edmonston; thereafter the virus strain was also named Edmonston
- Strains in use as measles vaccine are Schwarz, Moraten, Edmonston-Zagreb, etc.
- In liquid suspension the vaccine virus is very heat-labile. The vaccine may be stored frozen or refrigerated. But, after reconstitution, the vaccine should be injected within 4-6 hours
- Does not contain any antibacterial preservative. Bacterial contamination can lead to staphylococcal sepsis/toxic shock syndrome in rare instances. Unused vaccine should, therefore be discarded after 4 to 6 hours.
- *Route*: Subcutaneous
- *Site*: Right upper arm; this is only for uniformity. It can also be injected over the anterolateral thigh, but subcutaneously.

- Infants are protected from measles by the maternal antibodies upto 6-8 months and are susceptible from 9 months onwards. Vaccine virus is neutralized, if vaccine is given in the presence of measurable titres of maternal antibody, so 9 months of age is recommended as the ideal, in our country, 9 months means 370 days or more.
- In case of an outbreak (or impending out break) infants completed 180 days (6 months) may be given the vaccine, provided such infants (given vaccine below 9 months) are revaccinated after at least 3 months of interval.
- Being a live attenuated virus vaccine, it results in actual infection and multiplication of viruses within the body. This infection mimics the wild Measles virus infection, except, (a) the disease Measles is either totally absent or may occur in a very mild form and (b) the infection does not spread from the vaccinated child to anyone else.
- The response to the infection may present as a short fever of 2-3 days, starting from about 5-10 days after immunization. We could consider this is the "incubation period", which is shorter by about 4 days than the incubation period of measles itself.

Existing Coverage

According to recent countrywide National Family Health Survey (NFHS-3), about 58% of children aged 12-23 months had received measles vaccine. This figure is about 8% higher than NFHS-2 survey in 1998.

Immunogenicity

Measles vaccine given at 9-11 months, is 85-90% effective because of persistent measles maternal antibody in 5-10% of children of this age group. Serum measles antibodies develop in 95% of children immunized at 12 months of age and 98% of people immunized at 15 months of age. More than 99% of people who receive 2 doses separated by at least 4 weeks, with the first dose administered on or after their first birthday, develop serologic evidence of measles immunity. *Primary vaccine failure* (failure to generate antibody response after vaccination) is observed in up to 20% of children immunized before one year of age while *secondary vaccine failure* (waning of antibody levels after seroconversion) is rare (<0.2%).

Measles Vaccine Controversies

Anti-tubercular Therapy and Tuberculin Testing

Measles vaccine can be safely given to children receiving anti-tubercular therapy. Measles immunization temporarily may suppress tuberculin skin test reactivity. If tuberculin skin testing is indicated, it can be done on the day of immunization or otherwise, it should be postponed for 4 to 6 weeks.

Association with Encephalitis

There is no data to support causal relationship between measles vaccine and encephalitis, GBS, subacute sclerosing encephalitis and autism.

Role in Immunocompromised

The vaccine should be given to those with HIV infection irrespective of degree of immuno-compromise as here the benefits outweigh the risks.

History of Measles

The vaccine should be given irrespective of prior history of measles as any exanthematous illness is often confused as measles.

Catch up Immunization

Recently, various state governments have initiated campaign with a dose of measles vaccine to be given to all children 1-5 years of age, irrespective of previous immunization status. It is an attempt to increase measles vaccine coverage with one dose of vaccine and not an attempt to give a second dose as erroneously believed by some.

MMR VACCINE

- At present, IAP recommends a dose of MMR vaccine to all children.
- For infants given measles vaccine at 9 months, MMR vaccine may be given between 12 and 15 months of age. If measles vaccine is given later, a 3 months gap is advisable.
- If measles vaccine was missed altogether one MMR dose replaces it, when given at or after 12 months.
- The vaccine can be given along with any other vaccine like DPT, OPV but at different sites using different syringes and needles.
- The dose is 0.5 ml per dose, to be administered subcutaneously in the upper arm.
- The vaccine should be stored between +2° and +8° C in the ordinary compartment of the fridge.
- Reconstituted vaccine should be used within 6 hours.

Immunogenicity

Single dose of mumps vaccine is 95% effective in preventing mumps diseases. The duration of vaccine-induced immunity is prolonged (beyond 30 years) and probably lifelong. Similarly the protection offered by single dose of rubella vaccine is around 95% and long term probably lifelong.

MMR Vaccine Controversies

Second Dose of MMR

- For providing durable immunity against mumps and rubella second dose of MMR should be given.
- The second dose of MMR should be given at 4-5years of age at the time of school entry but it can be given at any point of time 8 weeks after the first dose.
- Catch up immunization with a total of two doses of MMR vaccine should be given to those children/ adolescents who have not received any dose of MMR in the past or who have received only one dose of MMR so far.
- The second dose of MMR vaccine is to protect children failing to seroconvert against primarily mumps and less commonly against rubella (primary vaccine failures).

Inclusion in National Immunization Schedule

MMR should be included in the national immunization schedule as it will

i. Provide protection from rubella and thus help in control of congenital rubella syndrome.
ii. Improve measles control by achieving seroconversion of those not protected by first dose and by giving a second opportunity to those who missed the first dose
iii Achieve control of mumps.

However, inclusion of the vaccine in the national immunization schedule may prove counter-productive in areas where the vaccine coverage is likely to be between 30%-60% by increasing the risk of congenital rubella syndrome in such areas due to epidemiologic shift.

In view of this Indian Academy of Pediatrics Committee on Immunization (IAPCOI) recommends:

- The vaccine should only be introduced in those districts where primary coverage with the measles vaccine is consistently more than 80%.

- In those areas where MMR is introduced in the national immunization schedule catch up vaccination of all adolescent girls (11-12 yrs age group) should be done to rapidly reduce the risk of congenital rubella syndrome and counter any epidemiologic shift.

MUMPS VACCINE

- Monovalent vaccine or as part of MMR vaccine.
- The mumps component in MMR vaccine contains live attenuated Mumps virus not less than 5000 $TCID_{50}$ (tissue culture infectious doses) per dose.

RUBELLA VACCINE

- Derived from *RA 27/3 vaccine* strain growth in human diploid cell cultures.
- Available either as a monovalent vaccine or as a part of combination vaccine-MMR.
- Contains live attenuated virus not less than 1000 $TCID_{50}$.
- Positive antibody response occurs in 95% of susceptible vaccinees.
- Provides long term and probably *life long protection* and vaccine failures are uncommon.
- Joint symptoms like arthralgia and arthritis may occur 1-3 weeks following vaccination especially in susceptible post pubertal female but is usually mild. Immune thrombocytopenic purpura may occur in frequency of 1 per 30,000 vaccinated children.
- Pregnancy should be avoided for 3 months after vaccination but babies born to women inadvertently vaccinated in pregnancy do not exhibit an increased risk of congenital malformations.

HEPATITIS-B VACCINE

- The World Health Organization recommends Universal Hepatitis B Vaccination.
- *Route*: Intramuscular.
- *Site*:
  - Anterolateral thigh in infants, avoiding the gluteal region.
  - Deltoid in older children/adults.
- As an adjuvanated vaccine, it should not be frozen. If frozen accidentally, the vaccine should be discarded.
- For children with bleeding diathesis, pressure should be applied for 5 to 10 minutes at the site of injection. It may be given subcutaneous in patients with Thrombocytopenia or bleeding disorders.
- Child born to carrier mother especially positive antigen must be protected with Hepatitis B immunoglobulin given within 12 hours of birth. When HBIG is not available, vaccine offers 95% of efficacy in terms of preventing either infection per se, or at least preventing chronic infection. Vaccine should be given as soon as possible, preferably within 12 hours of birth.
- Two alternate schedules are available:
- *For Infants:*
  - Birth, 6 and 14 weeks OR
  - 6, 10 and 14 weeks (Combined DTPw Hepatitis B vaccine can be preferred).
- *For older children, adolescents and adults:*
  - Elected date, 1 month and 6 months
  - Booster dose is not recommended as of date.
- *Contraindications*:
  - No adverse effects have been observed on the fetus, when pregnant women are vaccinated, however in low risk cases, immunization of the pregnant women should be deferred till after delivery.
  - Lactation is not a contraindication to vaccination.

Hepatitis B Vaccine Controversies

Schedule of Hepatitis B

Schedule of Hepatitis B has been modified (for developing countries) to 6, 10 and 14 weeks to ensure its incorporation in the UIP. It is another matter that no study in the world has shown the efficacy of this schedule in reducing perinatal transmission or in reducing prevalence of carrier states of Hepatitis B. Studies showing comparable percentage of seroconversion, have demonstrated that the levels of antibodies is lower than those achieved with classical 0,1 and 6 months of age. For optimal vaccine efficacy of Hepatitis B vaccine, the first dose must be given within 48 hours of birth, while a minimum of 4 months must separate second and third dose (which acts as a booster in the 3 dose schedule).

Estimation of Anti-HBsAg Levels and Nonresponders

Routine testing for anti-HBsAg levels 1 month after completion of the immunization schedule is recommended in children born to HBsAg positive mothers and health care workers. Antibody titers greater than 10 mIU/ml signify a response and are considered positive. Non responders should be tested for Hepatitis B carrier status. If found negative the same 3 dose schedule should be repeated.

Vaccine Resistance

Anti-HBs antibodies produced by vaccination generate an 'immune pressure' on HBV, which results in the emergence of mutant strains that have altered immunological characteristics of HBsAg, making the organism resistant to the currently available vaccine. A mathematical model suggests that owing to mutations, Hepatitis B virus strains will become resistant to the currently available vaccine in about 20 years. There is considerable effort towards the development of HB vaccine wherein the part of the genome coding for regions prior to the surface antigen, are also incorporated into the yeast DNA. These vaccines are at the research stage and may be beneficial where conventional vaccines fail.

Newer Hepatitis B vaccines

Single dose vaccine: Using controlled release microparticle technique in animal models, vaccine has been administered in a single dose within biodegradable polymer microsphere, from which it is released in different amounts at different time points.

Oral vaccines: HBV genes integrated with salmonella genome has been administered orally in mice to induce anti HBs response. Edible vaccines can be created from transgenic plants like banana that incorporate HBV genes within their genomes.

HEPATITIS B IMMUNOGLOBULIN

- Provides immediate passive immunity.
- After administration, detectable level of circulating anti-HbsAg antibody will persist for 3 months.
- HBIG does not interfere with generation of antibody response to hepatitis B vaccine.
- Ideally, persons known to be exposed to blood which is known to contain hepatitis B virus should be given combined passive-active immunization.
- *Adverse effects*:
  - Transient, mild pain at the site of injection, itching.
- *Contraindication*:
  - No specific contraindications.
- *Special precautions*:
  - Be careful in patients with history of previous systemic allergy to immuno-globin preparations
- Never administer intravenously. It should be always given *intramuscularly.*

- *Indications*:
  - Accident "needle-stick"/splash or oral ingestion (pipetting accident) involving HBsAg positive materials such as blood, plasma or serum.
  - Neonates born to HBsAg positive mothers.
- *Dosage*: Following exposure to HBsAg:
  - *Adults*: 1000-2000 i.u. Intramuscular
  - *Children*: 32-48 i.u./kg body wt. This should be administered within 7 days (preferably within 48 hrs) after exposure to HBsAg
  - *Neonates*: Initial dose is 100-200 i.u. The first dose should be administered within 5 days after birth. The booster dose should be 32-48 i.u./kg of body weight between 2 and 3 months after initial dose.

Management of an Infant Born to Hepatitis B Positive Mother

If the mother is HBsAg positive (and especially HBeAg positive), the baby should be given Hepatitis B Immune globulin (HBIG) along with Hepatitis B vaccine within 12 hours of birth, using two separate syringes and separate sites for injection. The dose of HBIG is 0.5 ml intra-muscular. HBIG may be given upto 7 days of birth but the efficacy of HBIG after 48 hours is not known. Two more doses of Hepatitis B vaccine at 1 month and 6 months are needed. The closely spaced schedule should not be used. If HBIG is not available (or is unaffordable), Hepatitis B vaccine may be given at 0, 1 and 2 months with an additional dose between 9-12 months. The efficacy of prophylaxis with both HBIG and Hepatitis B vaccine is 85-95% and that with Hepatitis B vaccine alone (1st dose at birth) is 70-75%. All infants born to HBsAg positive mothers should be tested for HBsAg and anti HBsAg antibodies at the age of 9-15 months to identify carriers/non responders.

MENINGOCOCCAL VACCINE

- For active immunization against *Neisseria meningitidis* infection which includes meningitis and septicemia.
- It is either a bivalent (A+C) or tetravalent (A, C, Y, W135) vaccine.
- Each 0.5 ml dose contains purified polysaccharide of *N. meningitidis* 50μg of the individual polysaccrides.
- Minimum recommended age of administration is usually 2 years because of poor immune response in younger infants.
- *Adverse Effects*:
  Low grade fever, pain at injection site.
- *Contraindications*:
  Acute infectious disease
- *Special Precautions*:
  - Meningitis caused by other meningococcal groups
  - Children below two years.

❖ *Indications*:
- Close contact of patient with the disease
- Complement deficiency
- Prior to splenectomy
- Sickle cell anemia
- During disease outbreak and prior to travel to endemic region.

- *Dosage*:
  - Single 0.5 ml subcutaneous or Intramuscular injection. Revaccination at 3-5 years if individual is still at risk.
- *Storage*:
  - 2-8°C

Meningococcal Vaccine Controversies

Immunogenicity and Efficacy

The efficacy of serogroups A and C polysaccharide vaccines has been estimated at 85% to 100% among older children and adults. Serogroup A induces antibody in children as young as 3 months of age and can induce short term protection in infants, but serogroup C is poorly immunogenic in children less than 2 years. Data on the serogroups Y and W 135 is not available but they have been shown to be safe and immunogenic in older children and adults. Antibody concentration declines markedly after 3 years in adults and even faster in children.

Chemoprophylaxis

Close contacts of patients are at an almost 1000 times increased risk of contacting the disease, most of the cases occurring in the first 4 days. Chemoprophylaxis has been recommended for close contacts, and the WHO recommendations for this are:

1. Early institution of rifampicin (drug of choice unless the organism is known to be sensitive to sulfadiazine) 600 mg twice daily for 2 days in adults.
2. Sulfadiazine 1 g twice daily for adults.

PNEUMOCOCCAL VACCINE

- Two types of vaccine are currently available– A 23 valent polysaccharide vaccine and a 13 valent conjugate polysaccharide vaccine.

23 valent polysaccharide vaccine

- 23-valent polysaccharide vaccine is capable of preventing 85% of meningitis and bacteremia caused by Pneumococcus.
- Each dose is 0.5 ml containing 25 μg of individual serotype polysaccharide.
- A single intramuscular injection is recommended after the age of 2 years with booster every 3 to 5 years till the age of 10 years.
- Immunization is *not effective against Otitis media* since prevalent serotypes causing ear infection is not included in the vaccine
- Not routinely recommended but is indicated in special situations because of several potential problems with the use of vaccine on a large scale.
- Mass use of this vaccine may result in high nasopharyngeal carrier rates and consequent disease with non-vaccine serotype.
- *Indications*:
  - Prior to splenectomy
  - Nephrotic syndrome (in remission)
  - HIV infection
  - Cerebrospinal fluid rhinorrhea
  - Sickle cell anemia
  - Chronic lung/heart disease, diabetes mellitus and, chronic renal failure.
- *Adverse reactions*:
  - Injection site soreness, malaise, low grade fever.

Pneumococcal Conjugate Vaccine

- 13 purified capsular polysaccharides
- Immunogenic in < 2 years
- Dose = 0.5 ml, Intramuscular

Advisory Committee on Immunization Practices (ACIP)

Table 4.3: ACIP recommends routine use of PCV-13 in < 2 years

Age at first dose	*Primary series*	*Additional dose*
2-6 months	3 doses, 1-2 months apart	1 dose at 12-15 months
7-11 months	2 doses, 1-2 months apart	1 dose at 12-15 months
12-23 months	2 doses, at least 2 months apart	—
24-29 months	Healthy child- 1 dose High risk group-2 doses, 2 months apart	

Newer Pneumococcal Conjugate Vaccines

- 9 valent vaccine
- 10 valent vaccine
- 11 valent vaccine
- 13 valent vaccine
- Combination vaccine with Hib, DPT, IPV, Hepatitis B, meningococcal being developed.

Difference between Conjugated and 23 Valent Polysaccharide Vaccine (Table 4.4)

23 Valent Polysaccharide Vaccine

- 23 serotypes covers 85% of pneumonia, meningitis and bacteremia caused by pneumococcus in western countries. It does not provide immunological memory and revaccination is required every 3-5 years in children <10 years. Due to poor / unpredictable response in children <2 years, it is recommended in children more than 2 years of age.

Pneumococcal Conjugate Vaccine

- 13 purified capsular polysaccharides (responsible for 65-80% of invasive pneumo coccal disease in west and 50% in India). This vaccine is immunogenic in children <2 years and has efficacy = 97% in preventing invasive disease due to these serotypes (serotype specific).

Pneumococcal Vaccine Controversies

Pneumococcal Vaccine for Indian Children

It is estimated that 25% of all child deaths in India are due to pneumonia. About 30-40% of all severe pneumonia in children is likely to be pneumococcal in origin.

In the United States and Canada, where the vaccine has been in use for over 5 years, impressive decline was seen in rates of invasive pneumococcal disease in immunized children, but also in unimmunized older age groups, including the elderly, through herd effect.

WHO considers the inclusion of this vaccine in national immunization programmes as particularly high priority in countries with under 5-mortality >50 per 1000 live births. With an infant mortality rate of >60 per 1000 live births India meets the WHO's criteria for countries where pneumococcal vaccination should be a priority for introduction.

Future Vaccine

Extensive search for a protein antigen that will be common to all 90 serotypes or at least the invasive serotypes is going on. Thiol activated toxin

Table 4.4: Difference between conjugated and 23 valent polysaccharide vaccine

	Conjugate	*Plain polysaccharide*
• Minimum age of vaccination	>6 weeks	>2 years
• Immune response		
– at 2 months of age	Strong	Absent to weak
– at 2 years of age	Strong	Moderate to strong
• Duration of immunity	Long term	Short term
• Vaccine efficacy – children < 2 years of age	Yes	None
• Important reductions in nasopharyngeal carriage	Yes	None
• Indirect protection	Reported	Unlikely
• Important reductions in the prevalence of antibiotic resistant isolates	Reported	Not established

pneumolysin, and pneumococcal surface protein A appear to be most promising candidate antigens.

INFLUENZA VACCINE

- The multivalent vaccine usually contain 3 virus strains (usually 2 type A and 1 type B) with composition changed periodically in anticipation of the prevalent influenza strains expected to circulate in the country.
- The vaccine is given in 2 doses in children 6 months to 9 years of age and one dose above 9 years of age.
- The dose is 0.25 ml between 6 months to 3 years intramuscular and 0.5 ml after the age of 3 years. The vaccine is not routinely recommended in India since the prevalent antigenic types are not known. However in some high risk children and adolescents, the vaccine may be helpful.
- The vaccine is effective for only short period (6 months to 1 year).
- *Indications*:
  - Chronic pulmonary and cardiac disease
  - Sickle cell disease
  - Immunodeficiencies/HIV infection
  - Systemic lupus erythematosus, diabetes mellitus
  - Long-term aspirin therapy.

Future Vaccine

Present influenza vaccines offer narrow spectrum of protection. There is a need to improve on the current egg-derived vaccines and to produce vaccines able to protect against the whole possible spectrum of influenza viruses. Production of cell culture vaccine would improve possibilities of upscaling of vaccine production capacities in face of a pandemic. A novel, live attenuated influenza vaccine, delivered by nasal spray is being commercialized. Lastly, many groups are concentrating on the evaluation of the potential of the DNA vaccines for influenza.

RABIES VACCINE

- There are 2 types of vaccines available in India
  1. Nerve tissue vaccine
  2. Tissue culture vaccines
     - Human diploid cell vaccine
     - Purified chick embryo cell vaccine
     - Vero cell vaccine.
- *Nerve tissue vaccine* is no longer recommended because of its poor efficacy and life threatening adverse reactions in the form of neuroparalytic conditions of 1:2000 to 1: 8000 doses.
- *Tissue culture vaccines*: All tissue culture vaccines are having almost equal efficacy and any one of them can be used.
- *Post exposure prophylaxis*
  - Wound thoroughly cleaned with soap and water.
  - Appropriate tetanus prophylaxis is given.
  - Rabies immunoglobulin either human or equine in the dose of 20 i.u. and 40 i.u./kg body weight respectively is infiltrated around the wound in case of severe bite or bites in the upper extremities, trunk, head and face. Currently Intramuscular injection of RIG is not recommended.
- *Route*: Intramuscular
- *Site*:
  - Deltoid region in infants > 2 years
  - Anterolateral aspect of thigh in infant < 2 years
  - Do not inject in gluteal region.
- *Dose*:
  - 1 ml/dose irrespective of age
  - Days 0, 3, 7, 14 and 28. Day of first injection is considered as 0

- For re-exposure, within 5 years –2 doses on Days 0 and 7 are given
- After 5 years –Full course of 5 injections or earlier whenever the antirabies titer falls below 0.5 IU/ml.

- *Pre-exposure prophylaxis*

1 ml of any of the tissue culture vaccine is given intramuscularly over the deltoid region on day 0, 7 and 28 for the high risk group.

Rabies Vaccine Controversies

Intradermal Route

DGHS issued a circular in 2006 permitting intradermal route for tissue culture vaccines. 0.1 ml intradermally of approved vaccine over deltoid area on days 0, 7 and 21 or 28 is to be given.

Revised Rabies Postexposure Prophylaxis Protocol - *Fifth Dose of Vaccine No Longer Necessary for Most Persons*

The Advisory Committee on Immunization Practices (On June 24, 2009) has advised that the 5-dose schedule be changed to four doses, eliminating the last dose administered on day 28.

RABIES IMMUNOGLOBULIN

- Liquid or freeze dried preparation containing immunoglobulins mainly IgG obtained from plasma or serum of at least 1000 donors immunized against rabies and contains specific antibodies that neutralize the rabies virus.
- Contains not less than 150 units/mL.
- It provides passive protection when given immediately to individuals exposed to rabies virus. This provides maximum circulating antibody with minimum interference of active immunization with human diploid cell vaccine.
- *Dose*:
  - 20 i.u. and 40 i.u./kg body weight respectively is infiltrated around the wound in case of severe bite or bites in the upper extremities, trunk, head and face. Currently Intramuscular injection of RIG is not recommended.
- *Adverse effects*:
  - Local tenderness, muscle soreness or stiffness at the injection site, low grade fever, sensitization to repeated injections of human globulin in immunoglobulin defi-cient patients.
- *Contraindications*:
  - Do not administer in repeated doses once vaccine treatment has been initiated.
- *Indications*:
  - All injuries even licks, on mucous membranes by wild animals (or even pet animals) suspected to be suffering from rabies.

H. INFLUENZAE-B CONJUGATE VACCINE

- Immunity is due to the presence of protective antibodies against the capsule (The type b capsular polysaccharide is known as PRP).
- Since polysaccharide antigens alone do not stimulate T-lymphocytes (thus leading to short-lived protection) and are not immunogenic in young children (the age at greatest risk), *PRP is conjugated with a carrier protein* which is immunogenic in nature.
- Conjugation provides:
  - Priming of Memory 'T' cells and
  - Good immune response in young infants
- *Hib Vaccines*

Type	*Carrier Protein*
HbOC	Mutant Diphtheria toxin (CRM197)
PRP–T	Tetanus toxoid
PRP–OMP	Outer Membrane protein of Neisseria *Meningitidis*

Table 4.5: Dosage schedule

Age of Immunization	*Number of doses required*	*Regimen to be followed*
From 2 months to 6 months of age	4	3 doses at interval of 1 month. Fourth dose (Booster dose) at 15-18 months of age
7-11 months of age	3	2 doses at interval of 1 month. Booster dose at 15-18 months of age.
12 -14 months of age	2	2 doses at 1 month interval. No Booster required.
> 15 months of age	1	A single dose of any vaccine type can be given

- Hib vaccine is for IM use only. In patients with Hemophilia it can be given subcutaneous like HBV and HAV.
- Immunological memory is insufficient for protection against Hib disease. Hence, a booster dose is mandatory for sustained protection.

Special Circumstances

- In patients with *progressive neurological disorders* or in whom DPT vaccine causes severe reaction such as hyperpyrexia or seizures, HbOC or PRP-D should not be given as the "carrier" protein is contraindicated in such cases. In these patients "PRP-OMP" can be used instead
- Patients who have developed *Invasive H. influenzae 'b' disease* when < 2 years of age any dose Hib vaccine given before *disease* development should be ignored and vaccination should be started as usual depending on the age of the patient.
- When invasive disease occurs after 24 months of age, the disease itself induces a protective immune response and hence, vaccination is not indicated.
- As Hib disease is essentially confined to infants and young children, catch up vaccination is not recommended for healthy children above 5 years. However the vaccine should be administered to all individuals with functional/anatomic hyposplenia irrespective of age.

Side Effects

Pain, Redness and Swelling.

H. influenzae–B Vaccine Controversies

Inclusion in UIP

Most studies show low rates of Hib isolation from invasive diseases such as pneumonia, meningitis etc. although high rates of carrier rates have been demonstrated. Even if 4% of meningitis and about 8% of pneumonias are due to Hib vaccination, it will justify inclusion of this vaccine in UIP.

TYPHOID VACCINE

- *Salmonella typhi* posses 3 major antigens.
- Envelop antigen (Vi antigen) – It is a heat labile antigen which is responsible for the virulence of the organism.
- Cell wall antigen (O antigen)
- Flagellar antigen (H antigen).

The new Typhoid vaccine is based on the concept of producing antibodies against the Vi antigen.

Types of Typhoid Vaccines

- Various types of Typhoid vaccines available are:
  - ❐ Parental vaccine
  - ❐ Oral vaccine
  - ❐ Conventional vaccine.

Parenteral Vaccine (Vi antigen)

It is a type of a subunit vaccine where only the Vi antigen (which is purified) is used as immunogenic material.

- *Composition*
  - ❐ A single dose of 0.5 ml of the vaccine contains 25 μg of purified and inactivated

Vi capsular polysaccharide of *S. typhi* with phenol as preservative.

- *Dosage*
  - 0.5 ml of the vaccine is to be administered intramuscularly as a single dose above the age of 2 years. The protective efficacy lasts for 3 years following which a Booster is recom-mended.
- *Contraindications*
  - Hypersensitivity to vaccine constituents
  - Pregnancy
- *Adverse reactions*
  - Local—Pain, swelling and redness at the injection site
  - Systemic – Fever, Headache and Malaise

Oral Vaccine (Ty 21a)

The oral vaccine (Ty 21a), mutant of *S. typhi* lacks UDP galactase-4-epimerase enzyme. Thus, the Galactose metabolism of the bacteria is disrupted, lysis of cell occurs releasing cell wall lipopoly-saccharide and other antigens which stimulates development of immunity, whereas continuous lysis due to impaired galactose metabolism leads to avirulence of the vaccine bacteria in the human host.

- *Composition of the vaccine*
  - The Ty21a vaccine is available as an enteric coated capsule containing about 10^9 viable bacilli of Ty21a strain in a lyophilized form.
- *Dosage Schedule*:
  - The capsule is to be taken on Day 1, 3 and 5 (i.e. on every alternate day) with lukewarm water or milk (Temperature of the liquid not exceeding 37°C).
  - The oral vaccine cannot be given to children below 6 years of age.
- *Adverse effects*:
  - Anorexia, nausea, vomiting
  - Diarrhea
  - Abdominal pain
- *Contraindications*:
  - Immunodeficient states
  - Pregnancy
- *Efficacy*:
  - Efficacy ranges from 67 to 96 percent and the duration of immunity is for 3 years after which a Booster is recommended.

Conventional Vaccines

These are the traditional whole cell vaccines which are prepared by inactivation of the *S. typhi* bacilli by either heat or acetone.

They are of 3 Types:

1. *TAB vaccines*:
   - Trivalent vaccine contains both *S. typhi* as well as *S. paratyphi* (A and B). The approximate composition of TAB vaccine is:
   - *S. typhi* – 1000 million bacilli/ml.
   - *S. paratyphi* A – 500 million bacilli/ml
   - *S. paratyphi* B – 500 million bacilli/ml
   - Paratyphi A and B antigens in the vaccine are thought to be responsible for the large number of reactions caused by adminis-tration of the vaccine. Also their effective-ness is also doubtful. Hence, the TAB vaccine is slowly losing favor and should be discontinued.
2. *Monovalent vaccine*:
   - It contains only *S. typhi* antigens (No paratyphi bacilli)
3. *Bivalent vaccine*:
   - It is also present in 2 types (i.e. phenol preserved and AKD type). It contains S.typhi and S. paratyphi A.

- Dosage Schedule:
  - *Primary Immunization:*
    2 doses of 0.5 ml given subcutaneously at an interval of 4 to 6 weeks in adults. In children < 10 years of age, 0.25 ml should be given.

- *Booster doses:*
  Booster doses should be given every 3 years. If more than 3 years elapse before administration of the booster dose, then the entire primary course needs to be repeated.
- Adverse Effects:
  - *Very common, they include*
    - Local reactions—pain, swelling, tenderness
    - Systemic reactions—fever, headache, malaise.

Typhoid Vaccine Controversies

Why Typhoid Vaccine was Withdrawn from EPI

Typhoid vaccine was withdrawn from the EPI because reported incidence of 1% of typhoid was not sufficient for a universal immunization against typhoid. Further emergence of MDR strains has increased the costs of care of typhoid cases without affecting the mortality from typhoid.

Role of Current Vi Vaccine

Currently available Vi vaccine has reasonable efficacy above 5 years of age and a possible efficacy above 2 years of age but does not qualify to be included in the UIP due to reason stated above.

Ideal Typhoid Vaccine

Epidemiological studies reveal that maximum incidence of typhoid is below 5 years of age with many cases occurring before 2 years of age and that paratyphoid A may constitute up to 20 % of all enteric fever cases in the country.

Recently, newer conjugate Vi vaccine has come which can be given below 2 years of age. This vaccine is more useful, but will not be helpful in preventing cases of paratyphoid fevers.

Role of TAB Vaccine

Ideal typhoid vaccine should be effective against both typhi and paratyphi strains and can be given before 2 years of age. None of the currently available vaccines meet these requirements.

We may need to go back to conventional TAB vaccine, which was immunogenic below 1 year of age although was withdrawn, because of unacceptable reactogenicity. Studies may be done with this vaccine (like reduced doses by ID route) or its modifications to try and reduce its reactogenicity, while retaining its efficacy.

HIV Infected Individuals

The polysaccharide (Vi) vaccine has been shown to be safe in HIV infected persons. However, the induction of protective antibodies is directly correlated with the levels of CD4 positive T-cells. The safety of the oral Ty21a vaccine has not been demonstrated in patients with an immunodeficiency condition. However, it can be safely administered to HIV–positive, asymptomatic individuals without risk as long as the CD4 is above 200/mm^3.

CHICKENPOX VACCINE

COMPOSITION

- Lysophilized preparation of live attenuated varicella vaccine containing at least 103.3 PFU (Plaque-forming units) of the attenuated OKA strain of Varicella Zoster virus. It is obtained by propagation of the virus in human diploid cell culture (MRC5).

Indications

- For adolescents and adult above 15 years of age (since symptoms are severe in adults).
- Immunocompromised children, malignancies, chronic renal failure and patient on steroids.

- Healthy close contacts of patients with Chickenpox not having history of Chicken pox affliction.
- Children from high socioeconomic strata who can afford.

- *Dose*: 0.5 ml
- Schedule and mode of administration:
  - *In children below 12 years of age:* A single dose given subcutaneously
  - *In children above 12 years of age*: 2 doses of given subcutaneously at an interval of 6-8 weeks.
- *Adverse reactions*:
  - Fever (5%)
  - Pain at injection site
  - Mild papulovesicular eruptions (4%) during 1st 2 weeks of immunization
- *Contraindications*:
  - Fever
  - Hypersensitivity to neomycin (systemic; not local hypersensitivity)
  - Pregnancy and lactation
  - Depressed cellular immunity
- *Efficacy*:
  - It prevents chickenpox in 70–90% of people who get it, and it prevents severe chickenpox in more than 95%. It is expected to provide life-long immunity.

Recent CDC Guidelines

Two doses of varicella vaccine are recommended for children. The first dose is recommended at 12–15 months of age. It is usually given at the same time as MMR vaccine. The second dose is recommended at 4-6 years, before entering kindergarten. It may be given sooner, as long as it is separated from the first dose by at least 3 months. Anyone who has had chicken pox does not need the vaccine.

Varicella Vaccine Controversies

Exposed to Varicella: Is Vaccination of Any Use Now?

Varicella vaccine used as post-exposure prophylaxis in children within 5 days of exposure significantly reduces the chance of developing clinical varicella infection. The effect is more pronounced if vaccine is given within 3 days of exposure and prevents nearly all cases of moderate to severe varicella.

Individuals with Altered Immunocompetence and Their Household Contacts

Varicella virus vaccine, like most other live viral vaccines, generally is contraindicated in children and adults with altered immunocompetence.

Shingles in Vaccinees

Reactivation of vaccine strain can cause shingles especially in immunocompromised patients. However, rates reported have been very low among the vaccinees.

Inclusion in UIP

The disease is highly infectious and there are no subclinical infections. The disease is severe in older individuals. It tends to infect children mostly in months of March and April which coincides with examination periods for school going children. Hence, Varicella vaccine should be considered for inclusion in UIP.

HEPATITIS A VACCINE

KILLED HAV VACCINE

- Hepatitis A virus vaccine contains inactivated Hepatitis A virus (Inactivated with formaldehyde) which are adsorbed onto Aluminium hydroxide.

- The virus is grown in human diploid cell culture (MRC5) and inactivated with formaldehyde.

Vaccine is available in 2 strengths:

Adult Vaccine – 1 ml dose contains at least 1440 EIU (Elisa Units) of viral antigens.

Junior Vaccine – 0.5 ml dose contains at least 720 EIU (Elisa units) of viral antigens.

Indications

- Patients suffering from chronic liver diseases
- HBV and HCV carriers
- Tribal communities with high HBV carrier rates
- Food handlers
- Sewage workers
- Recipients of blood products
  - Close contacts of infected persons
  - Medical and Paramedical personnel/ Sewage workers/Food handlers
  - Hemophiliacs/Drug addicts/Homosexuals.

Table 4.6: Dosage and mode of administration

Dose	*Age of immunization*	*Children*	*Adults*
1st Dose	Any age above 1 years of age	Single dose of 0.5 ml of Junior vaccine (720 EIU) given IM	Single dose of 1 ml of Adult vaccine (1440 EIU) given IM
Booster dose	6 months to 12 months after the 1st dose	As above	As above

- Vaccine is given intramuscularly
- Give vaccine subcutaneously in patients with bleeding disorders.
- For intramuscular use, avoid gluteal region.
- In infants, anterolateral part of thigh is the best site for administration of Intramuscular injections whereas in adults, deltoid is more preferable.

Adverse Reactions

- Pain, redness and swelling at injection site
- Fever, headache.

Contraindications

- Hypersensitivity to the vaccine
- Pregnancy and Lactation.

Efficacy of Vaccine

Seroconversion rates vary from 93 percent to more than 99 percent just 1 month after the 1st dose of the vaccine. Booster dose after 6 to 12 months gives long-term immunity.

A few experts do recommend an additional Booster dose 20 years after the 1st dose in order to obtain life-long immunity.

Live Hepatitis A Vaccine

- Single dose –1 ml subcutaneously
- No need of boosters presently
- Efficacy = 98%
- Side effects rare, No reversal to wild disease.

WHO Recommendation

In high endemicity regions large scale vaccination is not recommended.

In intermediate endemicity regions, it may be considered as a supplement to health education and improvement in sanitation.

Hepatitis A Vaccine Controversies

Inclusion in UIP

Unlike Varicella, most infections due to Hepatitis Aare subclinical or cause very mild symptoms.

Epidemiological studies from most parts of our country show that up to 80%, 90% and 95% children get infected by this virus before 5,10 and 15 years of age respectively. Natural infections besides being benign, lead to strong immunity providing life long protection. Although a few cases of fulminant hepatic failure in older children have been reported but this a rare phenomenon. Thus at present there are no reasons to incorporate Hepatitis A vaccine either in the UIP. If the seroprevalence goes below 50% at 5 years of age then we may consider including this vaccine in the immunization schedule.

ROTAVIRUS VACCINE

Six to forty five percent of all childhood diarrheas that need hospitalization are due to rotavirus. Currently two live oral vaccines are licensed and marketed worldwide, Rotarix and RotaTeq.

Rotarix: Rotarix is a monovalent (G3P8) attenuated human rotavirus vaccine to be administered orally in a 2-dose schedule to infants of approximately 2 and 4 months of age. The interval between the 2 doses should be at least 4 weeks. The 2-dose schedule should be completed by age 16 weeks, and no later than by 24 weeks of age. It is available as a lyophilized vaccine to be reconstituted with liquid diluent prior to administration. If the infant spits out or regurgitates the entire vaccine dose then the dose may be repeated at the same visit.

RotaTeq: The recommended schedule is 3 oral doses at ages 2, 4 and 6 months. The first dose should be administered between ages 6-12 weeks and subsequent doses at intervals of 4-8 weeks. Vaccination should not be initiated for infants aged >12 weeks. All 3 doses should be administered before the age of 32 weeks. The vaccine is available as a liquid virus mixed with buffer and no reconstitution is needed.

Rotavirus Vaccine Controversies

Rotavirus Vaccine and Intussusception

The first clinically licensed rotavirus vaccine (1998) was Rotashield, a live oral tetravalent vaccine. This vaccine was withdrawn soon after licensure due to occurrence of vaccine associated intussusception. Currently, two live oral vaccines are licensed and marketed worldwide, Rotarix and RotaTeq. Both vaccines have been demonstrated to be extremely safe with no increased risk of intussusception.

Inclusion in UIP

Rotavirus vaccine is expected to prevent only 8-12% of all diarrhoeas and may be about 40-45% of all severe diarrhea due to Rota virus. As such it is unlikely to be cost effective in our settings to introduce in the UIP.

HUMAN PAPILLOMA VIRUS (HPV) VACCINE

Background

Cervical cancer is responsible for significant morbidity/ mortality in Indian women and affects women of all socioeconomic strata.

Since protection is seen only when the vaccine is given before infection with HPV, the vaccine should be given prior to sexual debut.

The vaccine should preferably be introduced to parents as a cervical cancer preventing vaccine and not as a vaccine against a sexually transmitted infection.

Vaccines are not 100% protective against cervical cancer and not a replacement for periodic screening. Hence, screening programs should continue as per recommendations. Both the available vaccines are equally efficacious and safe for protection against cervical cancer and precancerous lesions as of currently available data.

The quadrivalent vaccine (Gardasil) has in addition, demonstrable efficacy against vaginal and vulvar cancers, and protects against anogenital warts.

Dose

The dose is 0.5 mL intramuscular in deltoid.

The recommended age for initiation of vaccination is 10-12 years. Catch up vaccination is permitted up to the age of 26 years.

Three doses at 0, 2 and 6 months are recommended with Gardasil (minimum interval between 1st and 2nd dose is 4 weeks and second and third dose is 12 weeks) and 0, 1 and 6 months with Cervarix.

Contraindications

Both vaccines are contraindicated in those with history of previous hypersensitivity to any vaccine component and should be avoided in pregnancy. The vaccines may be administered in the immunocompromised but immunogenicity and efficacy may be lower. At present there is no data to support use of boosters.

COMBINATION VACCINES

Definition

Vaccines which contain multiple antigens to prevent different diseases or to provide protection against multiple strains of infectious agents causing the same disease

Present Combinations

- DTaP (where aP stands for acellular pertussis)
- DTP-Hib (Diphtheria, Tetanus, Pertussis and *H. influenzae* B vaccines)
- Hib-Hepatitis B (*H. influezae* B and Hepatitis B vaccine)
- DTP-Hepatitis B (Diphtheria, Tetanus, Pertussis and Hepatitis B vaccine)
- HAV-HAB (Hepatitis A and B)
- Pentavalent vaccine (Diphtheria, Pertussis, Tetanus, Hepatitis B and *H. influenzae* B vaccines).

Future combinations which may be developed include Hexavalent and Septavalent vaccines containing IPV (injectable polio vaccine) and *Streptococcus pneumoniae*.

Advantages

- Improves vaccination coverage.
- Ensures the administration of different vaccines at the specified time with the minimum number of injection.
- Ideal for vaccinating children with delayed/ missed doses.
- Overcomes the problem of multiple injections
- Reduces the cost of extra visits

Disadvantages

- Incompatibility of different antigens when mixed together.
- Immunologic interference by the different antigens against each other.
- Decreased immunogenicity of individual vaccine components.
- Increased reactogenicity (increased incidence of adverse effects) of individual vaccine components.
- Decreased shelf-life of the vaccine.
- Patients may receive extra doses of vaccine antigens for disease to which they have already received the recommended number of doses.

COLD CHAIN

ORDER OF SENSITIVITY OF VACCINES TO HEAT

Most Sensitive

- BCG (after reconstitution)
- OPV
- Measles (both before and after reconstitution)

- Hepatitis B
- DTP
- DT
- BCG (before reconstitution)
- Tetanus toxoid.

Least Sensitive

- Sensitivity of vaccines to freezing

Vaccines damaged by freezing	*Vaccines that can be frozen without harm*
DTP	OPV
DT	Measles /MMR
TT	BCG (before reconstitution)
Hepatitis B	

The cold chain involves two complementary aspects:

- The set chain represented by the walkin cold rooms, deep freezers and refrigerators
- The mobile chain represented by isothermic boxes and vaccine carriers.

Equipment

- *Walk-in freezers (WIF)*:
  - Used for bulk storage of OPV and measles vaccines and for preparing frozen ice packs at state stores
  - Maintain a temperature of -20° C
- *Walk in cold rooms (WIC)*:
  - Used for bulk storage of vaccines at the manufacturer, state and regional levels which store vaccines for about 4-5 districts
  - Maintain a temperature of 2 to 8°C.
- *Deep freezers*:
  - Used for storage of OPV/Measles/MMR vaccines and for preparation of ice-packs
    - DTP/DT/TT/Hepatitis B vaccines should not be stored in deep freezers. Cabinet temperature is maintained between – 18 and -20°C.
    - In case of power failure these freezers can maintain the cabinet temperature for 18 to 26 hours, if not opened.
    - Vaccine diluents should never be kept in deep freezers.
- *Ice lined refrigerators (ILR)*:
  - Contains either ice cubes or ice packs filled with water upto 90% of their volumes; on freezing there is formation of an inner lining of ice; this enables the temperature to stay within a safe range even when there is electricity supply for only 8 to 12 hours in a day.
    - In top opening ILRs the lowest temperature are at the bottom – this should be used for storing OPV/Measles/MMR; DTP/DT/TT/Hepatitis B vaccines should kept near the top in a separate container to avoid accidental freezing.
- *Domestic refrigerators*:
  - Meant for vaccine storage, should not be used for any other purpose.
    - Should be kept away from heat and direct sunlight; should have ice-packs for freezer compartment and water bottles in the shelves, which help in maintaining low temperatures in case of power failure.
    - Periodic defrosting is necessary when the layer of ice exceeds 5 to 6 mm.
    - The usual temperature within the main compartment of a domestic refrigerator is between 4 and 10°C while that of the freezer compartment is between 0 and -4°C.
- *Cold boxes or isothermic boxes*:
  Are well insulated, sealed boxes packed with frozen ice packs at the bottom, sides and at the top.
  - These are supplied to all peripheral centers and are used for transportation of large amounts of vaccines to outreach facilities.

- Vaccines should be placed in cartons or polythene bags and then placed in the cold box; vials of DTP, DT and TT vaccines should not be placed in direct contact with frozen ice packs.
- In emergency situations, can also be used to store vaccines and frozen ice packs for up to 5 days.
- Ice packs should be made from tap water; water should be filled in the icepack up to the level marked.

- *Vaccine carriers*:
  - Are smaller versions of cold boxes and are used to carry small quantities of vaccines (e.g.16-20 vials).
    - Can maintain temperatures for 2 days if the packs are frozen and lid is kept tightly closed.
    - DTP/DT/TT/Hepatitis B vials should be wrapped in plastic to avoid direct contact with ice.
- *Day carriers*:
  - Are smaller versions of vaccine carriers and are used to carry still smaller quantities (e.g. 6-8 vials) of vaccine.
    - Have provision for only 2 frozen ice-packs.
    - Can be used to store vaccines for 6-8 hours.
    - Vaccines in day carrier should be issued on the day of immunization only; presently, the use of day carriers is not encouraged.
- *Ice packs*:
  - Are made of polyethylene and weight approximately 80 gms; the dimensions are 163 × 90 × 33 mm^3, contain 0.36 L of water; never add salt to the water.
    - Ice packs are used to line the sides of cold boxes, vaccine carriers and day carriers.

Vaccine Vial Monitor (VVM)

- Time and temperature sensitive colored label that provides the indication of the cumulative heat to which the vial has been exposed.
- The VVM warns the end user when exposure to heat is likely to have degraded the vaccine beyond and acceptable level.
- However, there may be other factors which can also affect the potency of vaccine (e.g. Storage beyond the expiry date) and these may not be reflected in the VVM.
- It is used especially for temperature moni-toring of OPV, which is the most thermolabile of all vaccines, it can be presumed that other vaccines would also be potent.

Interpretation of Color Changes of VVM

- *Inner Square is lighter than outer circle*: if the expiry date has not passed, vaccines can be used.
- *Inner Square matches the color of outer circle or is darker than outer circle*: Vaccine should be discarded.

The change in color is gradual but irreversible.

"T" Series of Vaccines

DPT, DT, TT, Typhoid Vi and also Hepatitis B vaccines should not be frozen since they contain aluminium salts which are used as adjuvants, which get desiccated and act as irritants which may result in sterile abscess. Hence, care should be taken not to allow these vaccines to come in direct contact with ice.

It is mandatory that shake test is done before the use of either of these vaccines to make sure that the solution is uniform. Generally, potency of the vaccine stored is tested by lifting a sample vial of OPV only. If this most thermolabile vaccine is found to be potent, the rest of the vaccines are presumed to be equally potent.

Vaccine Induced Diseases

BCG:	Tuberculosis BCG adenitis
OPV:	Vaccine induced poliomyelitis (1 in 3 million)
Pertussis:	Convulsion Encephalopathy Anaphylaxis Excessive crying
Measles:	Modified measles SSPE
Rabies:	Local pain, fever, neuroparalytic complications (with nervous tissue vaccines)

EDIBLE VACCINES

- Vaccines that are genetically implanted inside a food or plants
- Consumption results in immunity to specific diseases
- Scientists are hoping to wipe out enteric diseases, such as diarrhea and cholera, by using vaccines grown in specific foods that need no refrigeration.
- Genetically altered potatoes were used to produce vaccine against 'traveler's diarrhea'
- A tasty vaccine-containing food, particularly bananas, a favorite food among children, could be inexpensive and plentiful. Delivery of vaccines in plant cells also may protect the antigen as it passes through the acid environment of the stomach.
- Transformed plants with the gene encoding the hepatitis B surface antigen (HBsAg) have been used; this is the same antigen used in the commercial yeast-derived vaccine.

IMMUNIZATION IN SPECIAL CIRCUMSTANCES

PRETERM INFANTS

- All vaccines are safe
- All vaccines are given as per schedule irrespective of birth weight / period of gestation
- In VLBW – Immunize the child after initial stabilization.

On Steroid Therapy

- Topical/ Local Injection of steroids are not contraindications for vaccines
- At physiologic maintenance dose of steroids all vaccines are safe
- For patients on high dose oral steroids >2 weeks:
  - No live vaccines should be given until 4 weeks after stopping steroids.
  - Killed vaccines are safe but may not be completely effective.

On Immunosuppressive and Antimalignancy Drugs

- No live vaccines should be given
- Toxoids and inactivated vaccines are safe
- Preferably given 1 month after stopping treatment
- If planned therapy e.g. organ transplants- Complete Immunization schedule 4 weeks before initiating such therapy.

Bleeding Disorders on Anticoagulants

- Give all vaccines as per schedule
- Use ≤ 23 G needle
- Apply firm and sustained pressure without rubbing for 5 minutes.

Thalassemic Children

- All vaccines can be safely given
- Immune response is good
- Give hepatitis B Vaccine as soon as possible
- Give Hemophilus Infuenzae type B, Pneumococcal, Meningococcal vaccines at least 4 weeks prior to splenectomy.

Primary Immunodeficiencies

- No live vaccines should be given.
- Killed vaccines are safe but may not be completely effective.
- Exception – children with IgA deficiency.
- Phagocyte function disorders – all vaccines safe except live bacterial vaccines (BCG, Oral typhoid vaccine).

HIV Infection (Table 4.7)

Vaccine Safety

- Live Vaccines: Severe vaccine associated disease can occur.
- No reported increase of adverse reactions
- Disseminated BCG disease in infants with symptomatic HIV can occur.

Efficacy of Vaccines

- Satisfactory sero conversion in early stages, e.g. Polio and Tetanus Vaccine
- Gradual decrease with progression of infection e.g. Measles vaccine
- Lower antibody levels depending on severity of infection
- Rapid fall of antibody levels e.g. Hepatitis B vaccine.

Pregnancy and Lactation

- Vaccine to be given only if absolutely necessary
- No live vaccines should be given
- Accidental administration of vaccine – No reason for MTP
- Toxoids and killed vaccines are safe but should be delayed till second trimester
- Tetanus toxoid is safe and should be given
- All vaccines are safe during lactation.

Lapsed Immunization

- No need to restart regardless of the time elapsed.
- Give vaccine at the next visit.
- Complete the schedule at the earliest
- If immunization status uncertain / unknown – start schedule as for unimmunized child.

Simultaneous Administration of Vaccines

- Multiple vaccines can be given at the same time
- No major effect on efficacy of vaccines
- Use different sites using separate needles and syringes
- Do not mix vaccines unless specified.

Table 4.7: Recommendation for immunization in HIV infected children

	Symptomless HIV infection	*Symptomatic HIV infection*	*Children with HIV/AIDS*
BCG	Yes (at birth)	No	No
DTP	Yes (at 6,10,14 weeks)	Yes	Yes (But use DTPa)
OPV	Yes (at 0,6,10,14 weeks)	Yes	No (use inactivated polio vaccine)
Measles	Yes (at 6 and 9 months)	Yes	Yes (But contraindicated if CD4 + is <15%)
Hepatitis B	Yes (as for uninfected children)	Yes	Yes
Hib	–	–	Yes
Pneumococcal	–	–	Yes
Influenza	–	–	Yes (but not below 6 months of age)
Varicella	–	–	Yes
Meningococcal	–	–	Yes

Table 4.8: Schedule in adolescents

Vaccine	Age
1. Tetanus Toxoid/Td	Boosters at 10 and 16 years
2. Rubella vaccine or MMR vaccine	1 dose to girls at 12-13 years of age. If not given earlier
3. Hepatitis B vaccine	3 doses at 0,1 and 6 months, if not given earlier
4. Typhoid vaccine	Vi-polysaccharide vaccine every 3 years
5. Varicella vaccine	1 dose upto 13 years, and 2 doses (at 4-8 weeks interval) after 13 years of age (if not given earlier)
6. Hepatitis A vaccine	2 doses 0 and 6 months

Vaccination Schedule in Adolescents (Table 4.8)

- Three broad categories:
  - a. To boost waning immunity
  - b. To accelerate control or elimination
  - c. To counter specific risk, e.g. due to travel, their lifestyle, etc.

Immunization for Travelers

- No uniform recommendations
- Depends upon –Region /country to be visited and duration of trip:
  - ❐ Vaccine commonly recommended for Indians traveling abroad include:
    - ■ *Yellow fever* vaccine for those traveling to destinations in South America and Subsaharan Africa.
    - ■ The other vaccine that may be required is against *Tick born encephalitis* for travelers to Europe. However, this vaccine is not mandatory and not routinely available in India.

Vaccines to be recommended for children traveling from Western countries to India are *BCG, Typhoid* and *Hepatitis A* (if stay is prolonged).

CHAPTER 5

ANTIBIOTIC THERAPY

EMPIRICAL INITIAL ANTIMICROBIAL THERAPY (TABLE 5.1)

Broad guidelines for initial antibiotic therapy are:

Septicemia

First line: Third generation cephalosporin (Ceftriaxone/Cefotaxime) with aminoglycosides (Amikacin).

Alternative therapy: Quinolones (Ciprofloxacin) with Aminoglycosides (Amikacin), or Imipenem.

Pneumonia

Community acquired pneumonias tend to be due to Pneumococcus, Staphylococcus, or Atypical microbes such as Mycoplasma infections.

S. pneumoniae: Penicillin group of antibiotics (Ampicillin) or a second generation cephalosporin such as cefuroxime plus a macrolide (erythromycin, clarithromycin or azithromycin) to cover for Mycoplasma pneumonia.

Staphylococcal pneumoniae: Amoxycillin with clavulanic acid (Augmentin) or cloxacillin plus gentamicin for synergistic activity.

Aspiration pneumonia: Ampicillin, amikacin and metronidazole. Clindamycin has good anerobic and staphylococcal coverage.

Hospital acquired Staphylococcal pneumonias: Resistant to antistaphylococcal penicillins and therefore are best treated with vancomycin.

Hospital acquired Pseudomonas pneumoniae: Ceftazidime with quinolones (ofloxacin/ciprofloxacin/levofloxacin) or aminoglycoside such as amikacin may be appropriate.

Pneumonia in immunocompromized host: Third generation cephalosporin with Aminoglycoside empirically until culture results become available. One should consider adding acyclovir/antifungal therapy depending on clinical setting.

Abdominal Sepsis

Necrotizing enterocolitis, peritonitis due to gut perforation: Amoxycillin with Clavulinic acid or ceftriaxone/cefotaxime with metronidazole (both gram negative and anaerobic coverage). Alternatively ampicillin, gentamicin and clindamycin (or metronidazole).

Nephrotic syndrome with pneumococcal peritonitis: Amoxycillin with clavulanic acid.

Renal or urinary tract infections, such as pyelonephritis: Third generation cephalosporin with Aminoglycoside.

Enteric fever or colitis due to E. coli, Klebsiella, or Shigella: Ceftriaxone/quinolone and Metronidazole.

Central Nervous System (CNS) Infections: Meningoencephalitis

Therapy is based on suspected organisms:

- *Herpes simplex*: Acyclovir
- *Niesseria meningitis, H. Influenzae, Strep. pneumoniae*: Ceftriaxone
- *E.coli meningitis*: Cefotaxime & gentamicin
- *Brain abscess*: Ceftriaxone plus Vancomycin
- *Mastoid abscess*: Ceftazidime

Endocarditis

- *Strep viridans*: Penicillin and Gentamicin/ Amikacin therapy.
- *Staph. aureus*: Cloxacillin and Gentamicin/ Amikacin.
- *Methicillin resistant Staph. aureus (MRSA)*: Vancomycin (Hospital acquired infections).
- *Enterococcal endocarditis (Strep fecalis)*: Vancomycin and Gentamicin.

Table 5.1: Rational choice of antimicrobial agents

Site of Infection	Probable Organism	Antimicrobial of choice
i. Skin	Streptococcus, Staphylococcus	Penicillin, Erythromycin, Cephalexin*, Cloxacillin*
ii. Upper-respiratory tract	Streptococcus, Staphylococcus	Penicillin, Erythromycin, Cephalexin, Cloxacillin*
iii. Middle-ear	Pneumococcus, H.influenzae	Ampicillin, Amoxycillin, Cefaclor*
iv. Lower-respiratory tract		
<2 months	Esch.coli, Klebsiella	Ampicillin/Cefotaxime with gentamicin
2 months-3 years	H influenzae, Streptococcus, Staphylococcus	Ampicillin, Amoxycillin with or without clavulanic acid*, Chloramphenicol*, Cefaclor*
>3 years	Streptococcus, Pneumococcus, Staphylococcus	Penicillin, Ampicillin, Amoxycilliin, Cotrimoxazole Amoxicillin with clavulanic acid
v. Urinary-tract**	E. coli, Proteus, Klebsiella	Cotrimoxazole,Nitrofuration, Ampicillin, Amoxicillin, Nalidixic acid*
vi. Typhoid fever	Salmonella	Ciprofloxacin, Ceftriaxone
vii. Pyogenic meningitis***		
<3 months	E coli, Klebsiella, Staphylococcus, Psuedomonas	Ampicillin/Cefofaxime and Gentamycin/Amikacin
3 months-3 years	Pneumococcus, H. influenzae, Staphylococcus	Ampicillin and Chloramphennicol, Ceftriaxone* or Cefotaxime*
>3 years	Pneumococcus, Meningococcus	Crystalline penicillin and Chloramphenicol or Cefotaxime*
viii. Sepsis in newborn***	E.coli, Klebsiella, Stapylococcus	Ampicillin and Gentamicin/Cefotaxime and Amikacin

NB:

* These drugs should be considered as 2nd line of drugs, used only if other drugs have not been successful

** Culture and sensivity must be obtained before starting therapy

*** Would always require hospitalization.

POSTOPERATIVE EMPIRICAL ANTIBIOTICS

Urinary Catheter Infections

- Aminoglycosides until cultures are available.
- Catheter should be changed or removed.

Central Line Related Infections

Vancomycin with aminoglycoside to cover for Staph epidermidis and gram negative bacteria.

Peripheral intravenous line may be used for 48 hours or alternatively another central line should be placed at a different site. Guidewire change of central line is not routinely recommended for prevention of central line infections.

Ventriculoperitoneal Shunt Infection

Vancomycin (S. epidermidis and S. aureus coverage) and Ceftriaxone (gram negative coverage).

Remove shunt for resistant Pseudomonas infection.

Chest Infections

Augmentin and Ceftazidime, especially in patients with cystic fibrosis where *Pseudomonas aeruginosa* and *Pseudomonas cepacia*-lower respiratory tract infections are a common occurrence. Tobramycin by nebulizer may be indicated in such cases.

Empyema due to Staph aureus: Vancomycin/ Cloxacillin.

Empyema due to gram negative organisms: Cefotaxime/Gentamicin.

In case of resistant organisms imipenem may be required.

Neck Surgery

Amoxycillin with Clavulanic acid.

Heart Surgery

Ceftriaxone and Vancomycin.

Abdominal Surgery

Cefotaxime plus Metronidazole.

Orthopedics Surgery

Ceftriaxone with Aminoglycoside.

Septic arthritis or Osteomyelitis surgery: Vancomycin with Aminoglycoside.

FUNGAL INFECTIONS

Strongly suspected: Fever spikes and leukocytosis in patients on broad spectrum antibiotics longer than two weeks, as well as in immunocompromized children, children with malignancies, HIV and nephrotic syndrome.

Deep seated infections require Amphotercin B.

Urine culture may be positive for *Candida albicans* necessitating intravenous fluconazole in combination with Amphotericin B, bladder irrigation.

RENAL FAILURE

Antimicrobials needing dose reduction:

Even in mild failure	*Only in severe failure*
Aminoglycosides	Cotrimoxazole
Cephalexin	Carbenicillin
Ethambutol	Cefotaxime
Vancomycin	Norfloxacin
Amphotericin B	Ciprofloxacin
Flucytosine	Metronidazole
Acyclovir	

LIVER FAILURE

- Metabolism and elimination of some drugs (morphine, phenobarbitone, lidocaine, propranolol) are reduced so their dose should be reduced. Alternative drugs that should be preferred are oxazepam or lorazepam in place of diazepam, atenolol or sotalol as β blocker.

- Prodrugs needing hepatic metabolism for activation, e.g. prednisone, bacampicillin, sulindac are less effective and should be avoided.
- Due to reduced serum albumin, protein binding of acidic drugs is reduced and more drug is present in free form.
- Bioavailability of drugs having high first pass metabolism, e.g. phenobarbitone is increased due to loss of hepatocellular function.
- Avoid cephalosporins in general.
- Aminoglycosides, imipenem, quinolones are safe:

VANCOMYCIN

Indications

- Gram positive beta lactam resistant organisms (MRSA).
- Gram positive infections with allergy to beta lactam antibiotics.
- Second choice drug to metronidazole for antibiotic associated pseudomembranous enterocolitis caused by *C. difficile*
- Enterococcal endocarditis prophylaxis along with gentamicin.
- Prosthetic surgical procedure prophylaxis.

Vancomycin should *not be used* in the following situations:

- For routine surgical prophylaxis.
- Empirically if cultures negative for beta lactam resistant organism.
- For prophylaxis for central lines.
- For selective gastrointestinal decontamination.
- For eradication of MRSA colonization.

Alternative to vancomycin: Teicoplanin (same antibacterial spectrum to vancomycin but does not penetrate CNS so cannot be used in Staphylococcal meningitis).

CARBEPENEMS

Imipenem and Meropenem

- These are indicated for resistant hospital acquired gram negative infections such as Acinetobacter, Enterobacter, Klebsiella, Proteus, Pseudomonas species as well as aerobic gram positive bacteria such as Staphylococcus. These have good CSF penetration.
- Used in pediatric meningitis and severe infections in intensive care settings. It has also been used to treat septicemia, febrile neutropenia, lower respiratory tract infections including those in cystic fibrosis, and urinary tract infections.
- Not effective against methicillin resistant staphylococci (including MRSA) and enterococcus.
- Used as a reserve agent when the conventional therapy fails or when resistance to other antibiotics has been documented.
- With Meropenem there is lesser incidence of seizures when compared to Imipenem.
- Unlike Imipenem, Meropenem is stable against hydrolysis by human renal dehydropeptidase (DHP-1) and concomitant administration of cilastatin (DHP inhibitor) is not required.

Caution: These drugs do not cover Enterococcus, Chlamydia, Mycoplasma, Legionella and Listeria.

MONOBACTAMS

Monobactams such as Aztreonam are active against aerobic gram negative bacilli such as Pseudomonas, Serratia, Klebsiella and Enterobacter species.

NEWER MACROLIDES

Clarithromycin/Azithromycin

Useful for community acquired gram positive infections including Mycoplasma pneumonia.

QUINOLONES

Good broad spectrum gram positive and gram negative cover including enteric and urinary tract infections.

Indications

- UTI due to Pseudomonas
- Multidrug resistant enteric/gram negative bacterial infections
- Chronic suppurative otitis media
- Chronic osteomyelitis
- Cystic fibrosis exacerbation
- Oral therapy in immunocompromized host.

Alatrofloxacin, Trovofloxacin can cause acute liver failure.

Caution

Necrosis of developing cartilage arthropathy (Pefloxacin).

GRAM NEGATIVE RESISTANT INFECTIONS INCLUDING PSEUDOMONAS INFECTIONS

- Piperacillin and tazobactam
- Ampicillin and sulbactam
- Ticarcillin and clavulanic acid.

OTHER NEWER ANTIBIOTICS

Streptogramins (Quinapristin-dalfopristin): These antibiotics are meant for treating gram positive infection, especially Vancomycin resistant Strep faecalis (enterococcus), nosocomial pneumonia, central line related infections.

Everninomycin is used for gram positive nosocomial infections in intensive care units.

Telithromycin (a newer ketolide antibiotic) for respiratory infections.

Linezolid

- Outstanding activity against gram positive organisms including problem pathogens such as MRSA, penicillin resistant *Streptococcus pneumoniae* and Vancomycin resistant Enterococci, and against ciprofloxacillin resistant *S. aureus.*
- Acts early in protein synthesis, so cross resistance with other drugs acting on protein synthesis unlikely.
- 100% bioavailability allows rapid switch from intravenous to oral.
- No dose adjustment required in patients with hepatic and renal impairment.
- FDA approved for several indications like soft tissue infections with Vancomycin resistant enterococci and community acquired pneumonia.
- Safe and well tolerated.

CHAPTER 6

Differential Diagnosis of Abnormal Signs

BULGING ANTERIOR FONTANEL

The fontanel should be examined in a quiet child held in an upright position. The fontanel is normally flat and pulsatile. Bulging fontanel in infancy is a sign of raised intracranial tension:

- *Physiological:* Crying infant
- *Drugs:* Tetracycline/Vitamin A/Corticosteroid (following cessation)/Nalidixic acid
- *Metabolic Disorders:* Maple syrup urine disease/ Galactosemia
- Hyperparathyroidism/Vitamin D-dependent rickets/Congenital hypophosphatasia
- Raised intracranial tension (meningitis, intracranial bleeding, tumor, pseudotumor cerebri, etc.)
- Hydrocephalus.

CRANIOTABES

Craniotabes refers to softened bones which can be indented like a ping-pong ball. The sign should be elicited away from the suture line. It is normally elicitable in preterm babies.

- Physiological
- Rickets
- Congenital syphilis
- Hydrocephalus
- Osteogenesis imperfecta
- Lacunar skull.

BOSSING OF SKULL

Prominence of skull bones is called as bossing.

- Rickets
- Thalassemia major
- Congenital syphilis
- Achondroplasia
- Hurler's syndrome (mucopolysaccharidoses)
- Cleidocranial dysostosis
- Ectodermal dysplasia
- Ehlers-Danlos syndrome
- Pyknodysostosis.

PAPILLEDEMA

- *Intracranial space occupying lesions:* Tumor, abscess, tuberculoma
- Hydrocephalus
- Benign intracranial hypertension
- *Foster Kennedy syndrome:* Optic atrophy due to frontal lobe tumor pressing on optic nerve and contralateral papilledema secondary to raised intracranial pressure.

BLUE SCLERAE

- Normal newborn or small infants
- Osteogenesis imperfecta
- Glaucoma
- Ehlers-Danlos syndrome
- Marfan syndrome.

SETTING SUN SIGN

The eyes are rolled downward, iris is compeletely covered by the lower eyelids and upward sclera is visible. It occurs due to involvement of center of upward gaze which is located in the pretectal area of brainstem.

- Preterm infants
- Hydrocephalus
- Kernicterus
- Laron dwarfism.

CATARACT

- Prematurity
- Hereditary
- Chromosomal anomalies
  - ❐ 13, 18 and 21 Trisomy.
  - ❐ Turner's syndrome.
- *Developmental anomalies:* Persistent strand of papillary membrane
- *Intrauterine infections:*
  - ❐ Rubella.
- *Metabolic causes:*
  - ❐ Galactosemia, Juvenile Diabetes Mellitus, Hypoparathyroidism, Wilson's disease, Mucopolysaccharidosis.
- Miscellaneous: Steroids, Penetrating injury, Radiation.

CAT'S EYE

Normally when light shines through the pupil, red reflex is seen. Here it is absent and the pupil may appear white.

- *Lens:* - Cataract
- *Uveal tract:* - Persistent hyperplastic primary vitreous/Organized vitreous hemorrhage
- *Retina:*
  - ❐ Retinoblastoma
  - ❐ Retinal detachment
  - ❐ Retinopathy of prematurity
  - ❐ Endophthalmitis.

HYPERTELORISM

Increased interpupillary distance between the two eyes is called as hypertelorism. It occurs due to hypertrophy of the lesser wing of sphenoid.

Distance between the inner canthi divided by the distance between outer canthi > 0.38.

- Racial
- Down syndrome
- Cretinism
- Craniofacial dysostosis
- Thalassemia major
- Ehlers-Danlos syndrome
- Turner's syndrome
- Noonan syndrome.

Remember: Most of these are also causes of Depressed Nasal Bridge.

OCULAR HYPOTELORISM

Ocular hypotelorism is decreased distance between orbits. Distance between the inner canthus divided by the distance between the outer canthus < 0.33.

- Cyclops
- Ethmocephaly
- Cebocephaly
- Arrhinencephaly.

EXOPHTHALMOS

The sclera is visible above and below the cornea and lid lag is often present.

- Hyperthyroidism
- *Malignancies*: Neuroblastoma, Retinoblastoma, Teratoma
- *Nonmalignant masses*: Cavernous hemangioma, Optic nerve glioma
- *Orbital causes*: Retrorbital hemorrhage, Orbital cellulitis and abscess
- Crouzon's disease
- Chloroma (acute myeloid leukemia)
- Polyostotic fibrous dysplasia
- A.V. aneurysm
- Cavernous sinus thrombosis
- Neurofibromatosis.

PTOSIS

Ptosis is unilateral or bilateral drooping of eyelid

- Congenital
- Oculomotor palsy (ptosis with mydriasis)
- Horner's syndrome (ptosis, enophthalmos, miosis and lack of sweating)
- Myasthenia gravis
- Botulism
- Myotonic dystrophy
- Noonan syndrome
- Local lesion like edema of eyelid.

MONGOLOID SLANT (UP AND OUT)

- Racial
- Down syndrome
- Ectodermal dysplasia
- Prader-Willi syndrome.

ANTIMONGOLOID SLANT (DOWN AND OUT)

- Treacher-Collins syndrome
- Noonan's syndrome
- Mandibulofacial dysostosis
- Turner's syndrome
- Trisomy 18
- Apert's syndrome

LOW SET EARS

Imaginary line drawn between inner and outer canthi should bisect the ears into upper one-third and lower two third portions. Normally 1/3rd of the ear comes above this line. When less than 20% comes above this line, it is low set ear.

- Down syndrome
- Renal agenesis (Potter facies)
- Turner's syndrome
- Trisomy 17-18, 13-15
- Treacher-Collins syndrome
- Cri-du-chat syndrome
- Apert syndrome.

MICROGNATHIA (HYPOPLASIA OF MANDIBLE)

- Pierre Robin syndrome
- Cri-du-chat syndrome
- Fetal alcohol syndrome
- Rubinstein-Taybi syndrome
- Trisomy – 13 and 18
- Treacher-Collins syndrome
- Pyknodystosis

MACROGLOSSIA (BIG TONGUE)

- Cretinisim
- Down syndrome (tongue is normal but oral cavity is small)

- Glycogen storage disease (Pompe disease)
- Hurler's syndrome
- Generalized gangliosidosis
- Growth on tongue (lymphangioma, neurofibromatosis)
- Duchene's muscular dystrophy.

GUM HYPERPLASIA

- Poor oral hygiene
- Drug-induced Phenytoin
- Scurvy
- Acute monocytic leukemia
- Hurler's syndrome
- Epulis
- Diffuse fibromatosis
- Histiocytosis X.

DELAYED DENTITION

Eruption of primary dentition usually occurs around 6 to 8 months of age. Dentition is considered as delayed if there is no eruption of teeth by 12 months.

- Constitutional delay
- Protein-energy malnutrition
- Rickets
- Hypothyroidism
- Hypopituitarism.

TRISMUS (LOCKJAW)

There is inability to open the mouth.

- Tetanus
- Temporomandibular joint arthritis
- Part of dystonia (metaclopramide)
- Encephalitis
- Strychnine poisoning
- Tumor of the jaw (rhabdomyosarcoma)
- Anesthetic-induced malignant hyperthermia
- Infantile Gaucher's disease.

ORAL THRUSH

- Fungal infection
- Steroids
- Antibiotics
- AIDS
- Hypoparathyroidism.

LARGE HEAD (MACROCEPHALY)

- *Megalencephaly:*
  - Hydrocephalus, Storage disorders, Achondroplasia, Gigantism, Tay-Sachs disease, Neurofibromatosis.
- Subdural hematoma
- Intracranial SOL
- Arachnoid Cyst
- *Skeletal disorders:* Achondroplasia, Pyknodysostosis, Cleidocranial dysostosis, Hurler's syndrome.

SHORT NECK

Ratio of neck length (distance between external occipital protuberance and the C7 spine) and height is approximately 1:13, if it is more than 1:13 it suggests short neck.

- Down syndrome
- Hypothyroidism
- Hurler's syndrome
- Klippel-Feil deformity
- Turner's syndrome (Webbed neck)
- Sprengel's deformity
- Noonan syndrome.

NECK RIGIDITY

- Meningitis
- Subarachnoid hemorrhage
- Meningismus
- Space occupying lesions of brain

- *Local causes:* Retropharyngeal abscess, painful cervical adenitis
- *Neck retraction:* Tetanus, dystonia.

COSTOCHONDRAL BEADING

- Rickets (broad and dome-shaped)
- Scurvy (sharp like a bayonet due to posterior subluxation of sternum)
- Chondrodystrophy.

OPISTOTONUS

- Tetanus
- Kernicterus
- Dystonia (metaclopramide poisoning)
- Meningitis
- Infantile Gaucher's disease.

MICROPENIS

Micropenis is diagnosed when length of penis is less than 2.0 cm in infants (Normal length is 4-5 cm).

- Hypogonadotrophic hypogonadism (Kallmann's syndrome, Prader-Willi syndrome).
- Klinefelter's syndrome
- Down's syndrome
- Cornelia de Lange syndrome
- X-linked hypogammaglobulinemia
- Hypopituitarism
- CHARGE association.

ABNORMALITIES OF TESTICULAR SIZE

During pre-adolescence the size of testes are between 1.5-2.0 cm. The adult size of testes varies between 3.5-5.0 cm. Failure of testicular enlargement by the age of 14 years is suggestive of delayed sexual maturation or hypogonadism.

Micro-orchidism

- Hypopituitarism
- Hypothalamic disorder
- Rudimentary testis syndrome
- Klinefelter syndrome
- Laurence-Moon-Biedl syndrome.

Macro-orchidism

- Fragile-X syndrome
- Sexual precocity
- Hypothyroidism
- Testicular tumors

CAFË-AU-LAIT SPOTS

Café-au-lait spots are considered significant if:

- Prepubertal : > 5 mm in size and 5 in number
- Postpubertal : >15 mm in size and 6 in number
- Isolated Café-au-lait spot >15 cm in size
- Any Café-au-lait spot in the center of the body
- Café-au-lait spot associated with neurofibromatosis.

Causes

- Neurofibromatosis
- Tuberous sclerosis
- McCune-Albright syndrome
- Ataxia telangiectasia
- Gaucher's disease
- Chediak-Higashi syndrome
- Fanconi's anemia.

HEMIHYPERTROPHY

It is characterized by enlargement of one-half of the body or it may be limited to the face or one of the extremities.

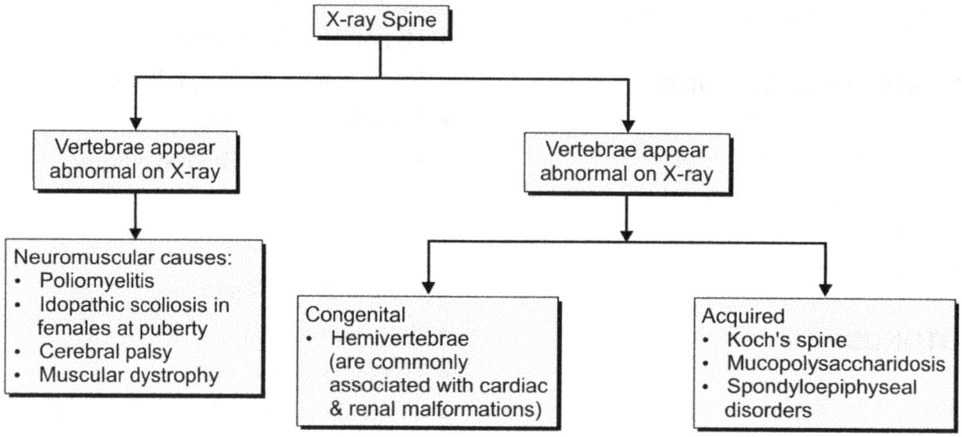

Fig. 6.1: Common causes of scoliosis

- Idiopathic
- Beckwith-Wiedemann syndrome
- Wilms tumor
- Neurofibromatosis
- Adrenocortical carcinoma
- Lymphedema
- Russell-Silver syndrome.

PIGEON–SHAPED CHEST

- Rickets
- Congenital
- Skeletal dysplasia
- Emphysema
- Mucopolysaccharidosis – Type IV
- Marfan's syndrome
- Noonan's syndrome.

SCOLIOSIS (FIG. 6.1)

Postural

- Commonest and disappears when the patient bends down.

Compensatory

- This occurs due to any cause which leads to shortening of one of the legs.

Structural

- Scoliosis which persists when the child bends down is known as Structural Scoliosis.

CHAPTER 7

DIETARY HISTORY

DIETARY HISTORY

Take dietary history specifying following points:

- Whether the child has been breastfed or not.
- Exclusively breastfed for what duration (how many months).
- If breastfeed:
  - ❒ Frequency
  - ❒ Duration of each feed
  - ❒ Adequacy of breastfeeding (child gaining weight; sleeps adequately between feeds with minimum interval of 2-3 hours between feeds; passes urine 6 to 8 times per day; Let down reflex occurs from the opposite breast on feeding).
- If top-fed:
  - ❒ Type of milk used
  - ❒ Dilution
  - ❒ Mode of feeding (bottlefed or katori spoon fed)
  - ❒ Whether bottle and nipple were washed regularly before each feed
  - ❒ Vitamin supplements given or not.
- Complementary feeds:
  - ❒ Age at which started
  - ❒ Nature
  - ❒ Amount of food given to the child
  - ❒ Frequency of food
- Dietary history:
  - ❒ Food intake during 24 hours prior to the onset of illness
  - ❒ Calculate the approximate calorie and protein intake per day
  - ❒ Compare the calorie and protein intake of child with that of normal child
  - ❒ Diet includes fruits and is rich in fiber or not.
- History of pica

Table 7.1: Comparison with human and cow's milk (100 ml)

Nutrient	*Human milk*	*Cow's milk*
Macronutrients		
Calories	67	67
Proteins	1.1 g	3.0 g
Casein	20% (β)	80% (α)
Whey	80% (lactalbumin and lactoferrin)	20% (lactoglobulin)
Lactose	7 g	4.5 g
Fat	3.5 g	4.5 g
Micronutrients		
Ca:P ratio	> 2	< 2
Sodium	0.9 mEq	2.2 mEq
Iron	30-50 µg (50% absorbed)	30-50 µg (20% absorbed)
Vitamins		
Vit. K	15 µg	60 µg
Vit. E	2 mg	0.4 mg
Osmolarity	7.9 mOsm	22.1 mOsm
Energy: Protein ratio	70:1	25:1

HEALTHY FEEDING HABIT FOR INFANTS

Breastfeeds

- Start immediately after birth.
- Exclusive breastfeed for 6 months (not even water, even in summer).
- Continue breastfeeds for 2 years.

Complementary Feeds

- Start at 6 months
- Soft, hygienic, home made, variety foods, culturally accepted
- By one and half years, child should be eating family diet.

  No bottle feeding, proprietary milk formula and proprietary weaning foods, refined food, egg, non-vegetarian, and limited salt and sugar.

  No superstitions like hot food and cold food, worm producing food (sugar), exclusion of colostrum, etc.

SIGNS THAT BREASTFEEDING IS GOING WELL

Remember the pneumonic **BREAST**

BODY POSITION

- Mother relaxed and comfortable
- Baby's body close, facing breast
- Baby's head and body straight
- Baby's chin touching breast
- Baby's bottom supported.

RESPONSES

- Baby reaches for breast if hungry
- Baby roots for breast
- Baby explores breast with tongue
- Baby calm and alert at breast
- Baby stays attached to breast
- Signs of milk ejection (leaking, after pains).

EMOTIONAL BONDING

- Secure, confident hold
- Face-to-face attention from mother
- Much touching by mother.

ANATOMY

- Breasts soft after feed
- Nipples stand out, protractile
- Skin appears healthy
- Breast looks round during feed.

SUCKLING

- Mouth wide open
- Lower lip turned outwards
- Tongue cupped around breast
- Cheeks round
- More areola above baby's mouth
- Slow deep sucks, bursts with pauses
- Can see or heard swallowing.

TIME SPENT SUCKLING

- Baby releases breast
- Baby suckled for _____ minutes.

CHARACTERISTICS OF IDEAL COMPLEMENTARY FOOD

- Timely introduction at 6 months
- Adequate and should provide sufficient energy, protein and micronutrients (Table 7.2).
- Hygenic and should be given in proper frequency according to age

Table 7.2: Holiday-Segar formula for calculation of calories

Up to 10 kg	– 100 kcal/kg
10 – 20 kg	– 1000 + 50 kcal for each kg above 10 kg
Above 20 kg	– 1500 + 20 kcal for each kg in excess above 20 kg

Table 7.3: RDA of vitamins and minerals

Vitamin A	1500 IU/day (500 μg)
Vitamin D	400 IU/day (10 μg)
Vitamin E	5-15 IU/day (5-15 mg)
Vitamin B complex	
B_1 Thiamine	0.5-1.5 mg/day (1 mg/1000 cal)
B_2 Riboflavin	0.5-1.5 mg/day
B_6 Pyridoxine	0.5-1.5 mg/day
B_3 Niacin	5-15 mg/day
B_{11} Folic acid	50-150 μg/day
B_{12} Cyanocobalamine	0.5-1.5 μg/day
Vitamin C	40-50 mg/day
Macroelements	
Calcium	500-1000 mg/day
Phosphorus	800-1000 mg/day
Magnesium	200-300 mg/day
Trace elements	
Iron	10-20 mg/day
Iodine	50-150 μg/day
Copper	0.5-1 mg/day
Zinc	5-15 mg/day
Fluoride	1-5 mg/day

Table 7.4: Some common foodstuffs supplying 100 Cals

	Amount	*Cooked Measure*
Cereals	30 gm	Approx. 1 katori or 2 chapati
Pulses	30 gm	Approx. 1 katori
Vegetables		
• Leafy	200 gm	Approx 1.5 katori
• Roots	100 gm	Approx ¾ katori
• Others	300 gm	Approx 2 katori
Nuts	15 gm	-
Fruits (Pulpy fruits)	125 gm	1 med size (raw)
Milk (Cow's)	150 ml	¾ - 1 cup
Egg	1 ¼	1 ¼
Meat	80 gm	2 big pieces
Sugar	25 gm	5 tsp
Butter	15 gm	3 tsp
Oil	10 gm	2 tsp
Sago seeds (Sabudana)	30 gm	1 medium katori (Cooked)

- 6-12 months—3 times/day if breastfeed and 5 times/day if not breastfeed;
- 12-24 months—5 times/day
- Soft, home made, easy to digest and culturally acceptable.

MILK PRODUCING REFLEXES (PROLACTIN REFLEX)

Suckling by baby stimulates sensory nerve endings in nipple
↓
Impulses travel along sensory nerve in vagus to hypothalamus
↓
Anterior pituitary releases prolactin into blood
↓
Prolactin acts on milk secreting cells to produce milk

MILK EJECTION REFLEX (OXYTOCIN REFLEX)

Baby sucks on nipple
↓
Sensory impulses act on post pituitary
↓
Post pituitary releases oxytocin
↓
Oxytocin acts on myoepithelial cells around alveoli, ducts and sinuses which contract to release milk

Important Points

- More prolactin production occurs at night
- Prolactin suppresses ovulation and helps spacing of births.
- Oxytocin contracts uterine muscle, preventing, causing leaking and milk from one breast when she feeds the baby at another.

FACTORS AFFECTING MOTHER'S REFLEXES

Acute (anger, shock, pain)
↓
Adrenaline released
↓
Vasoconstriction of vessels around alveoli
↓
Oxytocin does not reach myoepithelial cells
↓
No alveoli contraction
↓
No milk ejection

Chronic (anxiety, worry, lack of confidence and support)
↓
Inhibits both milk producing & milk ejection reflex

CHAPTER 8

DEVELOPMENTAL HISTORY

DEVELOPMENTAL HISTORY

Accurate history is often difficult to obtain due to poor observation and educational status of parents and early events in the life of child's development may be forgotten by the parents.

- Ask milestones in a chronological order in a simple and lucid manner
- Compare development of the index child with his siblings
- Ask whether the child interacts and plays with children of his age or likes the company of younger children
- Identify whether child is globally retarded or backward only in an individual or specific field
- Predominant speech delay: Hearing problem, autism, dyslexia
- Predominant motor delay
- Global delay that is nonprogressive (child is achieving milestones but at a later date than expected, child has not lost any achieved milestones)
- Global delay that is progressive (child was developing normally, has slowed down in development and ultimately stopped achieving milestones and has lost some of the milestones already achieved)
- Current social skills
- Participation in an early intervention program (if aged <3 years) or school support (if aged >3 years) should be reviewed, including resource room assistance
- Physical, occupational, speech and language therapy
- Adaptive physical education
- Standardized cognitive and educational testing can be asked.

  The developmental progress of older children is best evaluated by consideration of school performance, proficiency in games, motor dexterity and social behavior.

METHODS OF DEVELOPMENT ASSESSMENT

- *Below 3 years:*
  - Denver developmental screening test
  - Bayley scales of infant development
  - Phatak-Baroda Development Screening Tests
  - Trivandrum Draw-a-man test.
- *Above 3 years:*
  - Binet-Kamat test
  - Seguin form board
  - Goodenough's Draw-a-man test.

Tests of General Intelligence

- Stanford-Binet intelligence scale
- Wechsler intelligence scale for children
- Gesell developmental scale.

METHODS STANDARDIZED FOR ASSESSMENT OF DEVELOPMENT IN CHILDREN

Screening Tests

Denver Developmental Screening Test (DDST)

- To evaluate psychosocial status of children from birth to 6 years
- It contains about 125 items
- It contains range of developmental skills for gross, fine motor, language, adaptive and personal social milestones
- It does not quantitatively measure intelligence, motor development, communication skills or social competence
- It is only a screening test and does not measure IQ or DQ
- The test can be used by educated parents only or in office practice.

Bayley Scales of Infant Development (Motor and Mental)

- Most popular and widely practiced
- It requires the services covering mental, motor and infant behavior in children upto 30 months of age
- India's best known development testing system
- Test items arranged according to age.

Baroda Development Screening Test

- It is the Indian adaptation of Bayle scale of infant development
- It contains 22 motor items and 32 mental items
- Developmental age and quotient can be easily calculated
- Can be used by field workers and in office practice
- Sensitivity and specificity is >65%.

Trivandrum Developmental Screening Test

- It measures motor, mental, hearing and vision
- It contains 17 items from Baroda Scale
- Age range – 0-6 years
- Sensitivity – >66.7%
- Specificity – >78.8%
- If child fails to achieve any item 3rd percentile → developmental delay
- It does not require developmental kit.

Evaluation Tests

Development Assessment Scale for Indian Infants (DASII)

- It is revised Baroda scale by P Pathak (1997)
- It measures motor and mental development
- Age range – 0-30 months.

Gesell's Development Schedule

- Motor, adaptive language, personal and social development
- Age range – 0-6 years.

Amiel-Tison Method of Assessment

- Pays special attention to muscle tone (active and passive), neurosensory responses (visual and acoustic) and neurobehavioral assessment

Vineland and Raval's Social Maturity Scale

- Assess the social and adaptive mental development

INDICATIONS FOR DEVELOPMENT ASSESSMENT

- Follow-up of high risk neonates for early detection of cerebral palsy or mental retardation
- Complete evaluation of children with developmental, chromosomal and neurological disorders
- To differentiate children with retardation in specific fields of development as opposed to those with global retardation.

TARGET MILESTONES

The upper age limits for achievement of some of the target milestones are:

- Lack of social smile by 2 months
- Absence of stable head control by 4 months
- Inability to sit when pulled to sit by 6 months
- Lack of sitting without support by 8 months
- Inability to stand without support by one year
- Lack of pincer grasp by one year
- Inability to play interactive games by one year
- Inability to walk without support by 18 months
- Absence of syllabic babbling by one year
- Failure to make meaningful sentences by 3 years of age.

These children should be subjected to a detained developmental assessment.

Remember: A child who has attained social smile by 2 months, head control by 4 months, sitting by 8 months and standing by 10 months may be taken as grossly normal. Make sure the child sees, hears and listens. This helps in rapid assessment.

LAWS OF GROWTH

- Growth and development is *continuous* and *orderly* process
- Pattern of growth is *cephalocaudal*
- There is sequence of development within each development field, but development in one field does not run parallel with that in another field. This is called *dissociation.*
- Certain primitive reflexes have to be lost before corresponding voluntary movement is acquired.

MILESTONES

GROSS MOTOR

Ventral Suspension

4-12 weeks	Learns to lift and control his head in horizontal plane and then above horizontal plane

Supine Position

12-20 weeks	Control of head.

Prone Position

1 month	Lifts chin momentarily
3 months	Lifts head and upper part of forearm
6 months	Lifts head and greater part of chest
5-8 months	Supine to prone/prone to supine
8 months	Crawls
10 months	Creeps.

Sitting

8 months	Sits without support
9 months	Sits with support
10 months	Pulls from supine to sitting position.

Standing and Walking

9 months	Stand with support
10 months	Walking with support
11 months	Crawling
12 months	Stand without support
13 months	Walks without support with a broad based gait
15 months	Walks well without support
18 months	Creeps upwards and downwards in stairs
2 years	Climbs with both feet on one step
2-3 years	Kicks a ball
3 years	Climbs with one feet on one step/Pedaling tricycle
3-4 years	Standing on 1 foot
4 years	Goes down stairs one foot per step
5-6 years	Hopping
7-8 years	Skipping a rope

FINE MOTOR AND ADAPTIVE

Fine Motor

1 month	Hands remain closed
3 months	Grasp reflex disappears, opens hand spontaneously
4 months	Grasps ring when placed in hand. Initially object is held in ulnar side of hand (ulnar grasp)
5 months	Bidextrous grasp. Can grasp object voluntarily
7 months	Palmar grasp. Can transfer object from one hand to another
9 months	Pincer grasp
1 year	Releases object on command.

Feeding

15 months	With cup without spilling
18 months	With spoon with slight spilling

Picture Book

13 months	2-3 pages at a time
24 months	1 page at a time.

Scribbling

1-2 years	Scribbles spontaneously
2 years	Horizontal line
3 years	Copies circle
4 years	Copies square, rectangle
5 years	Copies cross, triangle
6 years	Copies hexagon
7 years	Copies kite
8 years	Copies double lined cross
9 years	Copies cylinder
11 years	Copies cube.

Tower of Cubes

18 months	Tower of 3 or 4
2 years	Tower of 6 or 7
2 ½ years	Tower of 8
3 years	Tower of 9

Vision

Binocular vision	2-3 months
Depth perception	6-8 months (begins); 5-7 years (accurate)

PERSONAL AND SOCIAL

1 month	Looks at face intently when spoken to
2 months	Social smile
3 months	Recognizes mother
6 months	Enjoys image in mirror, shows like and dislikes, stretches arms out when mother is going to lift him up
7-8 months	Stranger anxiety, Resists if toy pulled from hand
9 months	Waves bye bye, Enjoy peek a boo games

1 year	Comes when called, pulls mother's clothes to attract attention
1 ½ years	Mimics action of another
2 years	Wears simple garments/socks/shoes
3 years	Unbuttons dresses, dress and undress with help
4 years	Plays out with other children
5 years	Dresses without supervision, Domestic role play

LANGUAGE

1 month	Turns head towards sound
3 months	Cooing
6 months	Monosyllables
9 months	Bisyllables, responds to name
10 months	Understand spoken speech
1 year	Speaks 1-2 meaningful words
18 months	Speaks 6-20 words
2 years	Simple sentences without 2-3 nouns
3 years	Good vocabulary of 250 words, Knows age and sex
4 years	Coherent account of recent experience (story)
5 years	Names at least 4 colors

TOILET TRAINING

4 months	Gastrocolic reflex weekens
10 months	Placed on toilet seat
15-18 months	Walk to toilet, dry by day
2 years	Trainable, 50% dry by night
3 years	Withhold and postpones his bowel movement, 75% dry by night
5 years	90% dry by night

ERUPTION SEQUENCE OF TEETH

Primary Teeth

Lower central incisors	6-7 months
Upper central incisors	7-8 months
Lateral incisors	8-9 months
1st molar	12 months
Canine	18 months
2nd molar	24 months

Permanent Teeth

1st **M**olar (**M**other)	6-7 years
Central **I**ncisor (**Is**)	7-8 years
Lateral **I**ncisor (**In**)	8-9 years
1st **P**remolar (**P**ain)	9-10 years
2nd **P**remolar (**P**apa)	10-11 years
Canine (**C**an)	11-12 years
2nd **M**olar (**M**ake)	18 years
3rd **M**olar (**M**edicine)	24 years

DEVELOPMENT OF LOCALIZATION OF SOUNDS

Age	***Response***
3 months	Eyes move towards the side of sound
4-5 months	Eyes and head turn towards the side of sound.

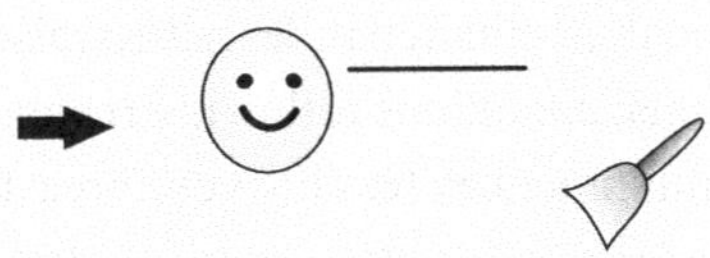

6 months	Eyes and head turn laterally and then drop to locate sound source in low position.

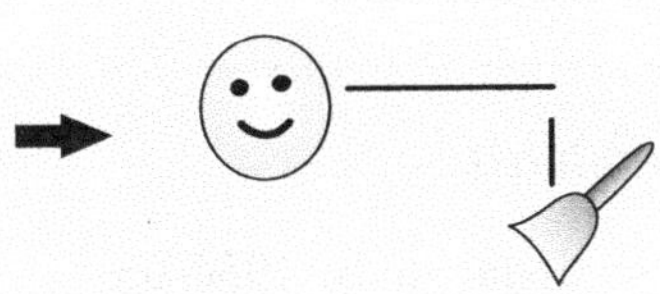

7-8 months	Eyes and head move in towards sound source.

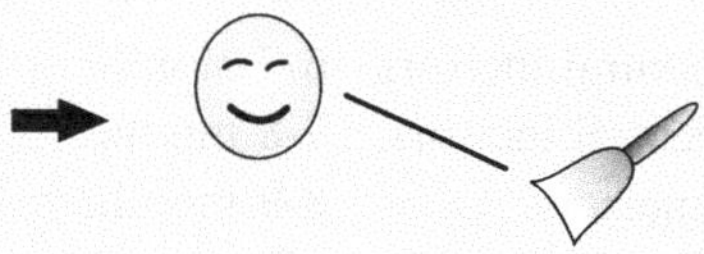

9 months	Eyes and head turn directly towards sound source. This occurs later to sounds in superior than in inferior positions. Visual searching for sound source may be seen.

GROWTH STANDARDS

International

1. *Harvard (Boston):* Longitudinal study from 1932-1956 in U.S.
2. *National center for health statistics (NCHS)*: Cross section study done in U.S. in 1977 using national health and nutritional examination survey
3. *Center for disease control (CDC):* Revised NCHS growth chart
4. WHO Standards
   - MGRS (Multicenter growth reference study), 1997-2003
   - Growth of children is described raised under optimal conditions following recommended health practices (exclusively breast fed)
   - 6 study sites in 5 continents: US, Brazil, Ghana, Norway, Oman, India
   - Longitudinal study: 0-6 years data available.

Indian Scenario

ICMR Standards

- Cross sectional study, 1956-65
- Studied lower socioeconomic class children.

Aggarwal et al

- 1989-91
- Affluent urban children from all major zones of India
- 0-18 years
- Recommended by Indian Academy of Pediatrics.

WHICH CHARTS TO USE

The Indian Council for Medical Research (ICMR) measurements were made on children of the lower socioeconomic class and hence cannot be used as a reference standard. The growth charts compiled by Agarwal, *et al* are based on affluent urban children from all major zones of India from birth to 18 years (unlike the new WHO standards providing data up to 5 years). Thus, in the present circumstances, these charts remain best option for growth monitoring in Indian children and are recommended for use by the Growth Monitoring Guidelines Consensus Meeting of the IAP. At the community worker level, the continued use of the Government charts for monitoring of weight is recommended.

IAP GUIDELINES FOR GROWTH MONITORING

Aim of Growth monitoring

Primary

- Identify children with growth deviation (under and over nutrition)
- Identify diseases.

Secondary

- Health promotion
- Education of parents
- Sensitize pediatrician to use chart.

RECOMMENDED INTERVALS AND PARAMETERS FOR GROWTH CHARTING

First visit

- Enter characteristics of child on chart
- Explain chart to parents
- Growth chart should be kept with parents
- Measure parent's height and enter it on chart
- Calculate mid parental height (child's target height), plotted at 18 years
- Target range 8 cm above and below the target height (3rd and 97th percentile).

Follow-up

- Immunization contact (6,10,14 weeks; 9 months, 15-18 months)
- Opportunistic monitoring (illness)
- After 18 months, 6 monthly till 8 years, then yearly
- Don't weight more than once in a fortnight in infants < 6 months of age and > once in a month thereafter as it increases parental anxiety.

GROWTH CHARTING

0-3 years

- Weight
- Height
- Head circumference (till 3 yrs), penile length and testicular decent in newborn period
- Done 6 monthly.

4-8 years

- Weight
- Height
- Body mass index and sexual maturity rating from 6 years onwards
- Done yearly

9-18 years

- Weight
- Height
- Body mass index and Sexual maturity rating
- Done yearly.

CONCEPT OF PERCENTILES

- Percentiles are used for all common parameters of growth assessment.
- All normal children of same age always vary in all proportions for each parameter.
- If hundred normal children of same age stand in a line with smallest child first in line and tallest child is last in the line. Then child standing 10th in the line signifies 10th percentile and the child standing 50th in the line signifies 50th percentile.
- All children in 3rd to 97th percentile are considered normal.

CHAPTER 9

FAMILY AND SOCIOECONOMIC HISTORY

SOCIOECONOMIC HISTORY

Take socioeconomic history specifying following points:

- Details of family:
  - Joint/nuclear
  - Number of family members
  - Literacy status and occupation of parents.
- Family income

  Per capita income = Total income of family/ Number of family members
- Is the mother employed
- Addiction in parents
- Housing details:
  - Owned/Rented
  - Type (Brick/mud)
  - Number of rooms
  - Details of environmental sanitation
  - Water supply and how water is stored in house.
- Sewage disposal/defaecation habits
- Birth order, spacing, sterilization
- Beliefs, customs, superstitions regarding child-rearing
- Marital harmony—divorce, second wife, alcoholism
- In laws and their dominance in house
- Details of schooling.

FAMILY HISTORY

Take family history specifying following points:

- Age of parents
- Number of siblings and their health status
- Death of sibling and its reason
- Ask about abortion and infant death specifically
- Familial and related illnesses
- History of contact with tuberculosis
- History suggestive of genetic disorders (inheritable illnesses) in family
- Consanguineous marriage
- Any pets in house
- Does child uses footwear while walking outdoors
- Make pedigree chart.

MORTALITY INDICATORS OF MCH CARE

Maternal Mortality Rate

$$\frac{\text{Total female deaths due to complication of pregnancy, or within 42 days of delivery from puerperal causes in an area during a given year}}{\text{Total number of live births in same area and year}} \times 1000$$

Stillbirth Rate

$$\frac{\text{Fetal deaths weighing over 1000 g at birth}}{\text{Total live + stillbirths weighing over 1,000 g at birth}} \times 1000$$

Perinatal Mortality Rate

$$\frac{\text{Late fetal deaths and early neonatal deaths weighing over 1000 g at birth}}{\text{Total live births weighing over 1000 g at birth}} \times 1000$$

Neonatal Mortality Rate

$$\frac{\text{Number of death in children under 28 days of age in a year}}{\text{Total live births in same year}} \times 1000$$

Postneonatal Mortality Rate

$$\frac{\text{Number of death in children between 28 days and 1 year of age in a year}}{\text{Total live births in same year}} \times 1000$$

Infant Mortality Rate

$$\frac{\text{Number of death in children less than 1 year of age in a year}}{\text{Total live births in same year}} \times 1000$$

TYPES OF FAMILIES

Nuclear: Mother, father plus children

Expanded: Mother, father, child plus grand-parents.

Combined: All above + uncle and aunt.

OVERCROWDING

- 1 Room: 2 Persons
- 2 Rooms: 3 Persons
- 3 Rooms: 5 Persons
- 4 Rooms: 7.5 Persons (Child between 1-10 years is counted as half)
- 5 Rooms: 10 Persons (Additional 2 person for each further room)

DEGREE OF RELATIONSHIP

- *1st degree consanguinity*: Dizygotic twins, siblings, parent-child. They share half of their genes.
- *2nd degree consanguinity*: Grandparents, Grand-children, nephew and neice, half siblings. They share quarter of their genes.
- *3rd degree consanguinity*: 1st cousins. They share one eight of their genes.

WHO CRITERIA FOR DIAGNOSIS OF ANEMIA

- Children 6 months to 6 years: Hb <11 gm/dl
- Children 6-14 years: Hb <12 gm/dl
- Mild anemia: Hb >10 g/dl
- Moderate anemia: Hb 7-10 g/dl
- Severe anemia: Hb <7 g/dl

MILLENIUM DEVELOPMENT GOALS (TARGET DATE 2015)

1. Eradicate extreme poverty and hunger
   - ❒ Reduce by half the proportion of people living on less than a dollar a day
   - ❒ Reduce by half the proportion of people who suffer from hunger.
2. Achieve universal primary education
   - ❒ Ensure that all boys and girls complete a full course of primary schooling.
3. Promote gender equality and empower women
   - ❒ Eliminate gender disparity in primary and secondary education preferaably by 2005 and at all levels by 2015
4. Reduce child mortality
   - ❒ Reduce by two-thirds the mortality rate among children under five.
5. Improve maternal health
   - ❒ Reduce by three quarters the maternal mortality ratio.

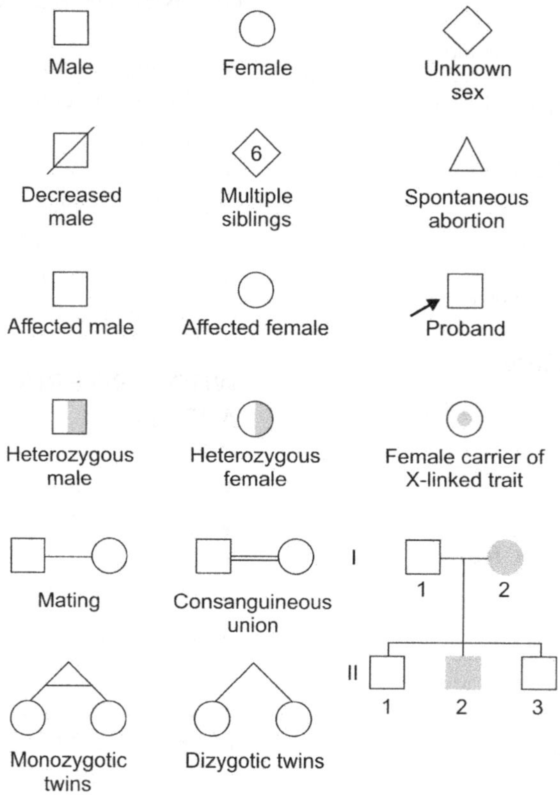

Fig. 9.1: Pedigree charts

6. Combat HIV/AIDS, malaria and other diseases
   - Halt and begin to reverse the spread of HIV/AIDS.
   - Halt and begin to reverse the incidence of malaria and other major diseases.
7. Ensure environmental sustainability
   - Integrate the principles of sustainable development into country policies and programs; reverse loss of environmental resources.
   - Reduce by half the proportion of people without sustainable access to safe drinking water.
   - Achieve significant improvement in lives of at least 100 million slum dwellers, by 2020.
8. Develop a global partnership for development
   - Develop further an open trading and financial system that is rule-based, predictable and, non-discriminatory includes a commitment to good governance, development and poverty reduction—nationally and internationally.
   - Address the least developed countries' special needs. This includes tariff and quota-free access for their exports; enhanced debt relief for heavily indebted poor countries; cancellation of official bilateral debt; and more generous official development assistance for countries committed to poverty reduction.

- Address the special needs of landlocked and small island developing states.
- Deal comprehensively with developing countries' debt problems through national and international measures to make debt sustainable in the long-term.
- In cooperation with the developing countries, develop productive work for youth.
- In cooperation with pharmaceutical companies, provide access to affordable essential drugs in developing countries.
- In cooperation with the private sector, make available the benefits of new technologies—especially information and communications technologies.

CHAPTER 10

General Physical Examination

COMPONENTS OF HEAD TO TOE EXAMINATION

Cranium

- Shape and size
- Sutures, fontanels
- Transillumination and crack pot sign (Macewan's sign) in hydrocephalus.

Face

- Any abnormal facies.

Eyes

- Intercanthal distance appears normal or not
- Slant in palpebral fissure (Downs' syndrome)
- Epicanthic folds
- Pupil—shape and size, reaction to light.

Ears

- Low set
- External ear abnormalities.

Nose

- Depressed nasal bridge.

Mouth and Oral Çavity

- Oral hygiene
- Any palate abnormalities like cleft lip or palate
- Tongue—pallor, cyanosis
- Tonsillar enlargement.

Neck

- Look for swelling or pulsations in neck.

Hands, Feet and Limbs

- Cyanosis or pallor in palm, rash in palms
- Any bony or joint abnormality.

Skin and Nails

- Color, texture, turgor of skin
- Rash, hemorrhages in skin
- Clubbing, koilonychia, splinter hemorrhages in nails.

Genitalia

- Males: Descent of testis in scrotum, scrotal rugosities, hypo/epispadius

- Females: Examine breast and see distribution of pubic and axillary hair (in front of female attendant).

CLUBBING

Definition

- Bulbous enlargement of soft parts of the terminal phalanges with both transverse and longitudinal curving of the nails.
- Probably caused by interstitial edema and dilatation of the arterioles and capillaries.

Causes

- *Pulmonary:* Bronchiectasis, lung abscess.
- *Cardiac:* Infective endocarditis, cyanotic congenital heart diseases.
- *GIT:* Inflammatory bowel disease, cirrhosis.
- *Endocrine:* Hyperthyroidism.
- *Miscellaneous:* Hereditary, idiopathic.
- *Uni digital:* Traumatic or tophi deposit in gout.

Grading of Clubbing

I. Softening of nail bed.
II. Obliteration of the angle of the nail bed.
III. Swelling of the subcutaneous tissues over the base of the nail causing the overlying skin to become tense, shiny and increasing the curvature of the nail, resulting in parrot beak or drumstick appearance.
IV. Swelling of the fingers in all dimensions associated with hypertrophic pulmonary osteoarthropathy causing pain and swelling of the hands, wrist, etc. and radiographic evidence of subperiosteal new bone formation.

Normal angle between the nail and nail bed: 180°

Severe clubbing: Angle > 180°

Schamroth's Sign

Normally when two fingers are held together with nails facing each other, a space is seen at the level of proximal nail fold. This is lost in case of clubbing.

Pseudoclubbing

This is due to subperiosteal resorption of terminal phalanges (there is no soft tissue proliferation) and is seen in:

- Scleroderma
- Acromegaly
- Hyperparathyroidism.

Possible Mechanisms of Clubbing

- Anoxia: It results in opening up of deep arteriovenous fistula (most acceptable), e.g. Fallot's tetralogy.
- Toxic, e.g. subacute bacterial endocarditis.
- Metabolic, e.g. thyrotoxicosis.
- Hormonal: Increased growth hormone, e.g. acromegaly.
- Reduced ferritin (may escape oxidation in lungs and leads to dilatation of arteriovenous anastomosis) may play an important role.

CYANOSIS

Definition

Cyanosis (Table 10.1) is a bluish discoloration of the skin and mucous membrane due to an increased quantity of reduced hemoglobin > 5 g per dl and PaO_2 < 85%, or due to the presence of abnormal hemoglobin pigments in the blood perfusing these areas.

Table 10.1: Differentiating features between central and peripheral cyanosis

Features	*Central cyanosis*	*Peripheral cyanosis*
Mechanism	Right to left shunts or lung disorders	Peripheral stasis
Site	Whole body	Nail bed, nose tip, earlobe, extremities
Associations	Clubbing Polycythemia	– –
Extremities	Warm	Cold
On warming the extremities	No change	Disappears
Oxygen inhalation	Slight improvement	No change
Arterial blood gas PaO_2	Low < 85%	Normal 85-100%.

Causes

Central

- *Cardiac:* Cyanotic congenital heart disease: Fallot's tetralogy, Eisenmenger's complex.
- *Pulmonary:* Interstitial pneumonia, ARDS.
- High altitude due to low partial pressure of oxygen.

Peripheral

- Cold (local vasoconstriction)
- Shock.

Abnormal Pigments

- *Methemoglobinemia:* Iron is in the ferric form, instead of usual ferrous form designated as MHb. Several substances like nitrite ingestion (well water), sulfonamide or aniline dyes oxidize Hb to MHb, but this is immediately reduced back to Hb by methemoglobin reductase I. If there is deficiency of methemoglobin reductase I, MHb circulates in blood, causing cyanosis.
- *Sulfhemoglobin (SHb):* It is formed by toxic action of sulphonamides, phenacetin and acetanilide. SHb forms an irreversible change in the Hb pigment that has no capacity to carry oxygen and causes cyanosis.

Absence of Cyanosis

- Severe anemia with hemoglobin < 5 gm%, even if all the hemoglobin is reduced in the capillaries, it will be less than the critical level of 5 gm% and cyanosis does not occur.
- Carbon monoxide poisoning, carboxyhemoglobin prevents reduction of oxyhemoglobin; the former has a cherry red color. Hence there is no cyanosis.

Pseudocyanosis

- Bluish tinge to skin or mucous membranes in absence of hypoxemia or peripheral cyanosis.
- Most causes are related to metals (silver, lead) or drugs (phenothiazine, amiodarone).

Differential Cyanosis

- *Upper limbs:* Coarctation of aorta with transposition of great arteries.
- *Lower limbs:* PDA with reversal of shunt.
- *Left upper limb and both lower limbs:* PDA with reversal of shunt and preductal coarctation of aorta.
- *Intermittent cyanosis:* Ebstein's anomaly.
- *Cyclical cyanosis:* Bilateral choanal atresia.

LYMPHADENOPATHY

Lymphadenopathy is inflammatory or non-inflammatory enlargement of lymph nodes.

Lymphadenopathy: Inflammatory or non-inflammatory enlargement of lymph nodes.

Generalized lymphadenopathy: Involvement of three or more non-contiguous lymph node areas.

Persistent generalized lymphadenopathy: Presence of enlarged lymph nodes (>1 cm) in two or more extrainguinal sites for more than 3 months.

Significant lymphadenopathy can be defined as:

- Axillary lymph node—1 cm in size
- Cervical lymph nodes—1 cm in size
- Inguinal lymph nodes—1.5 cm in size
- Palpable lymph nodes at multiple sites
- Lymph nodes which are red/tender/matted/ulcerated
- Enlarged lymph nodes associated with a focus of infection
- Enlarged lymph nodes associated with systemic signs and symptoms

Method of Lymph Node Examination

Nodes are palpated symmetrically on both sides of the body from above downwards.

Lymph Nodes in Neck

Palpated from 'behind' with child in sitting or standing with the head bending forward.

- The upper circular group is palpated by both hands in following order:
  - Submental
  - Submandibular
  - Preauricular
  - Postauricular and
  - Occipital.
- Lower horizontal or supraclavicular group of lymph nodes: They are further divided into medial, intermediate and lateral groups.
- The vertical chain in the middle of the neck: The glands in the anterior triangle, and posterior triangle are palpated (the triangles are divided by the sternomastoid muscle).

Axillary Lymph Nodes

The child sits on a stool and the examiner sits in front of the child (only subscapular group is palpated from behind).

- *Central group:* The child's arm is abducted and the hand of the examiner is placed in the axilla with palm directed towards the chest. Now the arm is adducted and allowed to rest on the examiner's forearm. The other hand of the examiner is placed on the child's opposite shoulder. The central group is palpated by sliding the fingers.
- *Apical group:* The same method is applied but fingers are pushed as high as possible.
- *Pectoral group:* These glands are situated under the anterior axillary fold. The nodes are palpated with the help of the thumb and fingers.
- *Brachial group:* Here the left hand is used for the left side and the right hand for the right side. This group is palpated against the upper part of the humerus with the examiner's palm directed laterally.
- *Subscapular group:* This group lies on the posterior axillary fold. It is a palpated from behind when the hand insinuates within the latissimus dorsi, keeping the child's arm horizontally forward.

Epitrochlear Lymph Nodes

Keep elbow of child slightly flexed, forearm supinated and wrist of child fixed by the examiners opposite hand. The glands are palpated in the anterior-medial region of the lower part of arm (in between the groove of biceps and brachialis muscle) adjacent to the elbow.

Inguinal Lymph Nodes

Examined in supine position after extending the thighs.

Popliteal Group of Lymph Nodes

Examined in supine position with flexed legs. The popliteal fossa is felt with the finger tips of either hand, the fingers of both hands being buried into the popliteal fossa.

Mediastinal Group of Lymph Nodes

Their presence can be detected indirectly by percussion of the sternum.

Abdominal Lymph Nodes

(Pre-and para-aortic, Retroperitoneal): This group will present as lump in the abdomen.

Causes of Lymphadenopathy

Inflammatory: Tuberculosis, syphilis and filariasis

Hematological: Hodgkin's disease, non-Hodgkin's lymphoma, AIDS.

Immunological: Serum sickness, drug reaction, SLE and rheumatoid arthritis.

TEMPERATURE

Body temperature is regulated by hypothalamus. Usually temperature is recorded in axilla.

The normal body temperature varies from 36°C to 37.5°C. There is normally a diurnal variation of 1°C, the lowest temperature being between 2-4 AM and highest in the afternoon.

Fever or pyrexia is an increase of more than 1°C or any rise above the maximal normal temperature.

Types of Fever

Continuous fever: Daily fluctuation does not exceed more than 1°C (1.5°F) and temperature never touches the baseline normal temperature.

Remittent fever: Daily fluctuation is more than 1°C and never touches baseline, e.g. typhoid.

Intermittent fever: The temperature touches the baseline in between febrile phases. When the spike occurs daily, it is quotidian, when every alternate day, it is tertian and when every third day, it is quartan.

Septic: The temperature variation between peak and nadir is very large and exceeds 5° C, e.g. septicemia.

Pel Ebstein type: There is a regular alternation of recurrent bouts of fever and afebrile periods. The temperature may take 3 days to rise, remains high for 3 days and remits in 3 days, followed by apyrexia for 9 days as seen in Hodgkin's lymphoma.

Definitions

Hyperpyrexia: Hyperpyrexia is said to occur when body temperature is more than 105°F. Causes: tetanus, malaria, septicemia, heat stroke, encephalitis.

Fever of unknown origin: Illness of more than three weeks duration; documented fever above 101°F (38.3°C) on multiple occasions; and lack of specific diagnosis after 1 week of admission and investigation in a hospital setting.

Nosocomial fever of unknown origin: Hospitalized patients in whom infection or fever were absent on admission but who have developed fever of 38.3°C or more on several occasions.

Neutropenic FUO: Patients with 500 neutrophils/mm^3 and multiple readings of more than 101°F are labeled as neuropenic FUO. 3 days of investigation and including at least 48 hours incubation of cultures are also required to justify the diagnosis.

Methods and Instruments to Measure Temperature

Mercury glass thermometer: Heat causes mercury to expand and rise in glass tube.

Oral temperature: Place under tongue in right or left posterior sublingual pocket, not in front of tongue for 2-3 minutes. Make the child keep the mouth closed without biting the thermometer.

Axillary temperature: Place under the arm with tip in the center of axilla and kept close to skin with no clothes in between for 3-5 minutes. Hold child arm firmly against side.

Rectal temperature: Place well lubricated tip not more than 2.5 cm into rectum. Place child in lying or prone with knees flexed position.

Appearance of Rash in Febrile Patient

Remember the pneumonic: Certain Silly People Make Typhus and Typhoral.

1st day	–	**V**aricella, i.e. chickenpox (mainly in trunk; all forms seen at a time; no umbilication of vesicle)
2nd day	–	**S**carlet fever (over chest, neck, scapula; mainly macular)
3rd day	–	**P**ox (smallpox)—not seen nowa days (peripheral disturbution; rashes come in a sequence; umbilication)
4th day	–	**M**easles (maculopapular; over forehead, hairline near ears, face and trunk)
5th day	–	**T**yphus (macular; over shoulders, chest, extremities, palms and soles)
6th day	–	**D**engue (morbilliform; over dorsum of hands and feet, trunk)
7th day	–	**T**yphoid or enteric fever (rose spots over abdomen, flanks and back; pale pink; fades on pressure)

PULSE

The normal pulse (Fig. 10.1) has a small anacrotic wave on the upstroke, which is not felt. This is followed by a big tidal or percussion wave which is felt by the palpating finger. On the following down stroke there is a notch (dicrotic notch) followed by a wave (dicrotic wave) both of which are not normally palpable.

Anacrotic Pulse

Anacrotic pulse is a slow rising and twice beating pulse where both the waves are felt during systole. The waves that are felt are the anacrotic wave and the tidal wave. It is best felt in the carotids in aortic stenosis. Typically the pulse in AS is known as *pulsus parvus et tardus.*

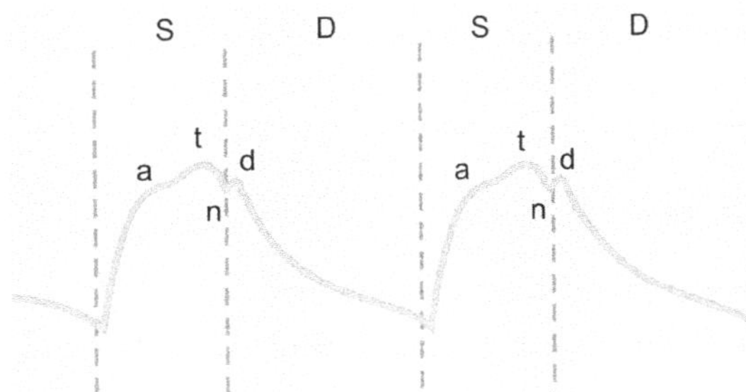

Fig. 10.1: Normal pulse wave, a: anacrotic wave; t: tidal wave; d: dicrotic wave; n: dicrotic notch; S: systole; D: diastole

Pulsus Bisferiens

Pulsus bisferiens is a single pulse wave with two peaks in systole.

Causes

- Aortic stenosis and aortic regurgitation
- Severe aortic regurgitation
- Hypertrophic obstructive cardiomyopathy (HOCM).

Dicrotic Pulse

It is a single pulse wave with one peak in systole and one peak in diastole due to a very low stroke volume with decreased peripheral resistance.

Causes

- Left ventricular failure
- Typhoid fever
- Dehydration
- Dilated cardiomyopathy
- Cardiac tamponade.

Pulsus Parvus Et Tardus

A low amplitude pulse (parvus) with a peak (tardus). It is seen in aortic stenosis.

Pulsus Alternans

Alternating small and large volume pulse in regular rhythm. It is best appreciated by palpating radial or femoral pulses, rather than the carotids.

Causes

- Severe left ventricular failure
- Following ventricular premature contraction.

Pulsus Paradoxus

It is an exaggerated reduction in the strength of arterial pulse during normal inspiration or an exaggerated inspiratory fall in systolic pressure of more than 10 mm Hg during quiet breathing.

Causes

- Superior vena cava obstruction
- *Pulmonary conditions:* Asthma, emphysema
- *Cardiac:* Pericardial effusion, constrictive pericarditis.

Reverse Pulsus Paradoxus

Reverse pulsus paradoxus is an inspiratory rise in arterial pressure.

Causes

- Hypertrophic obstructive cardiomyopathy.
- Intermittent positive pressure ventilation.

Pulsus Bigeminus (Coupling)

A pulse wave with a normal beat followed by a premature beat and a compensatory pause, occurring in rapid succession, resulting in alternation of the strength of the pulse.

In pulsus alternans, compensatory pause is absent, whereas in pulsus bigeminus, compensatory pause is present. Pulsus bigeminus is a sign of digitalis toxicity.

Causes

AV block, every third sinus impulse being blocked Sinoatrial block with ventricular escape.

Thready Pulse

The pulse rate is rapid and the pulse wave is small and disappears quickly. This is seen in cardiogenic shock.

Water Hammer Pulse

Large volume pulse with a rapid upstroke (systolic pressure is high) and a rapid downstroke (diastolic pressure is low). It is best felt in the radial artery with the patient's arm elevated. The rapid upstroke is because of an increased stroke volume. The rapid downstroke is because of diastolic run off into the left ventricle, and decreased peripheral resistance and rapid run off to the periphery.

Causes

- *Cardiac lesions:* Aortic regurgitation/patent ductus arteriosus/arteriovenous fistula/rupture of sinus of valsalva.
- *High output states or syndromes:* Anemia/beriberi/cor pulmonale/arteriovenous fistula/thyrotoxicosis.

Different Types of Double Beating Pulse

- Pulsus bisferiens

- Anacrotic pulse
- Dicrotic pulse.

Pulse Pressure and Mean Pressure

Pulse pressure is the difference between systolic and diastolic BP.

Normal pulse pressure is 30-60 mm Hg.

Mean arterial pressure is the product of cardiac output and total peripheral resistance. It is the tissue perfusion pressure.

Mean arterial pressure = Diastolic blood pressure + 1/3 of pulse pressure.

Normal Pulse Rate

Neonate	100-140 beats per minute
1 month to 1 year	80-120 beats per minute
1-5 years	70-100 beats per minute
5-10 years	60-80 beats per minute.

Description of Pulse

- Pulse rate: Measure pulse for whole 1 minute
- Rhythm: Regular/ irregular
- Volume: Volume is assessed in carotid artery
- Radio femoral delay: Feel radial and femoral pulses simultaneously. The beats should be felt together, otherwise there is coaractation of aorta.
- Character: Anacrotic/ bisferians/ dicrotic, etc.
- Presence of peripheral pulsations.

JUGULAR VENOUS PULSE (JVP)

Normal JVP

The normal JVP consists of three positive pulse waves (a, c and v) and two negative pulse waves (x and y).

Different Waves in Neck Vein

'a' wave	– Atrial contraction
'c' wave	– Closure of tricuspid valve (according to few clinicians, it is due to transmitted carotid impulse)
'x' descent	– Atrial relaxation with downward descent of tricuspid valve
'v' wave	– Atrial filling
'y' descent	– Right ventricular filling with atrial emptying

- a-wave coincides with S_1, v-wave with S_2
- x-descent follows S_1, y-descent follows S_2

Abnormalities of 'a' waves

- *Absent:* Atrial fibrillation
- *Giant 'a' waves:* Tricuspid stenosis/ tricuspid atresia/pulmonary stenosis/pulmonary hypertension
- *Cannon 'a' waves:* Complete heart block/ ventricular tachycardia.

Abnormalities of 'x' wave

- *Obliterated:* Tricuspid regurgitation
- *Prominent:* Constrictive pericarditis.

Abnormalities of 'v' wave

- *Giant 'v' waves:* Tricuspid regurgitation.

Abnormalities of 'y' descent

- *Rapid 'y' descent:* Constrictive pericarditis/ Severe heart failure/Tricuspid regurgitation.
- *Short 'y' descent:* Tricuspid stenosis.

Table 10.2: Differences between JVP and carotid pulse

	JVP	Carotid pulse
Appearance	Better seen than felt	Better felt than seen
Number of waves	Multiple	Single
Pressure below the angle of mandible	Obliterates the wave	No change
Changes with respiration and position	Present	Absent

Kussmaul's sign

Kussmaul's sign is an inspiratory increase in JVP.

Normally inspiration lowers the jugular venous pressure giving an inspiratory collapse, because intrathoracic pressure falls and there is increased blood flow into the thorax. In contrast, when the intrapericardial pressure is raised as in constrictive pericarditis there is a paradoxical increase in jugular venous pressure on inspiration. This is Kussmauls's sign.

Causes of Kussmaul's Sign

- Constrictive pericarditis
- Restrictive cardiomyopathy
- Right ventricle failure.

Friedreich's sign is the rapid fall (steep 'y' descent) and rise of JVP seen in constrictive pericarditis and tricuspid regurgitation.

JUGULAR VENOUS PRESSURE

Jugular venous pressure is expressed as the vertical height from the sternal angle to the zone of transition of distended and collapsed internal jugular veins. When measured with the patient reclining at 45°, is normally about 3-4 cm.

Procedure

- The patient is given a backrest to keep him at 45°. In this position, normally, the jugular vein is just seen above the clavicles.
- The upper level of the vein is noted and a ruler is kept at that level, parallel to the ground. Another rule is put perpendicular to the first ruler up to the angle of Louis.
- The distance from the angle of Louis to the first ruler gives the jugular pressure.
- At 45°, the vertical distance between the top of the oscillating venous column and the sternal angle is the jugular venous pressure (JVP) and is normally 3-4 cm.
- Thus, 3 cm + 5 cm = 8 cm of blood is the normal venous pressure or JVP or CVP.

Significance

The jugular veins are in direct continuity with the superior vena cava and the right atrium. Hence, it reflects pressure changes in the right atrium.

Elevated venous pressure occurs in:

- Right ventricular failure
- Cardiac tamponade
- Tricuspid stenosis
- Superior vena cava obstruction
- Hyperkinetic circulatory state
- Increased blood volume
- Pulmonary diseases like asthma, emphysema.

Causes of fall in JVP

- Hypovolemia
- Shock
- Addison's disease.

Importance of Hepatojugular Reflux

When gentle pressure is applied on any part of the abdomen for 30 seconds, especially over the right hypochondrium there is 'transient' rise in JVP as the hepatic venous reservoir is compressed. This is hepatojugular reflux (often called abdomino-jugular reflux).

Normally there is a 'less than 15 second rise' in JVP after abdominal compression and if it persists for more than 15 seconds, it suggests right ventricular dysfunction.

Importance

- Diagnosis of incipient (early stage) right heart failure (CCF)
- Differentiates between arterial and venous pulsation
- Differentiates between obstructive and non-obstructive causes of engorged neck vein (negative hepatojugular reflux is seen in SVC syndrome and Budd-Chiari syndrome).

PALLOR

Pallor is the paleness of skin or mucous membrane, which is usually due to diminished number of circulating red cells resulting in anemia and may also be a manifestation of shock.

Site of Pallor

Pallor is seen at the following sites:

- Lower palpebral conjunctiva (upper palpebral conjunctive may be scarred due to trachoma making assessment difficult)
- Dorsum of the tongue
- Palmar or plantar creases
- Nails.

Grading of Pallor

Severe pallor: Palmar creases become faint and pale.

Moderate pallor: Paleness of the mucosae, but pink hue of the palmar creases is maintained.

Prevalence of Anemia (NFHS 3 Data)

Any anemia: 79%
Severe anemia: 5%.

EDEMA

An excess of fluid in the subcutaneous tissues causes swelling of the tissues defined as edema. It may be *generalized* or *localized.*

Site of Edema

Press just above the medical malleolus of tibia or the sacrum for about 30 seconds and to allow a depression (pitting edema) to from. Wait for 15 seconds to allow the dimple to disappear. Edema due to lymphatic obstruction is usually non-pitting.

Common Causes of Edema

A. Generalized Edema

1. Nephrotic syndrome
2. Congestive heart failure
3. Kwashiorkor
4. Hepatic failure.

B. Localized Edema

1. Angioneurotic edema
2. Urticaria
3. Cellulitis
4. Filariasis
5. Congenital (Milroy diseases is congenital edema usually confined to the legs).

CHAPTER 11

ANTHROPOMETRY

ANTHROPOMETRY

Anthropometry is a tool for evaluating the nutritional status of the child.

Parameters to Assess Anthropometry

- Weight
- Length or Height
- Weight / Height
- Growth velocity
- Body ratio
- Head circumference
- Chest circumference
- Mid arm circumference
- Body mass index
- Dentition
- Growth chart.

WEIGHT

- Most reliable.

Formulas to Calculate Weight

3-12 months	$\frac{\text{Age in months} + 9}{2}$
1-6 years	Age (yr) × 2 + 8
7-12 years	$\frac{\text{Age (yr)} \times 7 - 5}{2}$

Simple Weight Calculation

- 4-5 months = 2 × birth weight
- 1 year = 3 × birth weight
- 2 years = 4 × birth weight
- 7 years = 7 × birth weight
- 10 years = 10 × birth weight.

Newborn

- 10% birth weight lost initially in first 5-7 days
- Regains birth weight by 10 days then,
- 1st three months—30 grams/day
- 3-6 months—20 grams/day
- 6-12 months—15 grams/day
- 1-3 years—3 kg/year
- 3-12 years—2 kg/year.

LENGTH OR HEIGHT

- <2 years—recumbent length using infantometer
- > 2 years—standing height using stadiometer.

Formulas to Calculate Height

- 2-12 years—age in years × 6 + 77 (in cms)
- In girls at 2 years—half of adult height obtained.
- In boys at 2½ years—half of adult height obtained.

Simple Length Calculation

- At birth—50 cm
- 1 year—75 cm
- 2 years—90 cm
- 4½ years—100 cm then,
- till 10 years—5 cm/year.

HEAD CIRCUMFERENCE

- Should not be measured within 24 hours after birth
- Should be measured using steel tape
- Bony landmarks—superior orbital ridge (anterior), external occipital proturbence (posterior).

Increments

- 1st 3 months—2 cm/month
- 3-6 months—1 cm/month
- 6-12 months—0.5 cm/month.

Simple Head Circumference Calculation

- Birth—35 cm
- 3 months—40 cm
- 12 months—45 cm
- 2 years—48 cm
- 12 years—52 cm.

Abnormal Increase in Head Circumference

- Hydrocephalus
  - Posthemorrhagic
  - Postmeningitic
  - Aqueductal stenosis
  - TORCH infections.
- Rickets.

Slow Growth in HC

- Microcephaly
  - Hypoxic ischemic injury
  - Meningitis
  - Intraventricular hemorrhage.

BODY RATIO—UPPER SEGMENT/ LOWER SEGMENT RATIO

The *lower body segment* is defined as the length from the symphysis pubis to the floor, and the *upper body segment* is the height minus the lower body segment.

The ratio of upper body segment divided by lower body segment (U/L ratio) equals approximately 1.7 at birth, 1.3 at 3 years of age, and 1.0 after 7 years of age.

Higher U/L ratios are characteristic of short-limb dwarfism or bone disorders, such as rickets.

ARM SPAN

- Distance between tips of middle fingers when arms outstretched at right angles to the body and measured across the back of the child.
- It is equal to height at 10 years
- In age < 10 years it is 1-2 cm less than height
- After 12 years it is 1-2 cm > height
- Abnormal large span:
  - Klinefelter's syndrome
  - Coarctation of aorta
  - Marfan's syndrome.

CHEST CIRCUMFERENCE

- Measured at level of nipple in a plane at right angle to the spine and at mid respiration

- At birth head circumference is more than chest circumference
- By 6-12 months—chest circumference is equal to head circumference
- At 1 year—chest circumference is more than head circumference.

MID ARM CIRCUMFERENCE

- Age independent criteria
- Measured at midpoint between acromian and olecranon process
- 1-5 years—arm circumference is constant
  - >13.5 cm—normal
  - 12.5-13.5 cm—moderate malnutrition
  - <12.5 cm—severe malnutrition.

Bangle Test

- Bangle made up of metal with a internal diameter of 4 cm (circumference 12 cm)
- If bangle crosses elbow, child is malnourished
- Simple but less sensitive.

Shakir's Tape

- **Shakir's tape** (Table 11.1) is used to measure nutritional status by measuring mid arm circumference:

Table 11.1: Shakir's tap

Color coding	*Markings*	*Interpertation*
Green	> 13.5 cm	Normal
Yellow	12.5-13.5 cm	Borderline malnutrition
Red	<12.5 cm	Severe malnutrition

QUAC Stick (Quacker Arm Circumference Stick)

- Rod with two sets of marking one indicating height and other for mid arm circumference for the corresponding height.
- MAC is measured, and QUAC stick is placed behind standing child.
- If height is more than the expected height for the measured arm circumference the child is malnourished.

SKIN FOLD THICKNESS

- Measured over the triceps or subscapular region with the help of herpenden's caliper.
- Measures subcutaneous fat and indirectly caloric reserve in body.

BODY MASS INDEX (TABLE 11.2)

$$\frac{\text{Weight in kg}}{(\text{Height in mtr})^2}$$

Table 11.2: Body mass index

Children's BMI	*Classification*	*Adult BMI*
<13	Severe malnutrition	
13-15	Moderate malnutrition	
18.5-25	Normal	
>22	Overweight	>25
>25	Obesity	>30

MID PARENTAL HEIGHT

$$\text{Boys}: \frac{(\text{maternal height} + \text{paternal height} + 13\text{ cm})}{2}$$

$$\text{Girls}: \frac{(\text{maternal height} + \text{paternal height} - 13\text{ cm})}{2}$$

CLASSIFICATION OF PEM

WHO Classification

	Moderate malnutrition	*Severe malnutrition*
Symmetrical edema	No	Yes
Weight for height (measure of wasting)	70-79% (wasting)	<70% (severe wasting)
Height for age (measure of stunting)	85-89% (stunting)	< 85% (severe stunting)

IAP Classification (Table 11.3)

- Based on NCHS standard
- Indian Academy of Pediatrics (IAP) classification based on Weight for age
- Children weighing more than 80% of the 50th percentile of the WHO/NCHS standards are considered normal
- Classification.

Table 11.3: IAP classification

Grade	*Percentage of standard weight for age*
I	70-80%
II	60-70%
III	50-60%
IV	<50%

If edema is associated with decreased weight, then "K" is added to the grade of malnutrition.

Advantage: Simple and the cut offs are suitable for Indian population.

Disadvantage: It does not take in account the child's height due to which children who are short statured (not necessarily due to nutritional deprivation) are also misclassified as PEM by this classification.

Wellcome Trust Classification (Table 11.4)

Based on standard weight for age (95th percentile ICMR value or 50th percentile Boston value) and presence or absence of edema.

Table 11.4: Wellcome trust classification

Weight for age	*80-60%*	*<60%*
With edema	Kwashiorkor	Marasmic kwashiorkor
Without edema (undernutrition)	Underweight	Marasmus

Gomez Classification (Table 11.5)

Based on Harvard standard.

Table 11.5: Gomez classification

Grades	*Percentage of standard weight for age*
I	76-90%
II	61-75%
III	<60%

Udani's Classification (Table 11.6)

Table 11.6: Udani's classification

Grades	*Loss of fat from*
I	Buttocks
II	Axilla/groin
III	Abdomen, chest, back
IV	Buccal pad of fat

AGE INDEPENDENT ANTHROPOMETRIC INDICES

Method	*Name of index*	*Normal (severely malnourished)*
$\frac{\text{Weight kg}}{(\text{Height cm})^{1.6}} \times 100$	Dugdale's	0.88-0.97 (< 0.79)
$\frac{\text{Weight kg}}{(\text{Height cm})^{2}} \times 100$	Rao's	0.15-0.16 (< 0.14)
$\frac{\text{Midaram circumference (cm)}}{\text{Head circumference (cm)}}$	Kanawati	0.32-0.33 (< 0.25)
Midarm circumference, between the ages of 1-5 years		>13.5cm (< 12.5 cm)

DENTAL DEVELOPMENT

Primary Teeth

Lower central incisors	6-7 months
Upper central incisors	7-8 months
Lateral incisors	8-9 months
1st molar	12 months
Canine	18 months
2nd molar	24 months

Permanent Teeth

1st **M**olar (**M**other)	6-7 years
Central **I**ncisor (**Is**)	7-8 years

Lateral **I**ncisor (**In**)	8-9 years
1st **P**remolar (**Pain**)	9-10 years
2nd **P**remolar (**Pa**pa)	10-11 years
Canine (**Can**)	11-12 years
2nd **M**olar (**M**ake)	18 years
3rd **M**olar (**M**edicine)	24 years

Delayed eruption is usually considered when there are no teeth by approximately 13 months of age. Common causes include hypothyroidism, hypoparathyroidism, familial, and idiopathic.

Individual teeth fail to erupt because of mechanical blockage (crowding, gum fibrosis).

Nutritional and metabolic disturbances, prolonged illness, and certain medications (tetracycline) commonly result in discoloration or malformations of the dental enamel. A discrete line of pitting on the enamel suggests a time limited insult.

HOW TO MENTION ANTHROPOMETRY IN EXAMINATION

In a Child < 1 Year of Age

Mention Following Parameters

- *Observed weight* of this child is ____kg (as against ____kg which is 50th centile of WHO growth chart). This is _____% of normal and falls between _______centile (e.g. 3rd) and ______ centile (e.g. 25th).
- *Observed height* of this child is _____cm (as against _____cm which is 50th centile of WHO growth chart). This is ___% of normal and falls between _____centile (e.g. 3rd) and ______ centile (e.g. 25th).
- Normal *Weight for Height* of ______cm is _____kg. Weight of this child is ____kg and height is _____cm. This is ___% of normal and falls between ______centile (e.g. 3rd)____ centile (e.g. 25th).
- *Observed head circumference* of this child is ____cm (as against _____cm which is 50th centile of WHO growth chart). This is ___% of normal and falls between ____ centile (e.g. 3rd) and ______ centile (e.g. 25th).

In a Child 1-5 Years of Age

Mention Following Parameters

- Weight
- Height
- Weight for height
- Mid arm circumference
- Head circumference.

In a Child > 5 Years of Age

Mention Following Parameters

- Weight
- Height
- Body mass index
- Head circumference (in patients of delayed developmental milestones, seizure disorder, meningitis or any CNS disorder).

CHAPTER 12

HEALTH INDICATORS

HEALTH INDICATORS

Indicators of Child Health

Mortality

Infancy:
- Infant mortality rate.
- Neonatal mortality rate.
- Perinatal mortality rate.

Childhood:
- Child mortality rate.
- Under-five mortality rate.

Wellbeing:
- Safe deliveries.
- Birth-weight.
- Safe water and sanitation.

Nutrition:
- Stunting/wasting prevalence.
- Night blindness.
- Goiter prevalence.

Immunization:
- Coverage.
- Completeness.
- Polio cases/ measles deaths.
- Child survival rate.

Disease:
- Vaccine preventable diseases.
- Acute respiratory infections.
- Acute gastroenteritis.
- HIV.
- PEM/vitamin deficiency.

Education:
- Literacy rates .
- School enrollment.
- School attendance.
- School drop-outs.

Social:
- Child labor.
- Child abuse.
- Addictions.

Health Care Service Utilization:
- ANC visits.
- Vaccine coverage.
- Supplementary feeds.

MORTALITY

Infancy

Infant Mortality Rate [57]

$$\frac{\text{Number of death in children less than 1 year of age in a year}}{\text{Total live births in same year}} \times 1000$$

Neonatal Mortality Rate [39]

$$\frac{\text{Number of death in children under 28 days of age in a year}}{\text{Total live births in same year}} \times 1000$$

Post-neonatal Mortality Rate [18]

$$\frac{\text{Number of death in children between 28 days and 1 year of age in a year}}{\text{Total live births in same year}} \times 1000$$

Perinatal Mortality Rate [49]

$$\frac{\text{Late fetal deaths and early neonatal deaths weighing over 1000 g at birth}}{\text{Total live birth weighing over 1000 g at birth}} \times 1000$$

Infant Mortality Continues to Decline

Infant mortality declined from 79 deaths per 1,000 live births in NFHS-1 (1991-92) to 68 in NFHS-2 (1998-99) to 57 in NFHS-3 (2005-06).

Childhood

Child Mortality Rate [18]
Under-Five Mortality Rate [74.3]
Child Survival Rate [92.6%]

LOW BIRTH WEIGHT (NFHS 3)

21.5% (Among recorded birth weights)
20.8 % (Among those with no weight record)

Among children for whom birth weight was reported, 22 percent had a low birth weight, that is, they weighed less than 2.5 kilograms. The proportion weighing less than 2.5 kilograms is slightly higher in rural areas (23 percent) than in urban areas (19 percent).

IMMUNIZATION COVERAGE (NFHS 3)

BCG 78%
Oral Polio drops (3 doses) 78%
Measles 59%
DPT (3 doses) 55%

- Children who received BCG, measles, and three doses each of DPT and polio (excluding Polio 0) are considered to be *fully vaccinated.*
- Nationwide, *only 44 percent* of children between 12-23 months are fully vaccinated and 5 percent have not received any vaccinations.
- Fifty-five percent of children have received three doses of DPT.
- Although DPT and polio vaccinations are given at the same time as part of the routine immunization programme, the coverage rates are higher for polio than for DPT (for all three doses), undoubtedly because of the Pulse polio campaigns.
- Not all children who begin the DPT and polio vaccination series go on to complete them. The difference between the percentages of children receiving the first and third doses is 21 percentage points for DPT and 15 percentage points for polio.
- Fifty-nine percent of children age12-23 months have been vaccinated against measles.
- The relatively low percentages of children vaccinated with the third dose of DPT and measles are mainly responsible for the low proportion of children fully vaccinated.
- The 12-23 months age group was chosen for analysis because both international and Government of India guidelines, specify that children should be fully vaccinated by the time they complete their first year of life.

CHILDREN WITH DISEASES TAKEN TO HEALTH FACILITY (NFHS 3)

- Diarrhea: 60 percent
- Acute respiratory infection (ARI): 69 percent
- Fever: 71 percent

- Sixty-nine percent of children received some advice or treatment from a health facility or health provider when ill with ARI.

TREATMENT OF CHILDHOOD DIARRHEA WITH ORS (NFHS 3)

Urban 33%
Rural 24%

- Children with diarrhea (overall) who received ORS (%) 26.2 %.
- Overall, 9 percent of all children under age five had diarrhoea, with 1 percent having diarrhea with blood.
- Among children 0-59 months, children 6-11 months are most susceptible to diarrhea (as is generally the case with ARI and fever as well).
- 39% of children under age 5 with diarrhea in the two weeks before the survey received some kind of oral rehydration therapy.
- 26% were treated with a solution prepared from oral rehydration salt (ORS) packets and 20% received gruel.
- More than one-quarter (26%) did not receive any kind of treatment.
- 16% received antibiotics, which are not normally recommended for treating childhood diarrhea.
- Knowledge of ORS among recent mothers in NFHS-3(73 percent) has increased by about 12 percentage points from its level in NFHS-2 (62 percent).

ANEMIA STATUS (NFHS 3)

Any Anemia: 79%
Severe Anemia: 5%

COVERAGE OF ANGANWADI CENTERS (NFHS 3)

- Overall, seventy-two percent of the sample enumeration areas are covered by an *anganwadi* center and 62 percent are covered by an AWC (*anganwadi* center) that had, existed for at least five years.
- Three-fourths of children age 0-71 months in areas covered by an *anganwadi* center did not receive any supplementary food from the center in the 12 months preceding the survey. Further, only a small proportion (12 percent) received supplementary food almost daily.
- It is recommended that children aged 0-35 months be weighed monthly and older children be weighed quarterly. The majority of children age 0-59 months (80 percent) in areas covered by an AWC were not weighed at all in an *anganwadi* center. Eighteen percent of children age 0-59 months in areas served by an *anganwadi* center have had their weight measured in an AWC.
- Overall, 20 percent of children age 0-71 months in areas covered by an *anganwadi* center received an immunization from an AWC in the 12 months preceding the survey.

HOUSEHOLD CHARACTERISTICS (NFHS 3)

- 68% of households have electricity, up from 60% in NFHS 2
- 88% of households use an improved source of drinking water
- Only 29% of households have improved toilet facilities
- 73% of urban households and 30% of rural households possess a TV.

EDUCATION (NFHS 3)

NFHS 3 shows that even among those in the age group 15-19, only 89% of men and 74% of women are literate.

CASTE/TRIBE STATUS (NFHS 3)

- Scheduled caste 19%
- Scheduled tribe 8%

Table 12.1: Mortality and nutrition indicators

Indicators	
Fertility Indicators	
Crude birth rate	22.8 (SRS 2008)
Total fertility rate	2.7 (NFHS 3)
Natural growth rate	15.4 (SRS 2008)
Mortality Indicators	
Crude death rate	7.4 (SRS 2008)
Infant mortality rate	57.0 (NFHS 3); 53 (SRS 2008)
Neonatal mortality rate	39.0 (NFHS 3)
Postneonatal mortality rate	18.0 (NFHS 3)
Perinatal mortality rate	33.0 (SRS 2003)
Stillbirth rate	09.0 (SRS 2003)
Child mortality	18.0 (NFHS 3)
Under 5 mortality	74.0 (NFHS 3)
Maternal mortality ratio	254 (SRS, 2004-06)
Life expectancy at birth	
Males	62.3 years
Females	63.9 years (2003)
Immunization coverage (12-23 months)	
Fully Immunized (BCG, Measles, DPT/OPV 3 doses)	43.5% (NFHS-3)
BCG	78.2% (NFHS-3)
DPT 3 doses	55.3% (NFHS-3)
OPV 3 doses	78.2% (NFHS-3)
Measles	58.8% (NFHS-3)
Nutrition Indicators	
Low birth weight newborns	21.5% (NFHS-3)
Children under 3 years breastfeed within 1 hour of birth	23.4% (NFHS 3)
Exclusive breastfeeding at 0-5 months	46.3% (NFHS-3)
Children age 6-9 months receiving solid or semi-solid food and breast milk	55.8% (NFHS 3)
% of underfives suffering from:	
Underweight	45.9% (NFHS-3)
Wasting	19.1% (NFHS-3)
Stunting	38.4% (NFHS-3)
Maternal Health	
Institutional deliveries	41.0% (NFHS-3)
Deliveries by skilled birth attendants	48.3% (NFHS-3)
At least three antenatal check ups	50.7% (NFHS-3)

- Other backward class 41%
- Others 32%.

MARITAL STATUS (NFHS 3)

Percent of women age 20-24 married by age 18: 45%.

CURRENT CONTRACEPTIVE USE (NFHS 3)

- Any method 56%
- Modern method 49%
- Female sterilization 37%
- Male sterilization 1%

ANTENATAL CARE (NFHS 3)

Percent of women who had any ANC: 77%

MATERNITY CARE (NFHS 3)

- 3+ ANC Visits: 52%
- Iron folic acid tablet for 90 days: 23%
- Postnatal care within 2 days: 37%

CHILD NUTRITIONAL STATUS (NFHS 3)

Percent of children age less than 3 years:

- Stunted (Low height for age) 45%
- Wasted (low weight for height) 23%
- Underweight (low weight for age) 40%

NUTRITIONAL STATUS OF ADULTS

Percent of women and men age 15-49.

	Male	*Female*
• Anemic	24 %	55%
• Obese	9%	13%
• BMI below normal	34%	36%

NATIONAL FAMILY HEALTH SURVEY (NFHS)

The National Family Health Survey (NFHS) is a large-scale, multiround survey conducted in a representative sample of households throughout India operational since 1992-93.

NFHS-3 (2005-06) is the third in the NFHS series of surveys, preceded by NFHS-1 in 1992-93 and NFHS-2 in 1998-99.

The survey provides state and national information for India on fertility, infant and child mortality, the practice of family planning, maternal and child health, reproductive health, nutrition, anemia, utilization and quality of health and family planning services.

NFHS surveys are conducted under the steward ship of MoHFW and all 29 states are covered.

SAMPLE REGISTRATION SURVEY

- Large-scale demographic survey for providing reliable annual estimates of birth rate, death rate and other fertility and mortality indicators at the national and subnational levels.

SECTION–II

LONG CASES IN PEDIATRICS

CHAPTER 13

PROTEIN ENERGY MALNUTRITION (PEM)

HISTORY

CHIEF COMPLAINTS

- Loss of weight
- Edema
- Fever/cough/difficulty in respiration/diarrhea.

HISTORY OF PRESENT ILLNESS

History of Disease

Fever

- Onset: Sudden, insidious
- Associated with chills and rigour
- Associted with sweating
- Documented or not
- Intermittent, remittent, continuous
- History of convulsions associated with fever
- History of immunization.

Diarrhea

- Acute onset or persistent
- Frequency of stools
- Accompanied by blood or mucus
- Presence of tenesmus (painful urgency is seen in invasive diarrhea)
- Presence of foul smelling, bulky stool difficult to flush (malabsorption, cystic fibrosis)
- Associated with abdominal pain or vomiting
- Ingestion of unusual food (food poisoning)
- Urine output (assess severity of dehydration)
- Use of antibiotics.

Vomiting

- Frequency
- Time of occurrence
- Projectile or non-projectile
- Antecedent symptoms:
  - Abdominal pain, diarrhea (GIT problem)
  - Headache (intracranial space occupying lesion, meningitis)
  - Cough (post-tussive vomiting)
  - Urinary symptoms (fever and vomiting may be due to urinary tract infection)
  - Ear symptoms (vertigo)
  - Abdominal distension (surgical cause).
- Content of vomitus
- Urine output
- Jaundice
- Association with history of drug intake.

Vitamin/Mineral Deficiency

- Night blindness/reduced vision (Vitamin A)

- Pain in lower limbs/bleeding from gums (Vitamin C)
- Polyuria (Vitamin D deficiency)
- Bleeding/bruising on skin (Vitamin K)
- Paleness of body (iron deficiency)
- Diarrhea with rash on extremities (pellagra).

History of Risk Factors

- Convulsions/unconsciouness/altered sensorium (CNS involvement)
- Pyoderma/Ear discharge
- Cough/breathlessness (respiratory tract infection)
- Vomiting/diarrhea (GIT involvement)
- Worms in stools (worm infestation)
- Rash (measles)
- Rash with itching (scabies)
- Fever with/without chills/rigors (urinary tract infection, malaria)
- Burning micturition (urinary tract infection)
- Contact with tuberculosis.

History of Differential Diagnosis

- Mental changes (decreased activity, lack of interest in surroundings), skin and hair changes [kwashiorkor]
- Past history of jaundice (hepatic cause)
- Palpitations/breathlessness/cyanosis/pain in abdomen/pedal edema (congestive cardiac failure)
- Hematuria /dysuria/oliguria (Urinary tract infection; nephritis).

ANTENATAL AND POSTNATAL HISTORY

Antenatal

- Prenatal exposure to illicit drugs, toxins or infections
- Acute maternal illness; trauma; radiation exposure
- Prenatal care and fetal movements
- Antepartum hemorrhage
- Premature onset of delivery or labor
- Frequent spontaneous abortions.

Postnatal

- Term/preterm
- Birth weight and subsequent weights
- American pediatric gross assessment record (APGAR) score
- Complications in the neonatal period
  - Time of onset of cry
  - Intubation time
  - Use of surfactant
  - Presence of ischemia or hemorrhage on neonatal ultrasound
  - Feeding difficulties, apnea
  - Infection
  - Hyperbilirubinemia.
- Duration of exclusive breastfeeding.

SOCIOECONOMIC HISTORY

- Details of family:
  - Joint/nuclear
  - Number of family members
  - Literacy status and occupation of parents.
- Total family income
- Is the mother employed?
- Addiction in parents
- Housing details:
  - Owned/rented
  - Type (brick/mud)
  - Number of rooms
  - Details of environmental sanitation
  - Water supply and how water is stored in house.

FAMILY HISTORY

- Birth order/spacing/contraceptive device or sterilization
- Number of siblings
- Death of sibling and its reason
- Comparison of child's nutritional status with his/her siblings.

DIETARY HISTORY

- Usual diet (before the current illness)
- Calculate calories and protein intake
- Exclusive breastfeeding done till what age
- Total duration of breastfeeding and adequacy
- Complementary feeding started at what age
- Type/dilution of feeds
- Method and frequency of feeding
- Whether vitamins/mineral supplements were given.

IMMUNIZATION/DEVELOPMENTAL HISTORY

- Detailed immunization and developmental history.

GENERAL PHYSICAL EXAMINATION

On General physical examination of malnourished child it is essential to look for:

- *General appearance:* Alert, irritable/lethargy, emaciated, loss of subcutaneous fat and sunken cheek.
- Posture
- Vital signs
- Anthropometry (detailed)—weight, height/length, mid arm circumference
- Signs of dehydration
- Shock (cold hands, slow capillary refill, weak and rapid pulse)
- Dysmorphic facies
- Dentition and oral hygiene— mouth ulcers or oral candidiasis
- Pallor/cyanosis/clubbing/icterus/lymphadenopathy/edema/JVP/pyoderma
- BCG mark.
- Localizing signs of infection, including ear and throat infections, or skin infection.
- *Hair changes:* Hypopigmentation/sparse hair/easily pluckable hair/flag sign.
- *Nail chages:* Brittle nails/paronychia/koilonychia/platynychia.
- *Skin changes:* Hypo/hyperpigmentation/violaceous spots/marbling/mosaic pattern/crazy pavement sign/flaky paint dermatoses/enamel paint dermatoses/edema/shiny skin/fissures/ulcers/petechiae.
- Bed sores/perianal excoriation.
- Signs of vitamin deficiency:
  - *Vitamin A deficiency:* Phrynoderma/corneal or conjunctival xerosis/Bitot spots
  - *Vitamin B deficiency:* Angular stomatitis/pellagra/glossitis
  - *Vitamin C deficiency:* Bleeding gums/pain in joints (however scurvy is rare in PEM)
  - *Vitamin D deficiency:* Bossing of skull/beading of ribs (rickets does not normally occur in PEM as it is a disease of growing bones and in PEM growth is retarded)
  - *Vitamin K deficiency:* Petechiae/purpura.
- Signs of HIV infection.

SYSTEMIC EXAMINATION

ABDOMEN

- Hepatomegaly (fatty liver in Kwashiorkor)
- Ascites
- Paralytic ileus (due to hypokalemia, muscle atrophy, sepsis)

- Rectal prolapse (due to wasting of fat in ischiorectal fossa).

CENTRAL NERVOUS SYSTEM

- Irritable/hypotonia.

RESPIRATORY SYSTEM

- Respiratory distress
- Any additional sounds.

CARDIOVASCULAR SYSTEM

- Cardiomegaly
- Murmur.

DIAGNOSIS

Protein energy malnutrition (Grade .... by IAP classification) with/without complications (Bronchopneumonia/meningitis/hypothermia/ tuberculosis); with/without vitamin/mineral deficiency; Probable etiology being inadequate diet/poverty/illiteracy and precipitating factors being diarrhea/measles/repeated LRTI's.

INVESTIGATIONS

- Hemogram with ESR.
- *Blood sugar:* Hypoglycemia.
- *Blood urea:* It increases in dehydration or renal disease.
- *S. electrolytes:* Hypokalemia.
- *S. bilirubin:* Increase suggests poor prognosis.
- *S. proteins:* Hypoproteinemia and hypoalbuminemia—beginning of kwashiorkor.
- *Liver function tests:* Liver enzymes—usually decreased.
- *Blood culture:* Septicemia.
- Peripheral smear for malaria.
- Urine routine and culture examination (urinary tract infection).
- *Stool routine examination:* Worm infestation.
- *Stool:* pH and reducing sugars (chronic diarrhea and malabsorption).
- *Arterial blood gases:* Acidosis.
- *X-ray chest* (pulmonary tuberculosis/bronchopneumonia).
- *Mantoux* test.

TREATMENT

IAP Guidelines 2006 on Hospital Based Management of Severely Malnourished Children (Adapted from the WHO Guidelines)

The treatment guidelines are divided into ten essential steps:

1. Treat/prevent hypoglycemia.
2. Treat/prevent hypothermia.
3. Treat/prevent dehydration.
4. Correct electrolyte imbalance.
5. Treat/prevent infection.
6. Correct micronutrient deficiencies.
7. Start cautious feeding.
8. Achieve catch-up growth.
9. Provide sensory stimulation and emotional support.
10. Prepare for follow-up after recovery.

Step 1: Treat/Prevent Hypoglycemia

Blood glucose level < 54 mg/dl is defined as hypoglycemia in a severely malnourished child.

Treatment

Conscious Child:

- Give 50ml of 10% glucose orally or by nasogastric tube
- Start feeding 2 hourly day and night
- Start appropriate antibiotics.

Symptomatic child (unconscious, lethargic or seizuring):

- Give 10% dextrose intravenously 5ml/kg
- Follow with 50 ml of 10% dextrose solution by nasogastric tube.
- Start feeding 2 hourly.
- Start appropriate antibiotics.

Step 2: Treat/ Prevent Hypothermia

If rectal temperature is less than 35.5°C or 95.5°F:

- Feed the child immediately (if necessary rehydrate first)
- Cloth the child with warm clothes and warm blanket. Ensure that the head is also covered well.
- Provide heat with an overhead warmer, an incandescent lamp or radiant heater.
- Or the child could be put in kangaroo mother care.
- Give appropriate antibiotics.

Treatment of Severe Hypothermia (Rectal Temperature < 32°C)

- Give warm humidified oxygen.
- Give 5ml/kg of 10% dextrose intravenously immediately or 50ml of 10% dextrose by nasogastric route (if IV access is difficult).
- Start IV antibiotics.
- *Rewarm:* Provide heat using radiation (overhead warmer), or conduction (skin contact) or convection (heat convector). Avoid rapid rewarming as this may lead to dysequilibrium.
- Give warm fluids.

Step 3: Treat/Prevent Dehydration

It is difficult to estimate dehydration status using clinical signs alone. Assume all children with watery diarrhoea may have dehydration. Use reduced osmolarity ORS with potassium supplements given additionally. Continue feeding.

Fluid Management for Severe Dehydration

Ideally, Ringer lactate with 5% dextrose should be used as rehydrating fluid. If not available, use half normal (N/2) saline with 5% dextrose. The other alternative is to use Ringer's lactate solution.

- Give oxygen
- Give rehydrating fluid at slower infusion rates of 15ml/kg over the first 2 hours with continuous monitoring (pulse rate, pulse volume, respiratory rate, capillary refill time, urine output).
- Administer intravenous antibiotics.
- If there is no improvement after the first hour of the fluid bolus, consider septic shock.

Step 4: Correct Electrolyte Imbalance

Give supplemental potassium at 3-4 mmol/kg/day for at least 2 weeks. Potassium can be given as syrup potassium chloride.

On day 1, give 50% magnesium sulphate intramuscular once (0.3 ml/kg up to a maximum of 2 ml).

Step 5: Treat/ Prevent Infection

In addition to complete clinical evaluation, following investigations may be done for identifying the infections:

- Hemoglobin, TLC, DLC, peripheral smear
- Urine analysis and urine culture
- Blood culture
- Chest X-ray
- Mantoux test
- Gastric aspirate for AFB
- Peripheral smear for malaria (in endemicareas)
- CSF examination (if meningitis suspected).

Choice of Broad Spectrum Antibiotics

Give parenteral antibiotics to all admitted children.

- Ampicillin and Gentamicin for seven days:

If the child fails to improve within 48 hours, change to Intravenous Cefotaxime/Ceftriaxone.

If meningitis is suspected, perform lumbar puncture and treat the child with intravenous Cefotaxime and intravenous Amikacin for 14-21 days. Moreover, if staphylococcal infection is suspected add intravenous Cloxacillin.

Add antimalarial treatment if the child has a positive blood film for malaria parasites.

Step 6: Correct Micronutrient Deficiencies

Although anemia is common, do not give iron initially. Wait until the child has a good appetite and starts gaining weight (usually by week 2). Giving iron may make infections worse.

Vitamin A orally on day 1 (if age >1 year give 2,00,000 IU; age 6-12 months give 1,00,000 IU; age 0-5 months give 50,000 IU) unless there is definite evidence that a dose has been given in the last month.

Give Daily

Multivitamin supplement containing Thiamin, Riboflavin, Nicotinic acid and vitamins A,C,D,E, and B_{12}.

- Folic acid 1 mg/day (give 5 mg on day 1).
- Zinc 2 mg/kg/day (can be provided using zinc syrups/ zinc dispersible tablets).
- Copper 0.2-0.3 mg/kg/day (will have to use a multivitamin/ mineral commercial preparation).
- Iron 3 mg/kg/day only once child starts gaining weight; after the stabilization phase.

Step 7: Initiate Re-feeding

Start feeding as soon as possible as frequent small feeds. Initiate nasogastric feeds if the child is not being able to take orally.

- Recommended daily energy and protein intake from initial feeds is 100 kcal/kg and 1-1.5 g/kg respectively.
- Total fluid recommended is 130 ml/kg/day; reduce to 100 ml/kg/day if there is severe, generalized edema.
- Continue breast feeding *ad libitum*
- The cereal-based low lactose (lower osmolarity) diets are recommended as starter diets.

Step 8: Achieve Catch up Growth

Once appetite returns, decrease frequency of feeds to 6 feeds/day and the increase volume offered at each feed.

- It is recommended that each successive feed is increased by 10 ml until some is left uneaten. Breast feeding should be continued adlibitum.
- Make a gradual transition from F-75 diet to F-100 diet. The starter F-75 diet should be replaced with F-100 diet in equal amount in 2 days.
- The calorie intake should be increased to 150-200 kcal/kg/day, and the proteins to 4-6g/kg/day.
- For children with persistent diarrhea, who do not tolerate low lactose diets, lactose free diet can be started.

Step 9: Provide Sensory Stimulation and Emotional Support

Delayed mental and behavioral development often occurs in severe malnutrition. Provide:

- A cheerful, stimulating environment.
- Age appropriate physical activity as soon as the child is well enough.
- Tender loving care.

Step 10: Prepare for Follow-up after Recovery

Review periodically after 1 week, 2 weeks, 1 month, 3 months and 6 months after discharge.

Progress is considered satisfactory, if the weight for height continues to be maintained at 90 percent of expected.

The aim is to prevent relapse and assure continued physical, mental and emotional development.

Advise Caregiver to

- Bring child back for regular follow-up checks.
- Ensure booster immunizations are given.
- Ensure vitamin A is given every six months.
- Feed frequently with energy and nutrient dense foods.
- Give structured play therapy.

DISCUSSION

CLASSIFICATION OF PEM

- **WHO classification (Table 13.1)**

Table 13.1: WHO classification of PEM

	Moderate malnutrition	*Severe malnutrition*
Symmetrical edema	No	Yes
Weight for height (measure of wasting)	70-79%	<70% (severe wasting)
Height for age (measure of stunting)	85-89%	< 85% (severe stunting)

- **IAP classification (Table 13.2):** Based on NCHS standard

Table 13.2: IAP classification

Grade	*Percentage of standard weight for age*
I	70-80%
II	60-70%
III	50-60%
IV	<50%

If edema is associated with decreased weight, then "K" is added to the grade of malnutrition.

- **Wellcome trust classification (Table 13.3):** Based on standard weight for age (95th percentile ICMR value or 50th percentile Boston value).

Table 13.3: Wellcome trust classification

Weight (percentage of standard weight) for age	*80-60%*	*<60%*
With edema	Kwashiorkor	Marasmic Kwashiorkor
Without edema	Underweight (undernutrition)	Marasmus

- **Gomez classification (Table 13.4):** Based on Harvard standard

Table 13.4: Gomez classification

Grades	*Percentage of standard weight for age*
I	76-90%
II	61-75%
III	<60%

- **Udani's classification (Table 13.5):**

Table 13.5: Udani's classification

Grades	*Loss of fat from*
I	Buttocks
II	Axilla/groin
III	Abdomen, chest, back
IV	Buccal pad of fat

- ***Shakir's tape*** to measure nutritional status by measuring mid arm circumference:

Green	> 13.5 cm	Normal
Yellow	12.5-13.5 cm	Borderline malnutrition
Red	<12.5 cm	Severe malnutrition

Table 13.6. Age independent anthropometric indices

Method	*Name of index*	*Normal (severely malnourished)*
$\frac{\text{Weight kg}}{(\text{Height cm})^{1.6}} \times 100$	Dugdale's	0.88-0.97 (< 0.79)
$\frac{\text{Weight kg}}{(\text{Height cm})^{2}} \times 100$	Rao's	0.15-0.16 (< 0.14)
$\frac{\text{Midarm circumference (cm)}}{\text{Head circumference (cm)}}$	Kanawati	0.32-0.33 (< 0.25)
Midarm circumference, between the ages of 1-5 years		>13.5 cm (< 12.5 cm)

Table 13.7: Classification based on NCHS (USA standard)

Deficiency status	*Test*	*Criteria for PEM*
Acute status	Weight for Height	<3rd centile
Chronic status	Height for age	<3rd centile
Fat deficiency	Triceps skin fold thickness	<5th centile
Somatic protein deficiency	Midarm muscle	<5th centile
Visceral protein deficiency	Albumin transferring ratio	< Std for age
Immune status	Total lymphocyte count	Reduced helper T-cell count

ETIOLOGY OF PEM

Classical Theory

Marasmus (Body Adapts)

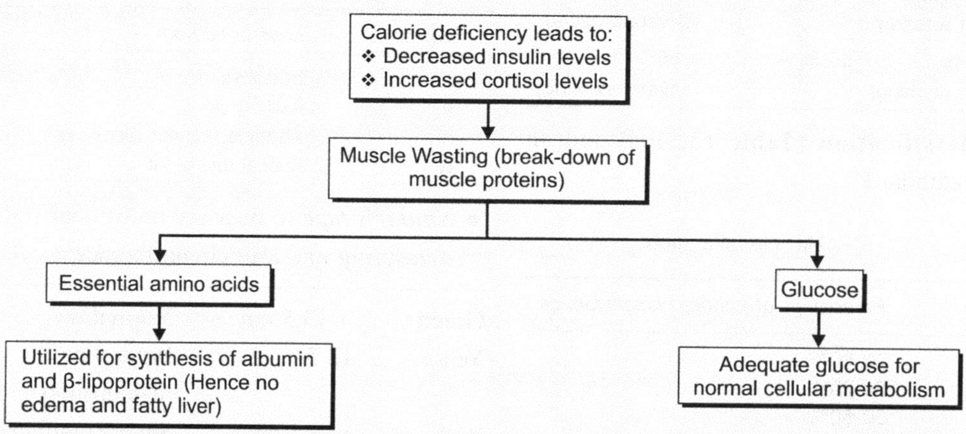

Kwashiorkor (Body Fails to Adapt)

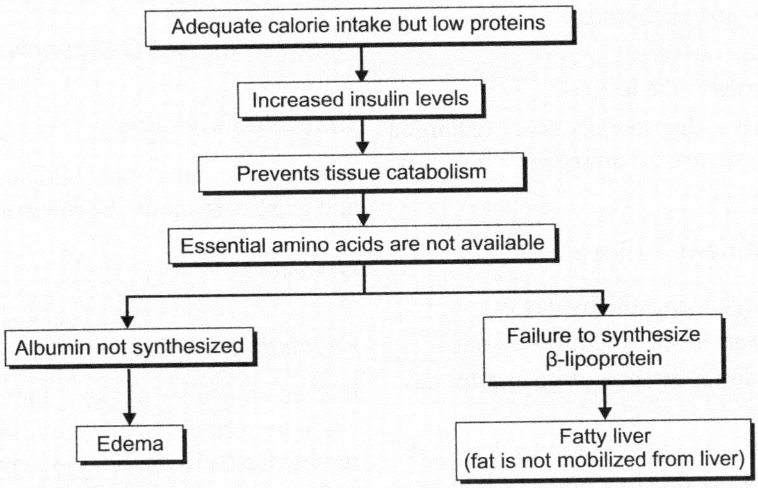

CLINICAL FEATURES OF MARASMUS

- Child is alert, irritable with voracious appetite.
- Body weight is less than 60% of expected weight for age
- The loss of subcutaneous fat gives rise to certain characteristic features:
  - Large head with depressed anterior fontanelle
  - Sunken, lusterless eyes
  - Prominent bony points
  - Loose folds of skin are prominent over gluteus and inner aspect of thigh
  - Contour of atrophic muscles is evident under skin.
- Hypopigmented hair
- Skin is dry, wrinkled, scaly and inelastic
- Distended abdomen with wasting and hypotonia of abdominal muscles.

CLINICAL FEATURES OF KWASHIORKOR

- *Mental changes:* Lethargic, listless, apathetic with little interest in surroundings and food.
- *Growth failure* is always present.
- *Edema:* Starts from lower extremities and later involves upper limbs and face.
  - Ascites is uncommon.
  - Face is moon shaped and puffy
- *Muscle wasting* is masked by edema
- *Hair changes:*
  - Thin, dry, easily pluckable, hypopigmented
  - *Flag sign*: Alternate band of hypopigmented and normal pigmented hair. It signifies alternate episodes of good and poor nutrition.
- *Skin changes:*
  - Dry and scaly skin
  - *Marbalization:* Soft and shiny skin with marble-like feel.
  - *Enamel paint dermatoses:* Hyperpigmented patches of skin in flexural areas and which desquamate.
  - *Flaky paint dermatoses*: When above areas becomes confluent.
  - *Crazy pavement dermatoses:* Seen in extensor surfaces (over shins); depigmen-

ted skin is covered with dark shiny patches which crack like parched earth.
- Petechiae and ecchymosis
- Hypopigmented areas
- Ecchymoses—like lesions.

- **Hepatomegaly**—due to fatty liver; enlarged with rounded lower margins and soft consistency.

Primary Treatment Failure

- Failure to regain appetite by day 4
- Failure to start losing of edema by day 4
- Failure of disappearance of edema by day 10
- Failure to gain weight at least by 5 g/kg of body weight per day by day 10 of therapy.

Secondary Treatment Failure

If the child does not gain > 5g/kg/day body weight for 3 consecutive days any time during the rehabilitative phase.

CRITERIA FOR DISCHARGE IN PEM

- Appetite should have returned and the oral intake is adequate
- Child is constantly gaining weight at normal rate
- All infections, vitamin and mineral deficiency have been treated
- Immunization initiated
- Mother educated regarding domiciliary care.
- Serum albumin should be more than 3.0 g/dl.

CAUSES OF POOR WEIGHT GAIN IN PEM

Inadequate Feeding

Check

- Night feeds have been given
- Target energy and protein intakes are achieved.
- Feeding technique
- All aspects of food preparation.

Specific Nutrient Deficiencies

Untreated Infection

Urinary tract infections, otitis media, tuberculosis and giardiasis should be ruled out.

HIV/AIDS

Psychological Problems

It is recommended to check for abnormal behavior such as stereotyped movements (rocking), rumination (self-stimulation through regurgitation) and attention seeking. These should be treated by giving the child special love and attention.

CAUSES OF ANEMIA IN PEM

It may be normocytic normochromic, microcytic hypochromic or dimorphic.

Mechanism

- Decreased intake
- Worm infestation
- Decreased absorption
- Protein deficiency (globin part of hemoglobin)/ Micronutrient deficiency (zinc, copper, selenium)/ Folate and iron deficiency
- Hemodilution (due to edema).

MANAGEMENT OF SEVERE ANEMIA IN MALNOURISHED CHILDREN

A blood transfusion is required on admission if:
- Hemoglobin is less than 4 g/dl
- If there is respiratory distress and hemoglobin between 4 and 6 g/dl. (In mild or moderate anemia, iron should be given for three months to replete iron stores but this should not be

started until after the initial stabilization phase has been completed).

Treatment

- Whole blood 10 ml/kg body weight slowly over 3 hours
- Furosemide 1mg/kg IV at the start of the transfusion.

It is particularly important that the volume of 10 ml/kg is not exceeded in severely malnourished children. If the severely anemic child has signs of cardiac failure, transfuse packed cells rather than whole blood.

MECHANISM OF IMMUNOSUPPRESSION IN PEM

- Decreased cell mediated immunity (explains negative tuberculin test in PEM despite active tuberculosis)
- Decreased humoral immunity (IgG, IgM, secretory IgA are not significantly affected in mild to moderate PEM, hence host responds well to bacterial infections and viral vaccines. But depressed in severe PEM)
- Decreased polymorphonuclear activity
- Decreased complement factors
- Decrease in lysozymes and interferon
- Decrease in transferrin level (in the absence of transferring free iron favours bacterial multiplication)
- Damage to epithelial barrier.

BIOCHEMISTRY IN PEM

Sodium	Decreased in the serum and increased within the cells. (sodium enters cells along concentration gradient due to activity of Na^+- K^+ ATPase)
Potassium	Low (decreased activity of Na^+ - K^+ ATPase so that intracellular K^+ enter the plasma), associated gastroenteritis increases hypokalemia
Magnesium	Low (dietary deficiency)
Serum albumin	Low (decreased synthesis)
Serum globulin	Increased (secondary to infection)
Blood glucose	Decreased
Serum amino acids	Essential amino acids (especially branched chain amino acids and threonine) decreased
Blood urea	Decreased (due to decreased synthesis—This is an adaptation mechanism to conserve nitrogen)
Urinary creatinine	Increased (increased production secondary to skeletal muscle atrophy)
Serum transferrin	Reduced (decreased synthesis)

Table 13.8: Composition of recommended ORS solution in severely malnourished (ReSoMal)

Component	*ReSoMal (mMol/L)*	*WHO ORS (mMol/L)*
Glucose	125	75
Sodium	45	75
Potassium	40	20
Chloride	70	65
Citrate	7	10
Magnesium	3	–
Zinc	0.3	–
Copper	0.045	–
Osmolarity	300	245

COMPLICATIONS OF PEM

Infective

- Septic shock
- Infections and associated nutrition deficiencies.

Metabolic

- Electrolyte disturbances:
  - Hypo- and hypernatremia
  - Hypo- and hyperkalemia
  - Hypomagnesemia
  - Hypocalcemia.
- Hypoglycemia
- Hypothermia.

Miscellaneous

- Dehydration
- Congestive heart failure
- Anemia
- Sudden infant death syndrome (SIDS)
- Delayed milestones.

POOR PROGNOSTIC FACTORS IN PEM

- Gross edema
- Hypothermia
- Hypoglycemia
- Jaundice
- Drowsiness
- Hyponatremia/Hypernatremia.

SEQUENTIAL ANTHROPOMETRIC CHANGES IN PEM

- Weight
- Skin fold thickness
- Mid-arm circumference
- Chest circumference
- Height
- Head circumference.

BODY MASS INDEX (BMI)

$$\frac{\text{Weight in kg}}{(\text{Height in mtr})^2}$$

- Ninty-five percentile for age or BMI more than 30 is considered as obesity. This is age independent index to assess nutrition.

Table 13.9: Composition of intravenous solutions (mEq per liter)

Fluid	Na^+	Cl^-	K^+	Ca^{2+}	*Glucose (g)*	*Others*
Normal saline (0.95% NaCl)	154	154				
N/2 (0.45% NaCl)	77	77				
Ringer lactate	131	111	5	3		29 (Lactate)
5% dextrose					50	
10% dextrose					100	
Isolyte P	25	20	22		50	Acetate 23 Phosphate 3 Magnesium 3

TREATMENT OF CONDITIONS ASSOCIATED WITH MALNUTRITION

Vitamin A Deficiency

If the child has any eye signs of vitamin A deficiency, give orally:

Vitamin A on days 1, 2 and 14 (if aged >1 year give 200,000 iu; if aged 6-12 months give 100,000 iu, if aged 0-5 months give 50,000 iu).

If there is inflammation or ulceration, give additional eye care to prevent extrusion of the lens:

- Instill chloramphenicol or tetracycline eye drops, 2-3 hourly as required for 7-10 days in the affected eye.
- Instill atropine eye drops, 1 drop three times daily for 3-5 days.
- Cover with saline-soaked eye pads and bandage.

Zinc deficiency is usual in affected children and the skin quickly improves with zinc supplementation. In addition:

- On affected areas apply 0.01% potassium permanganate solution.

- Apply barrier cream (zinc and castor oil ointment, or petroleum jelly or tulle grass) to raw areas.
- Omit nappies/diapers to keep perineum dry.

Parasitic Worms

If there is evidence of worm infestation, give mebendazole (100 mg orally twice a day) for 3 days. In areas where infestation is very prevalent, also add mebendazole to children with no evidence of infestation after day 7 of admission.

Tuberculosis

If TB is strongly suspected (contacts, poor growth despite good intake, chronic cough, chest infection not responding to antibiotics):

- Perform Mantoux test (Note false negatives are frequent).
- Chest X-ray.

If positive test or strong suspicion of Tuberculosis, treat according to national TB guidelines.

F-75 AND F-100 DIETS

- Two formula diets, F-75 and F-100, are used for severely malnourished children.
- F-75(75 kcal/100 ml), is used during the initial phase of treatment, while F-100 (100 kcal/100 ml) is used during the rehabilitation phase, after the appetite has returned.
- These formulas can easily be prepared from the basic ingredients: dried skimmed milk, sugar, cereal flour, oil, mineral mix and vitamin mix. They are also commercially available as powder formulations that are mixed with water.
- The mineral mix supplies potassium, magnesium and other essential minerals; it must be added to the diet. The potassium deficit, present in all malnourished children, adversely affects cardiac function and gastric emptying. Magnesium is essential for potassium to enter cells and be retained. The mineral mix does not contain iron as this is withheld during the initial phase.

Preparation of F-75 and F-100 Diets

Ingredient Amount

	F-75	*F-100*
Dried skimmed milk	25 g	80 g
Sugar	70 g	50 g
Cereal flour	35 g	—
Vegetable oil	27 g	60 g
Mineral mix	20 ml	20 ml
Vitamin mix	140 mg	140 mg
Water to make	1000 ml	1000 ml

- To prepare the F-75 diet, add the dried skimmed milk, sugar, cereal flour and oil to some water and mix. Boil for 5-7 minutes. Allow to cool, then add the mineral mix and vitamin mix and mix again. Make up the volume to 1000 ml with water.
- To prepare the F-100 diet, add the dried skimmed milk, sugar and oil to some warm boiled water and mix. Add the mineral mix and vitamin mix and mix again. Make up the volume to 1000 ml with water.
- If only small amounts of feed are being prepared, multivitamin supplement can be used instead of vitamin mix.

FEEDING ADVICE AT DISCHARGE

- Give appropriate meals at least 5 times daily.
- Give high energy snacks between meals (e.g., milk, banana, bread, biscuits).
- Assist and encourage the child to complete each meal.
- Give electrolyte and micronutrient supplements. Give 20 ml (4 teaspoons) of the electrolyte/mineral solution daily. Since it tastes unpleasant, it will probably need to be masked in porridge, or milk (one teaspoon/200 ml fluid).
- Breastfeed as often as child wants.

CHAPTER 14

Renal System

Nephrotic Syndrome

HISTORY

CHIEF COMPLAINTS

- Generalized body swelling
- Decreased urine output.

HISTORY OF PRESENT ILLNESS

History of Disease

- Onset of edema: Insidious/sudden
- Starts from face and gradually progresses to entire body
- Association with upper respiratory tract infection
- Associated with decreased urinary output
- Frothy urine
- Associated with increase in weight
- Ask about tightness of clothes and slippers, marks of undergarments over body
- Diarrhea (due to intestinal edema).

History of Complications

- Difficulty in respiration (hydrothorax/pericardial effusion)
- Cellulitis
- Abdominal pain, tenderness (subacute bacterial peritonitis).

History of Risk Factors

- Skin rash and joint pains (collagen vascular disease)
- Drug intake: NSAID's/penicillamine probenecid/captopril/hydralazine
- Jaundice and blood transfusion (hepatitis B)
- Fever with chills (malaria).

History of Differential Diagnosis

- Breathlessness, palpitations, fever with joint pains and sore throat (cardiac disorder)
- Oliguria, hematuria, dysuria (acute nephritis)
- Jaundice, hematemesis, malena, high-colored urine (hepatic cause)

- Dietary history, malnutrition (kwashiorkor)
- Measles/Tuberculosis
- Drug ingestion, insect bite, breathlessness associated with itching, fever, abdominal pain (allergic manifestations); sore throat (post-streptococcal).

TREATMENT HISTORY

- Past hospitalization
- Invasive procedures like ascitic tap/kidney biopsy.

DIETARY HISTORY

- Determine premorbeid caloric and protein intake.

IMMUNIZATION HISTORY

- In detail with special reference to *Streptococcus pneumoniae*, *Haemophilus influenzae*, Varicella and Hepatitis B.

GENERAL PHYSICAL EXAMINATION

- *General appearance:* The child appears alert, puffy and has generalized edema with periorbital puffiness.
- Bradycardia
- Blood pressure
- Jugular venous pressure
- Anthropometry: Growth failure is common in nephrotic syndrome
- Steroid facies
- Skin: Malar rash (SLE), pyoderma, purpura
- Assess edema: Ankle edema, ascites, abdominal wall edema, sacral edema, periorbital and scrotal edema
- Joint swellings
- BCG mark/Mantoux test.

SYSTEMIC EXAMINATION

ABDOMEN EXAMINATION

Inspection

- Skin and subcutaneous tissue
  - Ulcer, striae, pigmentation, puncture mark
  - Any breach of skin
  - If superficial veins are engorged – their location
- Umbilicus: Everted (ascites), displaced upwards or downwards by ascites or swelling
- Contour of abdomen
- Movements: Visible peristalsis, any pulsatile movement or respiratory movement
- Look for liver biopsy mark, ascitic tap mark, bone marrow biopsy mark
- Hernial sites like inguinal, femoral, umbilical
- Hair (secondary sexual hair—loss of pubic hair, virilization).

Palpation

Superficial

- Temperature
- Tenderness or hyperesthesia
- Consistency of feel (normal elastic feel, muscle guard or rigidity)
- Localized lump
- Fluid thrill with girth of the abdomen at the level of the umbilicus
- *Direction of blood flow in prominent veins:*
  1. Empty the vein of blood by placing two fingers side by side over the vein. Move one finger away while keeping the other fixed.
  2. Now, release the finger one by one to see the direction through which the blood fills

the vein. If direction of flow of blood is towards the umbilicus, it suggests inferior vena cava obstruction while the direction of blood flow away from the umbilicus suggests portal hypertension.

- Diverication of recti (if any) by rising test
- Pulsation (transmitted or expansile)
- Measure the girth of the abdomen with the help of a tape.

Deep

- Liver
- Spleen
- Gallbladder
- Kidneys
- Palpation of the testis (both sides)
- Any other lump in the abdomen
- Deep tender spots—McBurney's point, gall-bladder point, epigastric point, renal angle
- Rebound tenderness (pain elicited when pressure applied to the abdomen wall by the palpating hand is suddenly released. It is a sign that the underlying peritoneum is inflamed)
- Examination of hernia and external genitalia.

Percussion

- During abdomen percussion, always proceed from a tympanitic or resonant site towards a dull site. The middle finger should be positioned, so that it receives the strike parallel to the anticipated border and not perpendicular to it.
- To delineate the liver borders, start percussing along the midclavicular line at the 4th intercostal space. The percussion note will change from resonant to dull at the 5th intercostal space where the upper border of the liver normally lies. This dullness will continue till the lower border of liver which is just below the costal margin in a normal subject.

Puddle Sign

If the fluid in the peritoneal cavity is minimal, make patient prone so that he bears weight over his knees and elbows and the abdomen is off the couch. When the patient assumes this posture, the fluid gravitates down around the center and percussion over the umbilicus will give a dull note.

Fluid Thrill

Fluid thrill is demonstrable only if a large volume of ascitic fluid is present.

1. Lay the subject supine and place one hand flat against his flank on one side.
2. Ask an assistant to place the ulnar aspect of his hand firmly in the midline of the abdomen.
3. Now, tap the opposite flank of the abdomen with your other hand. If ascitic fluid is present, the impulse generated by the tap will be transmitted to your hand on the flank. The hand on the abdomen is to prevent transmission of the impulse through the subcutaneous fat of the abdominal wall.

Shifting Dullness

1. Expose the abdomen and ask the child to lie supine. Keep the plexor finger perpendicular to the midline at a point between the xiphisternum and umbilicus. Percussing here, normally elicits a resonant note.
2. Percuss downwards from this point towards the umbilicus up to suprapubic region. The note should remain resonant. A dullness suggests an underlying full urinary bladder. Ask the child to void so that the bladder becomes empty.
3. After the percussion note at the umbilicus is resonant, keep the plexor finger at the umbilicus in the direction of the mid-line.
4. Start percussing from the umbilicus and go laterally towards the right or the left flank.
5. If the note remains resonant throughout up to the flanks, this indicates absence of significant fluid in the peritoneal cavity. A dull note in the dependent flanks suggests presence of fluid because of gravitation.

6. If the flanks are dull, turn the patient towards the opposite side without removing your plexor finger. Wait for some time to let the fluid shift to the other flank because of gravitv. Percuss again over the same area. A resonant note now confirms that the fluid has shifted to the dependent area.

Auscultation

- Peristalsis
- Hepatic/splenic rub
- Venous hum
- Bruit.

RESPIRATORY SYSTEM

- Respiration is thoraco-abdominal in type
- Chest wall edema
- Bilateral hydrothorax
- Crepitations at lung bases.

CARDIOVASCULAR SYSTEM

- Pericardial rub (in renal failure)
- Pericardial effusion.

NERVOUS SYSTEM

- Patient may be lethargic or drowsy due to renal failure.

RETICULOENDOTHELIAL SYSTEM

- Lymphadenopathy.

DIAGNOSIS

Generalized edema with oliguria most probably of renal etiology, with/without hypertension or hematuria, with/without peritonitis; steroid responsive or unresponsive variety—most probably minimal change nephrotic syndrome.

DIFFERENTIAL DIAGNOSIS

NEPHROTIC SYNDROME

- Edema starts in face, arms and then descends. Swelling of scrotal sacs and lower eyelids are classical
- Edema is usually noticed in morning; pitting edema
- History of previous renal disease may or may not be elicited
- Presence of proteinuria, hypoproteinemia and hypercholesterolemia.

ACUTE NEPHRITIC SYNDROME

- Oliguria, hematuria, hypertension
- RBC and RBC casts in urine
- Proteinuria
- Tendency of early renal failure.

CONGESTIVE CARDIAC FAILURE

- Patient is dyspnoeic
- Tender hepatomegaly with engorged neck veins
- Cardiomegaly
- Edema starts in dependent parts and then ascends progressively, pitting edema.

CIRRHOSIS OF LIVER

- History of hematemesis and malena
- Ascites appears first, pedal edema appears next
- Splenomegaly with venous prominence
- Signs of hepatocellular failure.

ANEMIA WITH HYPOPROTEINEMIA

- Pallor
- Signs of malnutrition

- Edema appears first in ankle
- Systolic murmur over pulmonary area

MYXEDEMA

- Absence of urinary problem
- Horseness, constipation, cold sensitivity
- Bradycardia, hypertension
- Non pitting edema
- Delayed relaxation of ankle jerk

EPIDEMIC DROPSY

- Caused by contamination of cooking oil (especially mustard oil, rape seed oil) by toxic argemone oil.
- Characterized by nausea and diarrhea, followed by pitting edema of the extremities, extensive dilatation of vessels of the skin, subcutaneous tissues (including fat).
- Accompanied by right heart failure and painless hepatomegaly.
- *Detection of argemone oil in edible oil:* Take 2ml of oil in a test tube, add 2ml of concentrated HNO_3, heat and observe the colour. A red layer at the lower level in the test tube shows the presence of argemone oil.

INVESTIGATIONS

- Urine—Proteinuria (by dipstick or boiling method) [always ask for urine sample in test tube from patient for urine albumin analysis and show it to examiner after doing dipstick or heat coagulation test]
- Urine (24 hours)—Albumin > 1 gm/m^2 (nephrotic syndrome)
- Urine (24 hours)—Urine Protein/Urine Creatinine ratio: Best performed on first morning voided urine sample. Ratios < 0.5 in children younger than 2 years of age and < 0.2 in children more than 2 years of age suggest normal protein excretion. A ratio > 3 suggests nephrotic range proteinuria.
- Serum cholesterol and LDL—Elevated
- Serum albumin— < 3 gm/dl (Normal level is 3.5-5.5 gm/dL)
- Serum globulin—Normal, although α_2 and β globulin are elevated
- Urine culture (Urinary tract infection)
- Kidney function test—Normal but may be deranged in renal failure
- Serum electrolytes/blood gases/hemogram with ESR
- Mantoux test—To rule out tuberculosis before starting steroids as steroids can flare up Tuberculosis
- Chest X-ray —To look for pleural effusion or pulmonary tuberculosis
- USG abdomen—For kidney size or any organic pathology
- C3 levels— Serum C3 levels is determined in all patients of suspected acute glomerulonephritis because a low level narrows a differential diagnosis to certain forms of glomerulonephritis like post-streptococcal, lupus, membranoproliferative glomerulonephritis and chronic infection.
- Antinuclear antibodies/dsDNA/VDRL/HBsAg/peripheral smear—SLE/syphilis/hepatitis B/malaria
- Kidney biopsy.

TREATMENT

Specific Therapy

Steroids

Oral prednisolone is started in a dosage of 2 mg/kg/day (60 mg/m^2/day).

The total daily dose is usually split into two or three doses and given daily for 6 weeks.

For maintenance therapy prednisolone is given at ~1.5 mg/kg/day (40 mg/m^2/day) given on alternate days, as a single morning dose, for a 6-week period after which it is discontinued.

An antacid preparation may be given with prednisolone to reduce gastric irritation.

The earlier regimen (4 weeks daily and 4 weeks alternate days) employed by International Study Group for Kidney Disease in Children (ISKDC) is probably insufficient.

Treatment of Relapse

A relapse is treated with daily prednisolone until proteinuria resolves (it generally takes 14 days) and thereafter with the alternate day regimen for 4-6 weeks.

Frequent Relapser/Steroid Dependant

Start with 2 mg/kg/day till remission, followed by 1.5 mg/kg alternate day for 4 weeks.

- Prednisolone is tapered and maintained at 0.5-0.7 mg/kg/day on alternate days.
- Taper by 0.15-0.25 mg/kg/week till steroid threshold is achieved.
- Look for the steroid threshold lowest steroid dose to keep child in remission.
- Continue with low dose alternate day steroid for 9-18 months if child in remission and no steroid toxicity.
- Consider adding a second drug if
    - ♦ The child having features of toxicity
    - ♦ The child requires higher doses to stay in remission (> 0.5 mg/kg alternate day).

Immunomodulators

- Levamisole
- Cyclophosphamide
- Calcineurin inhibitors
    - ♦ Cyclosporin
    - ♦ Tacrolimus.
- Mycophenolate mofetil

Choice of Agent

- Benefits to be weighed against toxicity.
- Levamisole is preferred initial drug for patients with frequent relapses and steroid dependence.
- Cyclophosphamide is commonly used drug, preferred in severe steroid toxicity, severe relapses with thrombotic episodes and poor compliance, where long-term follow-up is unreliable.
- If both levamisole and cyclophosphamide fail to show response, cyclosporin or tacrolimus may be added.

Levamisole

- Dose: 2-2.5 mg/kg on alternate days.
- Duration: 12-24 months.
- Overlap with prednisolone: 1.5 mg/kg alternate day, followed by tapering of steroid, maintain at 0.25-0.5 mg/kg for 6 months or more.
- Side effects: Leucopenia, Rash, flue like symptoms, and rarely liver damage and seizures.

Cyclophosphamide

- Dose: 2-2.5 mg/kg/day orally for 12 weeks.
- Prednisolone overlap:
    - ❐ 1.5 mg/kg on alternate days for 4 weeks, followed by 1 mg/kg for the next 8 weeks; then tapered and stopped over next 2-3 months.
- Toxicity: Hemorrhagic cystitis, leucopenia, alopecia, gonadotoxicity.

Cyclosporine

- Dose: 4-5 mg/kg daily for 12-24 months.
- Prednisolone overlap: 1.5 mg/kg on alternate days for 2-4 weeks; taper and a maintenance dose of 0.25-0.5 mg/kg for six or more months.
- Side effects: Nephrotoxicity, hypertension, hyperlipidemia, hirsuitism, gum hypertrophy.

Failure of Treatment

If a patient has

- Two or more relapses over 6 months while on treatment with any of the above agents, its replacement with an alternative medication should be considered.

Steroid Resistant Nephrotic Syndrome

- Persistence of proteinuria despite of 4 weeks daily steroid.
- Causes
  - Focal segmental glomerulosclerosis 30-40%
  - Minimal change disease 30-35%
  - Membrano-proliferative GN 20%
  - Membranous GN
  - IgA nephropathy.
- Before labeling steroid resistance, rule out underlying infections like chronic UTI, respiratory tract infections
- Always perform kidney biopsy in all cases of steroid resistant nephrotic syndrome for:
  - Confirming the etiology
  - Document baseline renal damage
  - Monitor progression.
- Drugs used: Cyclosporine, tacrolimus, cyclophosphamide, IV methyl-prednisolone.

Recent Advances

- A low IgG/IgM ratio can be used as prognostic factor for poor outcome and more frequent and severe relapses
- Prolonged alternate day steroid for 6-7 months during 1st episode can significantly reduce the remission rates by 33% without significant increase in side-effects.

General Management

- *Diet:*
  - Diet with no added salt
  - Diet should provide adequate energy and protein
  - In case of severe edema, restrict fluids
  - High biological value protein (egg white most recommended protein but yellow part should be avoided due to high cholesterol levels)
  - Low saturated fatty acid and high PUFA may be useful
- Supplement calcium 250-500 mg and vitamin D if child is on steroids for more than 3 months
- Observation for infection
- *Home monitoring* of urine protein/albumin:
  - All parents should be trained to monitor random urine protein at home
  - Urine should be tested once each morning and the results recorded in the log book. This is particularly helpful during maintenance therapy and beyond since it helps to detect recurrences of the disease before edema occurs, thus allowing earlier initiation of treatment.
  - Ambulatory monitoring of the child's condition and response to management. Parents should keep an ongoing log (diary) of their child's treatment and progress.
- *Diuretics:*

  Indications
  - Scrotal edema
  - Recurrent skin infections especially peritonitis
  - Respiratory distress due to edema.
- Dose:
  - Furosemide: 1-2 mg/kg/day
  - Spironolactone: 2-3 mg/kg/day.

Human Albumin

Infusion when serum albumin falls < 1.5 gm% (other drugs are less useful when albumin level falls < 1.5 gm %).

Dose: 0.5-1 gm/kg over a period of 30 to 60 minutes followed by furosemide (after 1 hour) at 1-2 mg/kg intravenously.

Indications for Hospital Admission

- Massive edema with compromise of respiratory excursion due to ascites and/or pleural effusion
- Significant hypertension
- Anuria or severe oliguria or azotemia
- Peritonitis
- Significant respiratory infection.

DISCUSSION

DEFINITIONS

Nephrotic syndrome: Clinical state characterized by proteinuria, hypoalbuminemia, edema and Hypercholesterolemia.

Remission: Urine albumin nil or trace (or proteinuria < 4 mg/m^2/hour) for 3 consecutive days.

Relapse: Urine albumin 3+ or 4+ (or proteinuria > 40 mg/m^2/hour) for 3 consecutive days, having been in remission previously.

Frequent relapses: Two or more relapses in six months of initial response, or more than three relapses in any twelve months.

Steroid dependence: Two consecutive relapses when on alternate day steroids or within 14 days of its discontinuation.

Steroid resistance: Absence of remission despite therapy with 4 weeks of daily prednisolone in a dose of 2 mg/kg per day.

Late responder: Patient with initial resistance, who responds at some time after initial treatment.

Late resistance: Initial responder, who subsequently fails to respond to steroid therapy.

Congenital nephrotic syndrome: Nephrotic syndrome presenting within first 3 months of life.

Infantile nephrotic syndrome: Nephrotic syndrome presenting between 3 and 12 months of life.

Idiopathic nephrotic syndrome: Nephrotic syndrome of unknown origin

Secondary nephrotic syndrome: Nephrotic syndrome, accompanying or following a known disease.

PROTEINURIA

In nephrotic syndrome
Proteinuria is > 40 mg/m^2/hour or
>1 gm/m^2/day or
>3+ or 4 + by dipstick or sulfosalicylic acid method.

A reasonable upper limit of normal protein excretion in healthy children is 150 mg/24 hour. More specifically.

- Normal protein excretion in children is defined as ≤ 4 mg/m^2/hour
- Abnormal protein excretion is 4-40 mg/m^2/hour
- Nephrotic range proteinuria > 40 mg/m^2/hour.

HYPOALBUMINEMIA

- Serum albumin < 2.5 gm%
- Edema appears when serum albumin < 2 gm%
- With serum albumin < 1.5 gm%: Pleural and pericardial effusion appear.

HYPERCHOLESTEROLEMIA

Serum cholesterol > 250 mg% (Inverse relationship between serum albumin and serum cholesterol levels).

Lipid Profile

- VLDL and LDL increase
- HDL—normal or increased in minimal change nephrotic syndrome
- No treatment has been found to be specific and/ or successful.

METHODS FOR DETECTING PROTEINURIA

❖ *Heat coagulation method:*

Grade	
0 (Negative)	Urine clear
1+ (Trace)	Hazzy (lemon water)
2+	Cloudy (limca)
3+	Thick white (milk)
4+	White precipitate at the bottom (curd)

❖ *Dipstick test:*

Negative	0 mg/dl
Trace	0-29 mg/dl
1+	30-99 mg/dl
2+	100-299 mg/dl
3+	300-999 mg/dl
4+	>1 gm/dl

Dipsticks detect albuminuria and are less sensitive for other forms of proteinuria (low molecular proteins, Bence Jones proteins, gamma globulins). False positive test can be seen in gross hematuria, highly concentrated urine, and contamination with antiseptic agents like chlorhexidine.

Dipstick should be considered positive for protein if it is >1+ in a urine sample in which specific gravity is ≤ 1.015. If specific gravity is >1.015, the dipstick must be ≥ 2+ to be considered positive.

❖ *Sulfosalicylic acid test :* Add sulfosalicylic acid to urine (equal amounts)

Grade	
0 (Negative)	Urine clear
1+ (Trace)	Hazzy (Lemon water)
2+	Cloudy (Limca)
3+	Thick white (Milk)
4+	With precipitate at the bottom (Curd)

NEPHROTIC CHARTING

In a admitted patient for nephrotic syndrome, following should be looked for:

- Daily input/output charting
- Blood pressure monitoring
- Abdominal girth and weight
- Heat coagulation test
- Edema, facial puffiness.

CLASSIFICATION OF NEPHROTIC SYNDROME

Idiopathic nephrotic syndrome can be clearly separated into a 'minimal change steroid responsive type' and other with significant glomerular histologic lesions (focal segmental glomerulosclerosis, membranoproliferative GN, mesangial proliferative GN), mostly non-responsive to prednisolone.

In 3-5% cases nephrotic syndrome may be 'secondary' caused by systemic disorder (e.g. SLE, Henoch Schonlein purpura, Hepatitis B).

INDICATIONS FOR KIDNEY BIOPSY IN NEPHROTIC SYNDROME

At Onset

- Age < 1 year or > 8 years
- Persistent microscopic or gross hematuria, low serum C3
- Sustained hypertension (> 3 weeks)
- Renal failure not attributable to hypovolemia
- Suspected secondary causes of nephrotic syndrome.

After Initial Treatment

- Proteinuria persisting despite 4 weeks of daily corticosteroid therapy
- Before starting treatment with cyclosporine A
- Frequently relapsing or steroid dependant nephrotic syndrome (discretion of the pediatric nephrologist).

RECOMMENDATIONS FOR MANAGEMENT OF EDEMA IN NEPHROTIC SYNDROME

Furosemide 1-3 mg/kg/day
May add spironolactone 2-4 mg/kg/day

No response (no weight loss or diuresis 48 hours)

Hospital admission

↓

Double dose of furosemide until diuresis or maximum daily dose of furosemide (4-5 mg/kg/day) is reached

↓

No response

↓

Add metolazone 0.1-0.3 mg/kg/day

↓

No response

↓

Furosemide IV bolus 1-3 mg/kg/ per dose. or infusion 0.1-1 mg/kg per hour

↓

No response

↓

Albumin 20% 1 g/kg IV
Followed by IV furosemide

MANAGEMENT OF STEROID SENSITIVE NEPHROTIC SYNDROME

First episode of nephrotic syndrome
Absence of hypertension, hematuria, azotemia

↓

Prednisolone 2 mg/kg daily for 6 weeks,
1.5 mg/kg on alternate days for 6 weeks

- **Infrequent relapses** → Prednisolone 2 mg/kg daily until remission, then 1.5 mg/kg on alternate days for 4 weeks
- **Frequent relapses / Steroid dependence** → Refer for evaluation. Alternate day prednisolone to maintain remission. Assess steroid threshold
  - Threshold <0.5 mg/kg on alternate days → Alternate day Prednisolone for 9-18 months
  - Threshold >0.5 mg/kg on alternate days orsteroid toxicity → Levamisole, Cyclophosphamide, Cyclosporin A
- **Steroid resistance** → Refer for evaluation. Define therapy based on renal biopsy findings

VACCINATION IN NEPHROTIC SYNDROME

Live vaccines (measles, mumps, rubella, oral polio, Varicella): Should be avoided until steroid therapy has been discontinued for at least 4 to 12 weeks.

Other vaccines (pneumococcal, hepatitis B, Hemophilus Influenzae type B): May be given but vaccine response is often reduced.

These children are susceptible to infections, with encapsulated organisms, so immunize against Streptococcus pneumoniae, Haemophilus influenzae, Varicella and hepatitis B.

Pneumococcal vaccination is recommended in all children, especially those with a previous episode of peritonitis. 23 valent pneumococcal vaccine should be given.

Varicella vaccination: Patients in remission and not on corticosteroid therapy should receive varicella vaccine in a two – dose schedule, administered four weeks apart.

IMPORTANCE OF MANTOUX IN NEPHROTIC SYNDROME

Mantoux positive but show no evidence of disease: Prophylaxis with INH and rifampicin for six months.

Having active tuberculosis: Standard antitubercular therapy for two weeks before starting corticosteroid treatment for nephrotic syndrome.

COMPLICATIONS IN NEPHROTIC SYNDROME

- Infection: Spontaneous bacterial peritonitis is most frequent type of infection although Bacterial sepsis, cellulitis, pneumonia and UTI may also be seen.
- Flare up of tuberculosis
- Venous and arterial thromboembolism
- Acute renal failure: Severe hypovolemia leads to acute renal failure especially when complicated by gastroenteritis and other infections.
- Hypertension
- Tetany (due to hypocalcemia)
- Risk of collagen-vascular disease
- Hormonal and mineral alteration
- Abnormal growth
- Cataract, steroid facies.

CAUSES OF INCREASED SUSCEPTIBILITY OF INFECTIONS

- Commonest pathogen: *Streptococcus pneumoniae*
- Large fluid collections are prone to get infected
- Severe edema causes extreme stretching of skin, which may break spontaneously or after minor trauma and allow bacterial entry.
- Loss of Factor B in urine: Factor B is important for integrity of alternative pathway of complement activation, which is crucial in phagocytosis of encapsulated bacteria, such as *S.pneumoniae*.

STRESS DOSES OF STEROIDS

- Patients who have received prednisolone (>1mg/kg daily) for more than 2 weeks in the preceding 3 to 6 months have suppression of hypothalamopituitary axis.
- Such patients with serious infections, who require intravenous antibiotics or hospitalization should receive stress doses of steroids.

- Hydrocortisone is the preferred drug due to its short action and mineralocorticoid effects.
- Patient who can tolerate orally can be given prednisolone.

ADVICE TO PARENTS DURING DISCHARGE

- If respiratory tract infection/diarrhea occurs – patient can relapse, hence check urine protein
- Urine proteins should be checked weekly for 1st 3 months; then monthly for next 3 months; then 3 monthly for 6 months; then 6 monthly for 1 year; then yearly (unless patient relapses).
- Do not keep uristicks in bathroom (they adsorb water) and close the lid tightly after using it
- Side effects of steroid therapy should be explained.
- Ensure normal activity and school attendence
- Maintain a dairy showing proteinuria, medications received and intercurrent infections.
- Need for appropriate immunization and measures for protection against infections.

PROGNOSIS

Steroid Sensitive Nephrotic Syndrome

- The ultimate outcome in steroid sensitive nephrotic syndrome is excellent with majority of children cured by age of 10-15 years.
- In a given patient it is not possible to predict the course and age at which cure will take place.

Steroid Resistant Nephrotic Syndrome

These children are more prone to develop complications and end stage renal disease.

DIAGNOSIS OF CRF IN NEPHROTIC SYNDROME

- Beginning of polyuria
- Diminution of anasarca
- Appearance of hypertension
- Specific gravity of urine becomes low and fixed (1.010)
- Increase of blood urea and creatinine levels.

MARKERS OF ACUTE GLOMERULONEPHRITIS AND RPGN

- Serum C3 level
- Anti- GBM antibody
- ANCA serology.

CONGENITAL NEPHROTIC SYNDROME

- Defined as presence of nephrotic syndrome at time of birth or infants less than 3 months old.
- Autosomal recessive mode of inheritance.
- Gene defect localized to the long arm of chromosome 19.
- Histology: Marked cystic dilatation of the tubules (mostly proximal and cortical), with associated interstitial changes and immature glomeruli.
- Disease initiated *in utero*, because concentrations of alpha-fetoprotein in amniotic fluid are elevated by the 20th week of gestation.
- Hematuria and hypertension occur in 30 to 50% of these patients. Azotemia is unusual.

HOW COMMON IS RELAPSE

- 60-70% of newly diagnosed nephrotic syndrome have at least one relapse.
- Cochrane Database of systematic review 2008 mentions 80-90% relapse rates in steroid sensitive nephrotic syndrome.

- Relapse rate depends upon the dose and duration of steroid in initial therapy.

DIAGNOSIS OF URINARY TRACT INFECTION (TABLE 14.1)

Table 14.1: Diagnosis of urinary tract infection

Method of collection	*Colony count (per ml)*	*Probability of infection*
Suprapubic aspiration	Any number	99%
Urethral catheterization	$>10^5$	95%
	10^4-10^5	Very likely
	10^3-10^4	Suspicious; repeat
	$<10^3$	Unlikely
Mid-stream void		
Boy	$>10^4$	Very likely
Girl	$>10^5$	90-95%
	10^4-10^5	Suspicious; repeat
	$<10^4$	Unlikely

KEY POINTS: DIAGNOSIS OF UTI

- In infants and small children unexplained fever, diarrhea, vomiting, foul smelling urine suggest UTI; older children have dysuria, hypogastric flank pain.
- Fever, toxicity, leukocytosis indicate renal parenchymal involvement.
- Microscopic examination of fresh, mid-stream urine indicates UTI if bacteria and neutrophils are present.
- Report of a few "pus cells" in an asymptomatic child is insufficient to start antibiotics.
- UTI is confirmed on urine culture showing $>10^5$ organisms per ml; lesser numbers should be interpreted in relation to clinical features.

CHAPTER 15

CARDIOVASCULAR SYSTEM

CONGENITAL HEART DISEASE

HISTORY

CHIEF COMPLAINTS

- Cough/difficulty in respiration/fever
- Inability to gain weight
- Cyanosis
- Focal deficit
- Chest pain in adolescents.

HISTORY OF PRESENT ILLNESS

History of Disease

- Respiratory distress:
  - Rapid breathing
  - Nasal flaring
  - Chest retraction.
- Exercise intolerance:
  - Difficulty in keeping with peers in sports activities
  - Nap after coming from school.
- Cyanosis/cyanotic spells:
  - Blueness around lips, tongue, mucous membrane
  - When first noticed and time of day when it occurs
  - Length of episodes
  - Aggravating factors (crying/exercise)
  - Releiving factors.
- Squatting episodes
- History of drug intake (digitalis/furosemide)
- Syncope, faintness (aortic stenosis, pulmonary stenosis, primary pulmonary hypertension, coarctation of aorta)
- Increased precordial activity
- Dysphagia, leg fatigue and pain, claudication (coarctation of aorta).

History of Complications

- Congestive cardiac failure:
  - Breathlessness, cyanosis, excessive perspiration over forehead on feeding
  - Suck-rest-suck cycle

- Breathlessness gets releived on putting child to shoulders
- Decreased intake during feeds
- Swelling over body
- Repeated respiratory tract infections
- Inability to gain weight.

- Feeding difficulties
  - Frequency
  - Volume of each feed
  - Time spent on each breast
  - Gets diaphoretic or not
  - Will awaken for next feed after brief time.
- Infective endocarditis:
  - High fever with chills
  - Bleeding manifestations (petechial hemorrhages/hematuria/hemoptysis)
  - Convulsions/unconsciousness/altered sensorium
  - Tender pads of fingers (Osler's nodes)
  - Dental procedures/surgery.
- Cerebral abscess (in children > 2 years with cyanotic heart disease):
  - Fever/vomiting
  - Focal seizures
  - Hemiparesis/Focal neurological deficits.
- Cerebral infarct (in children < 2 years with cyanotic heart disease):
  - Vomiting
  - Focal seizures
  - Hemiparesis/focal neurological deficits.
- Impact on child:
  - Growth and development
  - Schooling (academic performance, sports restriction, teachers and peers attitude, school days lost).
- Horseness of voice (Large PDA)
- Pink frothy sputum.

History of Risk Factors

- Maternal risk factors:
  - Fever with rash in mother during pregnancy (Intrauterine infection)
  - Irradiation/alcohol intake
  - Drug intake (Phenytoin, steroids, lithium, carbamazepine, sodium valproate)
  - Diabetes mellitus (increased incidence of TGA and hypertrophic cardiomyopathy)
  - Hypertension in pregnancy
  - Fetal echocardiography done or not (essential in presence of suggestive history)
  - Affected siblings.
- Fetal risk factors:
  - Prematurity (increased incidence of VSD/ PDA)
  - Large baby (Transposition of great arteries)
  - Birth asphyxia and respiratory distress (persistent pulmonary hypertension and myocardial dysfunction)
  - Cyanosis/prolonged jaundice.

PAST HISTORY

- Previous hospitalization
- Previous surgery.

FAMILY HISTORY

- Diabetes in family members (TGA)
- Congenital heart disease in family (endocardial fibroelastosis)
- Parental consanguinity (autosomal recessive conditions, e.g. Friedreich ataxia).

GENERAL PHYSICAL EXAMINATION

a. Position of child—decubitus
b. Vitals:
   1. Pulse (in all 4 limbs)
      - Rate
      - Rhythm
      - Volume
      - Condition of the arterial wall
      - Comparison between two radial pulses
      - Radio-femoral delay
      - Any special character
      - Other peripheral pulses
   2. Respiration
   3. BP (in all 4 limbs in older child).
   4. Temperature
c. Anthropometry: Assess growth of child
d. Head to toe examination: Pallor/cyanosis/clubbing/hepatojugular reflux/pedal edema
e. Examination of neck veins:
   - Engorged or not
   - If engorged—pressure, pulsation, hepatojugular reflux
f. Signs of infective endocarditis:
   - *Osler's nodes* (pin head size tender papule seen in the pulp of fingers)
   - Petechiae
   - *Janeway's lesions* (nontender maculopapular lesion in palm)
   - *Roth spots* (seen on ophthalmoscopy)
   - *Splinter hemorrhages* (linear longitudinal. hemorrhage under the nail)
g. Signs to assess nutritional status:
   - Look for signs of malnutrition
   - Eye changes (vitamin A deficiency)
   - Bossing of skull/beading of ribs (vitamin D deficiency)
h. Dysmorphic facies:
   - Microcephaly
   - Cataract (rubella)
i. Other congenital anomalies
   - Vertebral, anal, renal, coloboma, atresia chonae, mental retardation, genital and ear anomalies
j. Scars of previous surgeries or other procedures.

SYSTEMIC EXAMINATION

CARDIOVASCULAR SYSTEM

Inspection

- Precordium
  - Deformity or bulging seen
  - Apical impulse; diffuse pulsation of precordium
  - Engorged superficial veins.
- Any pulsation present in aortic, pulmonary, parasternal areas, epigastrium, suprasternal area, carotid pulsation, inferior angle of scapula (*Suzman's sign* in coarctation of aorta).
- Inspection of the BACK
  - Scoliosis
  - Gibbus
  - Drooping of the shoulder
  - Winging of scapula.
- Skin for any sinus, ulcer, venous prominence, scar mark.

Palpation

- Aortic area:
  - Pulsation
  - Palpable heart sound (A_2)
  - Thrill.
- Pulmonary area:
  - Pulsation
  - Palpable hear sound (P_2)
  - Thrill.

- Mitral area
  - Apex beat for site and character
  - Palpable heart sound
  - Thrill.
- Tricuspid area
  - Left parasternal heave (its presence signifies right ventricular hypertrophy)
  - Palpable heart sound
  - Thrill.
- Direction of venous blood flow (in engorged superficial veins)
- Thrill in carotid arteries (carotid shudder)
- Pulsations:
  - Epigastric
  - Suprasternal pulsation (signifies aortic stenosis, PDA and rarely pulmonary stenosis)
  - Pulsation over the back
- Liver: Pulsatile due to gross tricuspid regurgitation
- Palpable pericardial rub
- Trachea position
- Pedal edema: Rarely seen, sacral and shin oedema should be looked for.

Percussion

Outer borders of heart

- Sequence of auscultation
  - Upper right sternal border (Aortic area)
  - Upper left sternal border (Pulmonary area)
  - Lower left sternal border
  - Apex
  - Apex—left lateral decubitus position
  - Lower left sternal border—sitting, leaning forward, held expiration

Auscultation

Aortic Area (2nd right intercostal space)

- Compare S_1 to S_2: S_1 should be softer. If the same, think Mitral Stenosis
- identify ejection murmur
- identify ejection click if present.

Pulmonary Area (2nd left intercostal space)

- listen for split S_2 (A_2/P_2)
- identify the intensities of A_2 and P_2
- time split S_2 with respiration
- normally widens with inspiration, closes with expiration
- wide split S_2-RBBB, RV volume overload, PS, RV failure
- wide fixed split = ASD
- paradoxical split = LBBB, severe AS, severe LV dysfunction, pacemaker.

Tricuspid Area (lower left sternal border)

- Listen for intensity of S_1
  - Soft: LV dysfunction, first degree heart block, severe AR/MR
  - Loud: Mitral stenosis.
- Identify quality, timing and intensity of systolic murmurs.
  - Ejection quality versus regurgitant quality
  - Pansystolic versus early or mid to late systolic murmur.

Apex

- Listen for S_3 and S_4
- Identify diastolic rumble
- Determine radiation of murmur, e.g. mitral regurgitation murmur to axilla
- Additional sounds like pericardial rub.

RESPIRATORY SYSTEM

- Crepitations/rhonchi

ABDOMEN

- Hepatomegaly/splenomegaly/Ascites

CNS

- Look for focal deficits.

DIAGNOSIS

Congenital, cyanotic/acyanotic heart disease with $L \rightarrow R$ or $R \rightarrow L$ shunt; with/without sinus rhythm; with/without CCF; with/without pulmonary hypertension; with/without Infective endocarditis; with/without failure to thrive; most probable diagnosis being.

DIFFERENTIAL DIAGNOSIS

VENTRICULAR SEPTAL DEFECT

- Age of presentation: 6-10 weeks
- History of dyspnea, feeding difficulty, poor growth, profuse perspiration, recurrent pulmonary infection
- CVS—hyperkinetic precordium, palpable parasternal lift, systolic thrill
- S_1S_2 masked by murmur at left lower sternal border, At 2nd left intercostal space S_2 widely split with accentuated P_2
- Pansystolic murmur best heard at left lower sternal border.

PATENT DUCTUS ARTERIOSUS

- Age of presentation: 6-10 weeks
- Retardation of growth with large shunt; older children—effort intolerance, palpitation, frequent chest infections.
- Wide pulse pressure
- CVS—apex prominent and heaving, thrill maximum at 2nd left intercostal space
- S_1 accentuated, S_2 difficult to appreciate due to murmur at 2nd intercostal space. S_2 in small shunt is normally split while in large shunt it is narrowly split.
- Continous murmur—onset after S_1, peaks at S_2 and disappears in late diastole. Best heard at 2nd left intercostal space and also below clavicle.

ASD (Ostium Primum and Endocardial Cushion Defect)

- Asymmetric or exercise intolerance, easy fatigability and recurrent pulmonary infections especially in large left to right shunt and mitral regurgitation.
- Hyperdynamic precordium
- Wide split S_2 and ejection systolic murmur are characteristic
- Holosystolic murmur—apical harsh radiating to left axilla.

ASD (Ostium Secundum)

- Generally asymptomatic. If symptomatic it leads to failure to thrive in young while in older children presents as exercise intolerance
- Mild left precordial bulge, palpable parasternal lift
- Wide split S_2 and ejection systolic murmur are characteristic
- Mild diastolic murmur (Increased flow across tricuspid valve) at left lower sternal border (Qp: Qs 2:1).

TETRALOGY OF FALLOT

- Cyanosis not present at birth, occurs later in 1st year. Most prominent in mucus membrane of lips, mouth, finger nails and toenail. With long standing cyanosis—dusky blue skin surface, gray sclera, engorged blood vessels and marked clubbing.
- Dyspnea on exertion. Infant plays for short time then sit or lie down. Older children walk a block or so before stopping to rest.

- Child assumes squatting position for relieving dyspnea and is usually able to resume activity in few minutes.
- *Cyanotic spell:* Onset is spontaneous and unpredictable, most frequent in morning on awakening/excessive crying. Child becomes hyperapneic, restless, cyanosis increases followed by gasping respiration. It could be short episode of generalized weakness and sleep or severe episode of unconsciousness, convulsion, hemiparesis.

INVESTIGATIONS

To Prove Heart Disease

- Chest X-ray: Look for:
  - Heart size—cardiothoracic ratio up to 55% is normal.
  - Pulmonary vascular markings—increased or decreased.
  - Any evidence of respiratory infection (infiltrates/consolidation).
  - Presence of thymus shadow.
- ECG: Look for:
  - Sinus rhythm
  - Heart rate
  - Axis
  - Chamber hypertrophy.
- Echocardiography
  - Pressure in chamber of heart
  - Position and size of defects
  - Vegetations (infective endocarditis).
- Color Doppler: Estimation of pressure in heart chambers
- Cardiac catheterization.

To Rule Out Complications

- Hemogram with ESR—infective endocarditis and respiratory tract infections.
- Blood culture—for infective endocarditis.
- CT Scan—if Abscess/Infarct in CNS.

To Look For Risk Factors

- TORCH titers (Intrauterine infection).

Investigations to Monitor Cyanotic Child

- Arterial blood gases
- Complete blood count
- Clotting studies—PT, PTTK, fibrogen levels
- Blood glucose and serum calcium levels
- Serum iron level
- Uric acid level in older cyanotic children since they are prone for hyperuricemia.

TREATMENT

Medical Management

- Treatment of chest infections
- Prevention and treatment of anemia
- Prevention and treatment of infective endocarditis
- Control of congestive cardiac failure—salt and fluid restricted diet, diuretics, digitalis, ACE inhibitors.
- Management of cyanotic spells—knee chest position, humidified oxygen, morphine, correction of acidosis, propranolol, vasopressors like methoxamine.

Surgical Management

- Depending upon the cause.

GUIDELINES OF WORKING GROUP ON MANAGEMENT OF CONGENITAL HEART DISEASES IN INDIA

Atrial Septal Defect (ASD)

Spontaneous closure: Rare if defect >8 mm at birth. Rare after age 2 years.

Patent foramen ovale: Echocardiographic detection of a asymptomatic patent foramen ovale is a normal finding in newborns.

Indication for closure: ASD associated with right ventricular volume overload.

Ideal age of closure:

i. In asymptomatic child: 2-4 years
ii. Symptomatic ASD in infancy (congestive heart failure, severe pulmonary artery hypertension): Early closure is recommended.
iii. If presenting beyond ideal age: Elective closure irrespective of age.

Ventricular Septal Defect (VSD)

Timing of Closure

- Large VSD with uncontrolled congestive heart failure: As soon as possible.
- Large VSD with severe pulmonary artery hypertension: 3-6 months.
- Small sized VSD with normal pulmonary artery pressure, left to right shunt >1.5:1: Closure by 2-4 years.
- Small outlet/perimembranous VSD with any degree of aortic regurgitation: Surgery whenever aortic regurgitation is detected.
- Small VSD with more than one episode of infective endocarditis: Early VSD closure recommended.

Patent Ductus Arteriosus (PDA)

Spontaneous closure: Small PDAs in full term baby may close up to 3 months of age, large PDAs are unlikely to close.

Timing of Closure

- Large/ moderate PDA, with congestive heart failure, pulmonary artery hypertension: Early closure (by 3-6 months).
- Moderate PDA, no congestive heart failure: 6 months to 1 year. If failure to thrive, closure can be accomplished earlier.
- Small PDA: At 12-18 months .
- Silent PDA: Closure not recommended.

Indomethacin/ ibuprofen not to be used in term babies.

PDA in a Preterm Baby

- Intervene if baby in heart failure (small PDAs may close spontaneously).
- Indomethacin or Ibuprofen (if no contraindication).
- Surgical ligation if above drugs fail or are contraindicated.
- Prophylactic indomethacin or ibuprofen therapy: Not recommended.

Obstructive Lesions

Coarctation of Aorta (CoA)

Timing of intervention:

- With left ventricular dysfunction / congestive heart failure or severe upper limb hypertension (for age): Immediate intervention.
- Normal left ventricular function, no congestive heart failure and mild upper limb hypertension: Intervention beyond 3-6 months of age.
- No hypertension, no heart failure, normal ventricular function: Intervention at 1-2 years of age.

Cyanotic Congenital Heart Disease

Tetralogy of Fallot (TOF)

Medical therapy: Maintain Hb >14 g/dL (by using oral iron or blood transfusion). Beta blockers to be given in highest tolerated doses (usual dose 1-4 mg/kg/day in 2 to 3 divided doses).

Timing of surgery: All patients need surgical repair.

- Stable, minimally cyanosed: Total correction at 1-2 years of age or earlier according to the institutional policy.

Transposition of Great Arteries (TGA)

Timing of Surgery

- TGA with Intact interventricular septum
  - If <3-4 weeks of age: Arterial switch operation immediately.
  - If >3-4 weeks of age at presentation: Assess left ventricle by ECHO. If the left ventricle is decompressed:Senning/ Mustard at 3-6 months, or rapid two stage arterial switch. If the left ventricle is still prepared, very early arterial switch operation is indicated.
- TGA with ventricular septal defect: Arterial switch operation, by 3 months of age.

Total Anomalous Pulmonary Venous Connection (TAPVC)

Types of TAPVC

- *Type I:* Anomalous connection at supracardiac level (to innominate vein or right superior vena cava).
- *Type II:* Anomalous connection at cardiac level (to coronary sinus or right atrium).
- *Type III:* Anomalous connection at infradiaphragmatic level (to portal vein or inferior vena cava).
- *Type IV:* Anomalous connection at two or more of the above levels.

Each type can be obstructive (obstruction at one of the anatomic sites in the anomalous pulmonary venous channel) or non-obstructive. Type III is almost always obstructive.

Timing of Surgery

- Obstructive type: Emergency surgery.
- Non obstructive type: As soon as possible (beyond neonatal period if baby is clinically stable) .
- Those presenting after 2 years of age: Elective surgery whenever diagnosed, as long as pulmonary vascular resistance is in operable range.

Guidelines for Infective Endocarditis Prophylaxis

1. Maintain good oral hygiene and a regular dental check up.
2. Unrepaired cyanotic heart diseases are high-risk conditions for infective endocarditis, therefore prophylaxis is mandatory.
3. Atrial septal defect (secundum type) and valvular pulmonic stenosis are low-risk conditions for infective endocarditis and prophylaxis is not recommended.
4. Other acyanotic congenital heart diseases including a bicuspid aortic valve are moderate risk and prophylaxis is recommended.
5. Repaired congenital heart diseases with prosthetic material need prophylaxis for the first six months after the procedure.
6. Device placement by transcatheter route also requires prophylaxis for the first six months.
7. Prophylaxis is recommended for residual defects after a procedure.

DISCUSSION

LOCATION OF APICAL IMPULSE

- Up to 4 years: Left 4th intercostal space lateral to midclavicular line

- 4-8 years: Left 5th intercostal space lateral to midclavicular line
- 8-12 years: Left 5th intercostal space medial to midclavicular line

NADAS DICTATUM

Diagnosis of a patient over 2 years of age with cyanotic heart disease as Fallot's tetrology is 75% correct.

Table 15.1: Nadas criteria (to determine the presence or absence of congenital heart disease)

Major criteria	*Minor criteria*
❖ Systolic murmur >Grade III	❖ Systolic murmur <Grade III
❖ Diastolic murmur	❖ Abnormal 2nd heart sound
❖ CCF	❖ Hypertension (with absent femorals)
❖ Cyanosis	❖ Abnormal chest X-ray
	❖ Abnormal ECG

Presence of one major or two minor criteria is essential for indicating the presence of heart disease.

CLASSIFICATION OF CONGENITAL HEART DISEASES

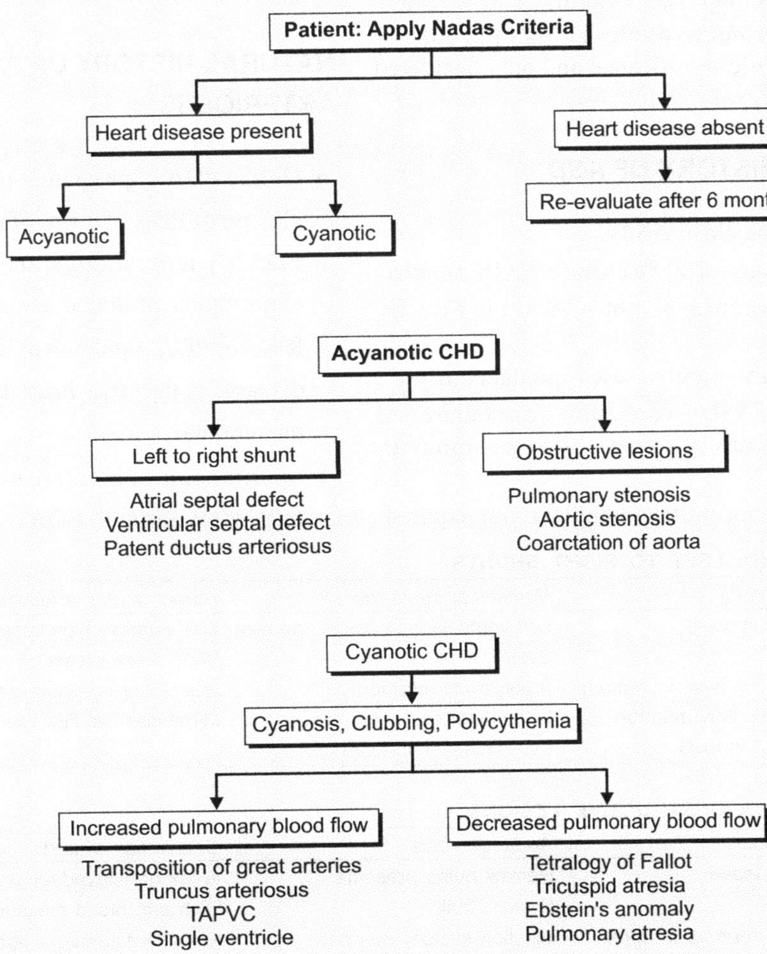

PATHOLOGY OF ASD

- Three types: Secundum, primum and sinus venosus.
- Ostium secundum is most common (50-70%). The defect is present in fossa ovalis, causing shunting from left atrium to right atrium.
- Ostium primum seen in 30% of all ASD's including those as a part of atrioventricular canal defects.
- Sinus venosus seen in 10% cases is commonly seen at entry of superior venae cavae into right ventricle and sometimes at entry of inferior venae cavae into right atrium.
- Patent foramen ovale is usually of no hemodynamic significance and not considered ASD.

NATURAL HISTORY OF ASD

- Spontaneous closure 87%
- ASD < 3 mm—100 % closure by 18 months
- ASD between 3-8 mm—80% closure by 18 months
- ASD >8 mm—rarely closes spontaneously
- In untreated ASD—congestive heart failure and Pulmonary artery hypertension develops in adults.
- Infective endocarditis prophylaxis not required.

NATURAL HISTORY OF VSD

- Spontaneous closure in 30—50% most frequently during 1st 2 years of life.
- Small muscular VSD are more likely to close (up to 80%) than membranous.
- VSDs (up to 35%) majority of defects that close do so before age of 4 years.
- Risks of unoperated VSD—infective endocarditis, arrhythmia, subaortic stenosis and exercise intolerance.

NATURAL HISTORY OF PATENT DUCTUS ARTERIOSUS

- Unlike PDA of premature infants, spontaneous closure of PDA of term infants does not occur. PDA of term infants are due to structural abnormality of ductal smooth muscle.
- Risks of PDA—pulmonary vascular obstructive disease, congestive heart failure or recurrent pneumonia.
- Spontaneous bacterial endocarditis, more frequent with small PDA.

ACYANOTIC CHD: LEFT TO RIGHT SHUNTS

Atrial septal defect	*Ventricular septal defect*	*Patent ductus arteriosus*
Left parasternal impulse	Left ventricle type apical impulse	Left ventricle type impulse
Wide, fixed S_2	Systolic thrill	Wide pulse pressure
Pulmonary ejection systolic murmur	Pansystolic murmur	Systolic or continuous thrill
Tricuspid diastolic flow murmur	Mitral diastolic flow murmur	Mitral diastolic flow murmur
rSR pattern in V1 in ECG	LV dominance in ECG	

ACYANOTIC CHD: OBSTRUCTIVE LESIONS

Pulmonary stenosis	*Aortic stenosis*	*Coarctation of aorta*
Left parasternal leave	Narrow pulse pressure	Weak or delayed femoral compared to radial
Systolic thrill	Systolic thrill	High arm blood pressure
Ejection systolic murmur in upper left sternal border	Ejection systolic murmur radiating to neck	Prominent carotid, palpable aorta in suprasternal notch, palpable collaterals
Wide split second sound, delayed well heard P_2	Delayed A_2	Ejection systolic murmur in interscapular region

HEMODYNAMICS OF SPELL

- Increased activity
- Increased respiration
- Increased venous return
- Fixed pulmonary blood flow
- Increased right ventricle to left ventricle shunt
- Increased cyanosis.

HEMODYNAMICS OF SQUATTING (KNEE CHEST POSITION)

- Decreased venous return
- Increased systemic vascular resistance
- Increased pulmonary blood flow
- Decreased cyanosis

CLASSIFICATION OF VSD

Clinical Classification

- *Mild VSD*:
  - Asymptomatic
  - Loud, harsh, blowing holosystolic murmur frequently accompanied by thrill.
- *Moderate to large VSD*:
  - Failure to gain weight, repeated pulmonary infections, decreased exercise tolerance
  - Mild pulmonary hypertension (S_2 loud, right ventricular heave, pulmonary heave, mild systolic murmur in pulmonary region) may be present.
- *Large shunt with severe pulmonary HT*:
  - Poor growth, recurrent pulmonary infection and congestive heart failure in early infancy
  - Duskiness, Clubbing (in view of Eisenmenger's complex)
  - P_2 may be single and loud in view of pulmonary artery hypertension
  - Right pulmonary heave
  - Pulmonary midsystolic murmur.

Classification Based on Site of Lesion

Ventricular septum is divided into a small membranous portion and a large muscular portion. The muscular portion has 3 components—inlet, trabecular septum and outlet (infundibular) septum. The trabecular septum has 3 components—central, marginal and apical.

- *Perimembranous* (80%): Most common defect.
- *Inlet* (5-8%): Posterior and inferior to perimembranous defect.
- *Muscular* (5%-20%):
  - Central: Mid-muscular.
  - Apical.
  - "Swiss cheese" septum: Large number of muscular defects.
  - Marginal: Along RV septal junction.
- *Outlet* (5-7%): Situated just beneath the pulmonary valve (synonyms:supracristal, conal, infundibular, subpulmonary)

ECHO Based Classification

Defect size is often expressed in terms of the size of the aortic root:

- *Large*: Lesions that approximate the size of the aorta
- *Moderate*: Lesions one-third to two-thirds of the diameter of the aorta
- *Small*: Lesions less than one-third the aortic root diameter
- *Pinhole*: Lesions detected only by color-flow mapping (< 2 mm in diameter).

INDICATIONS FOR SURGICAL CLOSURE OF VSD

- Any age with large VSD in whom clinical symptoms is not controlled medically.
- Infant between 6 and 12 months of age with large VSD associated with pulmonary artery hypertension.
- Supracristal VSD of any size
- Age > 24 months with Qp:Qs ratio>2:1.

Contraindication to Surgery: Severe pulmonary vascular disease.

SUDDEN IMPROVEMENT IN SYMPTOMS OF VSD

- Closure of VSD
- Development of Eisenmenger's complex.

CAUSES OF NONCLOSURE OF PDA IN PRETERM CHILD

- Anemia
- Acidosis
- Infection
- Hypoxia
- Congestive heart failure.

Before administration of prostaglandin inhibitors (like indomethacin) these conditions should be treated first and investigations like Bleeding time/ Clotting time/Prothrombin time/PTTK/platelet count/urea/electrolytes/serum creatinine should be normal.

IMPORTANCE OF CYANOSIS IN CHD

- Determine whether cyanosis appeared at birth or later:
  - *Cyanosis at birth:* Transposition of great arteries (TGA), Tricuspid atresia, pulmonary atresia.
  - *Cyanosis appears after 6-8 weeks:* Fetralogy of Fallot (TOF)
  - *Cyanosis appears after feed or during crying:* Large VSD (shunt temporarily reverses).
- Differential diagnosis of cyanosis

2 As – Pulmonary Atresia
Aortic Atresia

5 Ts – Transposition of great arteries (TGA)
Tricuspid atresia
Tetralogy of Fallot (TOF)
Total anomalous pulmonary venous return (TAPVC)
Truncus arteriosus

APPROACH TO CHD IN A NEWBORN

- *Cyanosis:* TGA, Right sided obstruction (Pulmonary atresia, Tricuspid atresia)
- *Mild Cyanosis with CCF:* TAPVC, Truncus arteriosus
- *Shock:* Hypoplastic left heart syndrome, Aortic stenosis
- *Late onset CCF (> 2 weeks):* VSD, PDA, Cardiomyopathy
- Asymptomatic: Small VSD, mild pulmonary stenosis

DIFFERENTIAL DIAGNOSIS OF FALLOTS PHYSIOLOGY

- Fallot's tetralogy
- Transposition of great arteries
- Tricuspid atresia
- Single ventricle
- Double outlet right ventricle
- Atrioventriclar canal defect.

VARIANTS OF TOF

Fallot's Tetralogy—Ventricular septal defect + Right ventricular outflow tract obstruction + Overriding of aorta + Right ventricular hypertrophy.

Fallot's Triology—Pulmonary stenosis + Atrial septal defect + Right ventricle hypertrophy.

Fallot's Pentalogy—Fallots tetralogy + Atrial septal defect.

Acyanotic (pink) Fallot (Fallots Duology)—Right ventricular tract obstruction is mild so clinical picture resembles VSD.

Fallot's Monology (atretic Fallot)—Pulmonary atresia +/–VSD.

CCF EXCLUDES TOF EXCEPT WHEN COMPLICATED BY

- Anemia
- Infective endocarditis

- Valvular regurgitation
- Large left to right shunt
- Systemic hypertension.

COMPLICATIONS OF TOF

- Erythrocytosis
- Brain abscess
- Acute arthritis
- Infective endocarditis
- Cerebrovascular infarct/abscess
- Delayed puberty.

SYNDROMIC ASSOCIATION OF CHD

- Down's syndrome: Endocardial cushion defect
- Rubella syndrome: Patent ductus arteriosus
- Turner's syndrome: Coarctation of aorta
- Trisomy 13: Ventricular septal defect, atrial septal defect, patent ductus arteriosus, dextrocardia
- Trisomy 18: Ventricular septal defect.

FEATURES SUGGESTIVE OF INNOCENT OR FUNCTIONAL MURMUR

- Normal blood pressure
- No cardiomegaly or congestive cardiac failure
- No cyanosis
- Normal S2
- Normal chest X-ray and ECG.

CLINICAL FINDINGS IN CHF

Signs of Impaired Myocardial Performance

- Cardiomegaly
- Tachycardia
- Gallop rhythm
- Arterial pulsations—cold extremeties, pallor, feeble peripheral pulses, low BP
- Pulsus paradoxus
- Pulsus alterans
- Growth failure
- Sweating.

Signs of Pulmonary Congestion

- Wheezing
- Rales
- Cyanosis
- Dyspnea
- Cough.

Signs of Systemic Venous Congestion

- Hepatomegaly
- Neck vein distension
- Peripheral edema.

3-Minute Examination in CHF

- Take sleeping or resting respiratory rate for 1 full minute (of the 3 minutes).
- After the count patient's general appearance, distress, color and perfusion are noted.
- Patient's forehead is palpated for diaphoresis, capillary refill is checked, and the tibial and other areas are examined for edema.
- The precordium is palpated to assess its activity.
- The abdomen is examined for hepatomegaly and the edge of the liver is measured below the costal margin.
- The pulses are palpated. The right arm pulse is felt simultaneously with a leg pulse and carotid pulses are palpated.
- Then the stethoscope is used to listen to the head and abdomen for bruits, the heart for murmurs or gallops, and the lungs for rales or rhonchi.
- If the diagnosis of CHF is made or even suspected, then referral and treatment should be instituted.

Table 15.2: Time of onset of CHF in congenital lesions

Age	*Lesion*
Birth to 72 hours	Pulmonary, mitral and aortic atresias
4 days to 1 week	Hypoplastic left heart, TGA
1 to 4 weeks	Endocardial fibroelastosis, coarctation of the aorta, transposition complexes
1 to 2 months	Endocardial cushion defects, VSD, PDA, TAPVC, Anomalous left coronary artery

CAUSES OF NONIMPROVEMENT OF CCF DESPITE TREATMENT

- Anemia
- Infection
- Infective endocarditis
- Associated cardiac anomalies
- Poor compliance.

EISENMENGER'S SYNDROME

Left to right shunt gets reversed (right to left) with the development of severe pulmonary hypertension, resulting in central cyanosis, clubbing, and secondary polycythemia.

Pulmonary artery hypertension is due to development of pulmonary vascular obstructive disease which is acquired complication in patients with congenital heart disease who have increased pulmonary blood flow.

Patients with left to right shunt and increased pulmonary blood flow are potential candidates for development of Eisenmenger's physiology.

DEVELOPMENT OF EISENMENGER'S COMPLEX

- PDA—11 years (2nd decade)
- VSD—22 years (3rd decade)
- ASD—33 years (4th decade)

HYPEROXIA TEST

- Differentiates shunt cyanosis and pulmonary cyanosis
- Give 100% oxygen to patient for 10 minutes:
- If $PaO_2 > 200$ mm Hg, congenital heart disease is ruled out
- If $PaO_2 < 100$ mm Hg, possibility of congenital heart disease.

PERSISTENCE OF FETAL CIRCULATORY PATTERN

A PaO_2 gradient between preductal (right radial artery) and postductal (umbilical artery or left radial artery) blood sampling greater than 20 mm Hg suggests persistence of fetal circulatory pattern.

CAUSES OF FAILURE TO THRIVE IN CONGENITAL HEART DISEASE

- Hypoxia (hence development is more delayed in cyanotic as compared to acyanotic heart disease)
- Increased basal metabolic rate
- Congestive heart failure
- Acidosis
- Infections: Repeated respiratory tract infection, infective endocarditis
- Feeding difficulties.

RHEUMATIC HEART DISEASE

HISTORY

CHIEF COMPLAINTS

- Difficulty in respiration on exertion (dyspnea)
- Palpitations/chest pain
- Joint pains.

HISTORY OF PRESENT ILLNESS

History of Disease

- Dyspnea:
  - Note onset, progression, duration
  - Relation to activity and position
  - Progression
  - Orthopnea
  - Associated features like cough, palpitation, chest pain, sweating, edema
- Palpitation—also note associated features like sweating, chest pain, choking
- Recurrent bleeding from nose, mouth
- Fatigue and decreased exercise tolerance
- Chest pain
- Carditis:
  - Breathlessness
  - Palpitation/syncope
  - Cough
- Arthritis:
  - Joints involved
  - Nature of involvement—migratory or not
  - Pain, swelling, redness and restriction of movement (to differentiate arthritis from arthralgia)
  - Rash on trunk and proximal limbs, exacerbated by heat (erythema marginatum).
- Chorea:
  - Purposeless movements of the arms and legs
  - Difficulty in writing
  - Involuntary grimacing
  - Speech impairment
  - Generalized weakness
  - Emotional liability (chorea).
- Firm, nontender nodules on extensor surfaces
- Regular drug intake (penicillin injection)
- Awareness of pulsation in neck (primary pulmonary hypertension, severe pulmonary stenosis).

History of Complications

- Infective endocarditis:
  - Fever with chills
  - *Osler's nodes* (pin head size tender papule seen in the pulp of fingers).
  - *Janeway's lesion* (non-tender maculopapular lesion in palm)
  - Hemoptysis/hematuria
  - *Petechial hemorrhages* (linear longitudinal hemorrhage under the nail)
- Congestive cardiac failure:
  - Swelling, breathlessness
  - Abdominal pain, anorexia, vomiting
  - Repeated respiratory tract infection.
- Impact on child:
  - Growth and development
  - Schooling (academic performance, sports restriction, teachers and peers attitude, school days lost).
- Lower respiratory tract infection:
  - Fever
  - Cough
  - Difficulty in respiration.

History of Differential Diagnosis

- Congenital heart disease
  - Cyanosis
  - Symptoms from birth
  - Repeated respiratory tract infection and breathlessness
  - Inability to gain weight.
- Systemic lupus erythematosus (mainly in female patients):
  - Facial rash
  - Fever with joint pain.

- Juvenile rheumatoid arthritis
  - ❖ Morning stiffness
  - ❖ Involvement of small joints, pain in spine and temporomandibular joint
  - ❖ Joint stiffness increases after prolonged use.
- Reactive arthritis
  - ❖ Fever
  - ❖ Loose motions with blood in stools.
- Leukemia
  - ❖ Progressive weight loss
  - ❖ Paleness of body with bone pain
  - ❖ Bleeding manifestation.

PAST HISTORY

- Similar history before (joint pain, abnormal movements)
- Previous history of hospitalization
- Any previous surgery.

SOCIAL HISTORY

- Living conditions, upbringing
- Economic and cultural background.

OCCUPATIONAL HISTORY

- Relevant in days of child labour in poor and underprivileged.

GENERAL PHYSICAL EXAMINATION

a. Vitals
  - ❖ *Pulse* (in all 4 limbs)
    - ○ Rate
    - ○ Rhythm
    - ○ Volume
    - ○ Condition of the arterial wall
    - ○ Comparison between two radial pulses
    - ○ Radio-femoral delay
    - ○ Any special character
    - ○ Other peripheral pulses
  - ❖ *Respiration*
  - ❖ *Blood pressure* (in all 4 limbs in older child)
  - ❖ Temperature

b. Anthropometry: Assess growth of child
  - ❖ Head to toe examination: Pallor/cyanosis/icterus/hygiene/clubbing/hepatojugular reflux/lymphadenopathy/pedal edema

c. Examination of neck veins:
  - ❖ Engorged or not
  - ❖ If engorged—pressure, pulsation, hepatojugular reflux.

d. Signs of infective endocarditis:
  - ❖ Osler's nodes (pin head size tender papule seen in the pulp of fingers)
  - ❖ Janeway's lesions (non-tender maculopapular lesion in palm)
  - ❖ Roth spots (seen on ophthalmoscopy)
  - ❖ Splinter hemorrhages (linear longitudinal hemorrhage under the nail)

e. Hepatojugular reflux is obtained with pressure over the liver for 30 seconds; there is a > 1 cm rise in JVP column which does not fall immediately (elicit this reflex even with normal JVP, since it is a sign of incipient failure).

f. Nodules:
  - ❖ Firm
  - ❖ Nontender
  - ❖ Free from attachments to the overlying skin
  - ❖ Size: Few mm to 1-2 cm
  - ❖ Vary in number

g. Arthritis

h. Hyperextended joints, hypotonia, diminished deep tendon reflexes, tongue fasciculations and a relapsing grip demonstrated by alternate increases and decreases in tension when the patient grips the examiner's hand (chorea)

i. Erythema marginatum: Pink-to-red nonpruritic macules or papules located on the trunk and proximal limbs (never on the face)

j. Peripheral signs of aortic regurgitation if present

k. Congestive heart failure.

SYSTEMIC EXAMINATION

CARDIOVASCULAR SYSTEM

- As described in congenital heart disease.

RESPIRATORY SYSTEM

- Crepitations/rhonchi.

ABDOMEN

- Hepatomegaly/splenomegaly/ascites.

CENTRAL NERVOUS SYSTEM

- Look for involuntary movements (chorea)
- Decreased movement of any part of body (emboli).

DIAGNOSIS

Mitral stenosis/mitral regurgitation/aortic regurgitation/aortic stenosis with/without sinus rhythm with/without CCF with/without infective endocarditis with/without pulmonary hypertension with/without active signs of rheumatic fever.

Most probable diagnosis being________.

DIFFERENTIAL DIAGNOSIS

MITRAL STENOSIS

- Low volume pulse
- Hypotension
- Tapping apex beat
- Diastolic thrill, best palpable in left lateral position
- *Auscultation*
  - S_1 – Loud
  - S_2 – Normal
  - Opening snap – Audible, just after S_2
  - Murmur – Diastolic murmur.

MITRAL REGURGITATION

- Tachycardia
- Engorged JVP and pedal edema (CCF)
- Epigastric pulsation and left parasternal heave– present (Right ventricular hypertrophy)
- Hyperdynamic apex shifted down and out; systolic thrill is present in apical area.
- Palpation of pulmonary area – Diastolic shock (palpable P_2) present.
- Auscultation
  - S_1 – Soft
  - S_2 –Audible
  - High-pitched, soft blowing pansystolic murmur. The murmur radiates towards the left axilla and inferior angle of left scapula **("hallmark of diagnosis")**
  - Pulmonary area – Ejection systolic murmur (different from pansystolic murmur at apex) with loud P_2.

AORTIC STENOSIS

- Low v\olume pulse 'anacrotic' in type. 'Carotid shudder', i.e. a systolic thrill in carotid artery is felt.
- Low pulse pressure.
- Apex beat—Heaving in character (though there is Left ventricular hypertrophy, apex is usually not shifted because aortic stenosis causes concentric hypertrophy).

- Palpation of the aortic area—Systolic thrill with radiation to the carotid artery.
- Auscultation of aortic area.
  - S_1 – Audible
  - S_2 (A_2) – Muffled
  - Ejection click – Present
  - Harsh midsystolic ejection murmur with direction of selective propagation towards the carotids is heard
  - Murmur of AS is known as *crescendo-decrescendo murmur.*

AORTIC REGURGITATION

- All the peripheral signs are present
- Hyperdynamic apex with downward and outward shift
- Ausculation of the aortic area
  - S_1 – Audible
  - S_2 (A_2) – Muffled
  - High pitched, soft blowing early diastolic decrescendo murmur. The murmur is radiated towards the apex and is best heard at neoaortic area (left 3rd ICS).

INVESTIGATIONS

- Throat culture: Taken before initiation of antibiotic therapy
- Antistreptococcal antibody testing: Anti-streptolysin O (ASO), anti-deoxyribonuclease (DNAse) B, antihyaluronidase, antistreptokinase, antistreptococcal esterase and anti-DNA. Antibody titers should be checked at 2-week intervals in order to detect a rising titer.
- Acute phase reactants: The C-reactive protein and erythrocyte sedimentation rate
- Rapid detection test for D 8/17: Immunofluorescence technique for identifying B cell marker D 8/17 in rheumatic fever
- Chest roentgenogram: To look for cardiomegaly, pulmonary congestion.
- Doppler-echocardiogram: To look for severity and type of cardiac lesion
- ECG: To look for severity and type of cardiac lesion
- Heart catheterization: Not indicated in acute rheumatic heart disease. Required in chronic disease to evaluate mitral and aortic valve disease and to balloon stenotic mitral valves.
- Repeated blood culture/urine routine for hematuria and proteinuria: To look for infective endocarditis.

TREATMENT

Consensus Guidelines on Pediatric Acute Rheumatic Fever and Rheumatic Heart Disease (Cardiology Chapter of IAP' 2007)

Management of Streptococcal Pharyngitis (Table 15.3)

Group A beta hemolytic streptococcal (GABHS) sore throat: Clinically patient has high fever, sore throat with pustules, strawberry tongue, petechiae on palate and tender anterior cervical lymph nodes.

Management of Acute Rheumatic Fever

Diagnosis

Diagnosis is based on recognition of major and minor criteria supported by evidence of preceding streptococcal infection.

First episode: Two major or one major and two minor criteria plus supportive evidence of previous streptococcal throat infection.

Recurrence in a patient without established heart disease: Two major or one major and two minor criteria + supportive evidence of previous streptococcal throat infection.

Recurrence in a patient with established heart disease: Two minor criteria and supportive evidence of previous streptococcal throat infection.

Table 15.3: Drugs for the treatment of Streptococcal pharyngitis and secondary prophylaxis

Drugs	*Dose*	*Sore-throat treatment (duration)*	*Secondary prophylaxis (interval)*
Benzathine Penicillin G (deep IM injection)	1.2 million unit (> 27 Kg) after sensitivity test (AST)	single dose*	21 days
	0.6 million unit (<27 Kg) (after sensitivity test) contraindication: penicillin allergy	single dose*	15 days
Penicillin-V (oral)	Children: 250 mg qid	10 days	twice a day
	Adult: 500 mg tds contraindication: penicillin allergy	10 days	twice a day
Azithromycin (oral)	12.5 mg/kg/day once daily	5 days	not recommended
Cephalexin (oral)	15-20 mg/kg/dose bd	10 days	not recommended
Erythromycin (oral)	20 mg/kg/dose max 500 mg contraindication : liver disorder	not recommended	twice a day

*only one dose is sufficient for GABHS pharyngitis.

Rheumatic chorea and insidious onset rheumatic carditis: No requirement of other major manifestations or supportive evidence of streptococcal sore throat infection:

Indicators of recurrence of rheumatic fever in established heart disease:

i. New murmur/change in pre-existing murmur;
ii. Pericardial rub (and other evidence of pericarditis); and
iii. Unexplained congestive heart failure (CHF), including cardiomegaly.

Terminology

Recurrence: A new episode of rheumatic fever following another GABHS infection; occurring after 8 week following stopping treatment.

Rebound: Manifestations of rheumatic fever occurring within 4-6 week of stopping treatment or while tapering drugs.

Relapse: Worsening of rheumatic fever while under treatment and often with carditis.

Sub clinical carditis: When clinical examination is normal but echocardiogram is abnormal. Around 30 percent of patients having chorea present as sub clinical carditis.

Indolent carditis: It is a common entity in our country. Patient presents with persistent features of CHF, murmur and cardiomegaly. There are no or very few features of carditis.

Treatment

General Measures and Symptomatic Relief:

- Treatment for pain relief should be given (codeine or paracetamol till diagnosis is confirmed and aspirin after the diagnosis is confirmed).
- For arthritis, rest for two weeks is adequate. Carditis without congestive heart failure (CHF) needs 4-6 weeks of rest. In cases of CHF, rest must be continued till the CHF is controlled. Appropriate diet is a must for a growing child with cardiac involvement.

Management of Inflammatory Process—Therapy to be continued for 12 Weeks (Table 15.4)

- Aspirin and steroids are primarily used to control inflammation. Naproxen and methylprednisolone can be used alternatively. Therapy to be continued for 12 weeks (Table 15.4).

Management of Chorea

Mild chorea is treated with quite environment, and sedatives like oral phenobarbitone or diazepam.

If there is no response, then one may use haloperidol (0.25-0.5 mg/kg/day), sodium valproate (15 mg/kg/day), or carbamazepine (7-20 mg/kg/d) may be used.

Resistant cases can be treated with plasmapheresis or pimozide. Treatment should be continued for 2-4 weeks after clinical improvement.

If there are laboratory features of rheumatic activity (ESR, CRP, ASO), anti-inflammatory drugs must be given.

Management of Cardiac Complications

Management of congestive heart failure: Restrict physical activities to reduce or eliminate symptoms. Monitor the weight and fluid balance (input /output charting). Treat anemia with iron and/or packed cells, as and when indicated.

Interventions in Valvular Heart Disease

A. *Mitral Stenosis:* Pure mitral stenosis must be treated with balloon mitral valvuloplasty.
The patients unsuitable for BMV may need valve repair or replacement.

B. *Mitral Regurgitation:* Acute rheumatic fever with acute severe mitral regurgitation and uncontrolled congestive heart failure, secondary to chordal rupture, is an indication for urgent surgical intervention.
Symptomatic chronic MR is treated with either valve repair or replacement.

C. *Aortic stenosis:* Treatment with ballooning procedures is usually not helpful. Surgical intervention is done in symptomatic patients.

D. *Aortic regurgitation:* Aortic regurgitation presenting as isolated or combined lesion, is treated with prosthetic valve replacement.

Endocarditis

Treatment of endocarditis needs prolonged administration of recommended IV antibiotics.

Duration differs according to status of patient (with native or prosthetic valve) and the type of organism.

Secondary Prophylaxis

The purpose is to prevent colonization or infection of the upper respiratory tract with group A beta-hemolytic streptococci and the development of recurrent attacks of rheumatic fever.

After surgery or intervention secondary prophylaxis should be continued.

Duration of Secondary Prophylaxis

i. No carditis: 5 years/18 years of age, whichever is longer.
ii. Mild to moderate carditis and healed carditis: 10 years/25 years of age, whichever is longer.
iii. Severe disease or post intervention patients: Life long. One may opt for secondary prophylaxis up to the age of 40 years *(see Table 15.3).*

Drugs Recommended for Secondary Prophylaxis (See Table 15.3)

Sensitivity Testing for Penicillin

- Ideally sensitivity test has to be done with major and minor allergen supplied separately (not available in India).
- Benzathine penicillin is unsuitable for skin test.
- Intradermal test must be done with both benzyl penicillin, i.e. crystalline penicillin and control saline (0.02-0.05 ml at volar surface of forearm or lateral surface of arm).
- Positive test is indicated by formation of a wheal, 2 mm more than control or 4 mm more than initial edema (test time 20-30 min).

Table 15.4: Drugs for control of inflammation in acute rheumatic fever

Inflammation	*Doses*
Arthritis ± mild carditis **Aspirin**	*Regime I* Starting doses: children 100 mg/kg/day for 2-3 weeks Adult 6-8g/day: divide in 4-5 doses Tapering doses: once symptoms resolved, taper to 60-70 mg/kg/day. For older children 50 mg/kg/day *Regime II* 50 to 60 mg//kg /day for total 12 weeks
No response to aspirin in four days	Switch over to steroid. Rule out other conditions like chronic inflammatory/ myelo-proliferative disorders before switching over to steroids.
Moderate to severe carditis **Steroids**	*Regime I* Prednisolone: 2 mg/kg/day, maximum 80 mg/day till ESR normalizes—usually 2 weeks. Taper over 2-4 weeks, reduce dose by 2.5-5 mg every 3rd day. start aspirin 50-75mg/kg/day simultaneously, to complete total 12 weeks *Regime II* Prednisolone same doses × 3-4 weeks. taper slowly to cover total period of 10-12 weeks
Nonresponders Methyl Prednisolone (Intravenous)	If no response to oral steroid therapy then start IV methylprednisolone 30 mg/kg/day for 3 days

DISCUSSION

LUTEMBACHER'S SYNDROME

Atrial septal defect (ASD) plus mitral stenosis (of rheumatic origin).

CRITERIA FOR DIAGNOSIS OF RHEUMATIC FEVER (JONE'S CRITERIA)

Major Criteria C^2ASE

- Carditis
- Arthritis
- Subcutaneous nodules
- Chorea
- Erythema marginatum.

Minor Criteria

Clinical

- Fever
- Arthralgia
- Previous rheumatic fever or rheumatic heart disease.

Laboratory

- Increased TLC
- Increased PR interval
- Increased ESR
- Positive CRP.

Essential Criteria

- Increased ASO titre
- Positive throat culture
- Recent scarlet fever

Presence of **2 major or 1 major and 2 minor criteria** are required in the presence of **at least 1 essential criteria.**

DIFFERENTIATION BETWEEN RHEUMATIC ARTHRITIS AND RHEUMATOID ARTHRITIS

Rheumatic Arthritis

- Major joints affected

- Migratory polyarthritis
- No diurnal variation in joint pain observed
- Fifty percent have associated carditis
- Dramatic response within 48 hours after administration of salicylates
- No residual defect after recovery
- ASLO test positive.

Rheumatoid Arthritis

- Minor joints affected (Spine/Temporomandibular joints/finger joints)
- Symmetric involvement of joints is common and pain is not migratory
- Morning stiffness is common
- Less than 10% have associated carditis
- Response to analgesics is not so fast
- Residual defect in the joint persists after recovery
- Rheumatoid factor may be positive.

SUBCUTANEOUS NODULES IN RHEUMATIC FEVER

- Appears by 6 weeks after onset of rheumatic fever
- Small, pea sized 0.5-2 cm in diameter
- Firm, mobile, painless
- Seen over extensor surface of wrist, elbow and spine
- *Importance:* Patients with subcutaneous nodules almost always have carditis
- Biopsy differentiates subcutaneous nodule from lymphadenitis as the subcutaneous nodule contains *Aschoff bodies*
- Lasts for few days to weeks.

SYDENHAM'S CHOREA

- Usually delayed and often the sole manifestation of rheumatic fever
- Fast and involuntary
- Quasi-purposive
- Jerky
- Exacerbated by stress
- Disappears during sleep (myoclonus is unaffected by sleep)
- Involves proximal joints
- Associated with poor school performance, emotional labiality and hypotonia
- Rarely leads to permanent neurological squeal.

Cardinal Signs of Chorea

- *Hypotonia*
- *Milkmaid's grip*—Ask the patient to grasp or squeeze the examiners hand. There is waxing and waning of grip.
- *Pronator sign*—Patient tends to pronate his hand while extending the hand above the head.
- *Jack-in-the box tongue/Lizard tongue*—Ask the patient to protrude the tongue. The patient protudes it momentarily and takes it back within the oral cavity immediately.
- *Spooning sign*—The patient is asked to stretch out the hand and spread the fingers. Elbow is hyperextended, forearm will be hyperpronated, wrist joint is flexed and metacarpophalangeal joints are extended with the separation of fingers (dinner fork deformity). This is a manifestation of hypotonia. This will be more obvious if the patient is asked to raise the hands above his head.
- *Hung–up reflexes*—Knee jerk is pendular due to hypotonia. It is called hung up reflex due to superimposition of choreic movement on tendon reflex at times.
- On attempting to button a shirt, they become fidgety.

ERYTHEMA MARGINATUM

- Rare
- Erythematous, serpiginous, macular rash with pale centre.

- Nonpruritic, no induration
- Seen over trunk and extremeties.

AREAS OF AUSCULTATION OVER PRECORDIUM

- *Mitral area:* Cardiac apex.
- *Tricuspid area:* Lower left parasternal area.
- *Aortic area:* Second right intercostal space close to the sternum.
- *Pulmonary area:* Second left intercostal space close to the sternum.
- *Erb's area (second aortic area):* Third left intercostal space close to the sternum.
- *Gibson's area:* Left first intercostal space close to sternum. PDA murmur is best heard here (Gibson's murmur).

LEVINE AND FREEMAN'S GRADING OF MURMURS

Systolic Murmur Grading

I. Very soft (heard in a quiet room)
II. Soft
III. Moderate
IV. Loud with thrill
V. Very loud with thrill (heard with stetho-scope)
VI. Very loud with thrill (heard even when stethoscope is slightly away from the chest wall).

Diastolic Murmur Grading

I. Very soft
II. Soft
III. Loud
IV. Loud with thrill.

ASSESSMENT OF SEVERITY OF MITRAL REGURGITATION

- Apical displacement
- Palpable S_3
- Loud MR murmur
- Widely split S_2 (early A_2).

ASSESSMENT OF SEVERITY OF MITRAL STENOSIS

Clinical

- Proximity of S_2 – OS gap, and
- Longer duration of mid diastolic murmur.

Gradient

Normal valve gradient	0 mm Hg
Mild MS	< 5 mm Hg
Moderate MS	5 to 15 mm Hg
Severe MS	> 15 mm Hg

Opening Snap

- Produced due to bellowing down of the closed mitral valve cusps at the onset of ventricular diastole (i.e. mitral valve will open just now but has not opened yet).
- Sharp and high pitched, best heard after expiration and present in early diastole
- It indicates:
  - Organic cause
  - Pliable valve cusps
  - Significant mitral stenosis
  - High atrioventricular pressure gradient
  - Severe aortic regurgitation, gross pulmonary hypertension, atrial fibrillation, left atrial failure or subacute bacterial endocarditis is absent.

DIASTOLIC MURMUR IN MITRAL REGION IN CASE OF RHEUMATIC FEVER

- Carey-Coombs' murmur (active carditis)
- Flow murmur
- Mitral stenosis.

PERIPHERAL SIGNS OF AORTIC REGURGITATION

Peripheral signs are produced as a result of *'wide pulse pressure'*

- Visible capillary pulsation *(Quincke's sign):*
  - When pressure is applied to the tip of fingers or nails, there is alternate flushing and pallor of the nail bed, or
  - When a glass slide is pressed on the everted lower lip, it produces alternate redness and blanching.
- Prominent digital artery pulsation—Hold the fingers of the patient with your fingers in flexed position to feel the pulsation
- High volume collapsing pulse *(water hammer pulse)*
- Blood pressure—Wide pulse pressure with low diastolic pressure (even Korotkoff sounds may continue up to 200 mm of Hg)
- *Corrigan's sign*—Dancing carotids in neck
- *de Musset's sign*—To and fro head-nodding along with carotid pulsation
- Pulsation in the suprasternal (Jugular) notch
- Pistol shot sound or *Traube's sign*—Booming sound produced after pressing the stethoscope over femoral artery.
  - Systolic murmur on compression of the femoral artery proximally.
  - *Duroziez's murmur*—Diastolic murmur on distal compression of the femoral artery.
- *Hill's sign*—Increase in the femoral artery systolic BP > 20 mm Hg above the brachial artery systolic BP. The normal difference is within 20 mm of Hg. In severe AI, the increase is > 60 mm of Hg. It is a very important and specific sign of AI
- Pulsation in uvula, liver and enlarged spleen is respectively known as *Muller's sign*, *Bosenbach's sign* and *Gerhardt's sign.*

NEW YORK HEART ASSOCIATION (NYHA) CLASSIFICATION FOR GRADATION OF DYSPNEA

Grade I	No limitation of activities with ordinary physical activity, i.e. asymptomatic though the patient is suffering from organic heart disease.
Grade II	No limitation under resting condition but symptoms appear on ordinary activity.
Grade III	Limitation of activities on mild exertion of less than ordinary acitivity.
Grade IV	Limitation of activities at rest, restricting the person to bed or chair.

This functional classification refers not only to dyspnea but to symptoms like fatigue, palpitation, angina pectoris, etc. This is actually a classification of cardiac disability.

'SEVERITY' OF AORTIC STENOSIS

Clinical

- Low pulse volume.
- Systolic decapitation of BP (low systolic pressure due to low and fixed cardiac output; in a patient with Aortic stenosis, systolic BP never goes above 150 mm of Hg).
- Paradoxical splitting of S_2—When the splitting happens to occur only during expiration (When the splitting is present only during inspiration, it is known as physiological splitting)
- S_4—Absence of systolic thrill often tells against a severe stenosis.

Gradient

Normal	0 mm Hg
Mild AS	< 30 mm Hg

Moderate AS	30-50 mm Hg
Severe AS	> 50 mm Hg

According to Valve Area

- Normal 3-4 cm^2
- Severe AS < 0.75 cm^2/m^2 body surface area
- Critical AS < 0.5 cm^2/m^2 body surface area.

BEDSIDE DIAGNOSIS OF ACUTE RHEUMATIC CARDITIS

The features of *'pancarditis'* are:

a) *Pericarditis:* Pericardial rub/Pericardial effusion.

b) *Myocarditis:*
- Relative tachycardia
- S_1 – Muffled (due to prolonged PR interval in ECG)
- Congestive heart failure
- Cardiomegaly
- Conduction defects – Dropped beat in pulse due to heart block.

c) *Endocarditis:* The appearance of:
- Soft systolic murmur of mitral incompetence
- Soft early diastolic murmur of aortic incompetence
- *Carey-Coombs' murmur*: Due to mitral valvulitis (oedema of mitral valve cusps results in development of MS)
- Change in the character of existing organic heart murmur.

SIGNS OF ACTIVITY OF RHEUMATIC FEVER

- Active carditis (described above)
- Fever lasting more than 14 days and no cause
- Subcutaneous nodules
- Migratory polyarthritis
- Chorea
- Erythema marginatum
- Raised ESR/CRP.

APPEARANCE OF MURMUR IN RHEUMATIC CARDITIS

In Order of Sequence

- Mitral regurgitation murmur (due to maximum pressure gradient)
- Aortic regurgitation murmur
- Carey-Coombs' murmur.

NEGATIVE ASO TEST IN RHEUMATIC FEVER

- In 20% patients
- In 1st week and after 5th week
- Mild carditis/chorea/treated case

In such cases, Anti- DNAse B and Streptozyme test should be carried out (> 98% Positive).

NORMAL ESR IN RHEUMATIC FEVER

- Chorea
- Mild carditis
- Congestive cardiac failure (in such cases CRP is positive).

CAUSES OF MIGRATORY ARTHRITIS

- Rheumatic arthritis
- Systemic lupus erythematosus
- Drug reaction/serum sickness
- Meningococcal bacteremia
- Viral arthritis (lyme arthritis)
- Inflammatory bowel disease.

INDICATIONS OF STEROID IN RHEUMATIC FEVER

- Carditis
- Congestive cardiac failure
- Aspirin intolerance or nonsettlement of ESR following aspirin treatment.

IMPORTANT RULES

- In mitral area—Diastolic thrill is very common
- In all other areas—Systolic thrill is more common
- In pulmonary area—Thrill may be continuous or systolodiastolic, e.g. PDA
- Thrill is usually present in stenotic lesions and generally absent in regurgitant lesions of the heart
- Difference between a conducted murmur and transmitted murmur:
  - Conducted murmur—is of the same intensity and duration
  - Transmitted murmur—is of decreased intensity and of duration.

OPENING SNAP AND S_3

	Opening Snap	S_3
Disease	Mitral stenosis	Heart failure
Best audible	At left parasternal region	At apex
Pitch	High-pitched	Low-pitched
Palpability	Not palpable	Often palpable
Timing	Early diastole	Mid-diastole
Treatment of heart failure	OS becomes louder	S_3 vanishes

FINDINGS SUGGESTIVE OF PULMONARY HYPERTENSION

Normal pulmonary artery pressure: 25/10 mm of Hg. Pulmonary artery hypertension: > 30/15 mm Hg.

- Visible pulmonary artery pulsation in left 2nd ICS
- P_2—Palpable (diastolic shock)
- Auscultation (pulmonary area)—The classical sequence of events are:
  - S_1—Audible
  - Pulmonary ejection click
  - Ejection systolic murmur (due to relative obstruction)
  - Close splitting of S_2 with loud P_2
  - *Graham-Steell murmur*—An early diastolic murmur due to functional pulmonary incompetence
  - Right sided S_3 (right ventricular gallop)—Heard at the lower left sternal border.

INFECTIVE ENDOCARDITIS (IE)

Acute infective endocarditis: Caused by highly virulent organisms mainly *S. aureus* (20-30%), seeding a previously normal valve.

Subacute infective endocarditis: Caused by organisms of moderate or low virulence mainly *Streptococci* (60-70%), seeding an abnormal or previously injured valve.

Endocarditis occurring in IV drug abusers: Caused predominantly by organisms found on the skin (*S. aureus, Candida)* and affecting the valves on the right side of the heart.

Prosthetic valve endocarditis: This may be early (symptoms appearing within 60 days of valve insertion) due to intraoperative infection of the valve or insertion of an infected valve or late (symptoms appearing after 60 days of valve insertion) due to late bacteremia or earlier infection with micro-organisms having a long incubation period.

Nonbacterial thrombotic endocarditis (Marantic endocarditis): Nonbacterial thrombotic vegetations seen in malignancy or wasting disorders which are prone for bacterial seedling.

Endocarditis associated with SLE (Libman-Sachs endocarditis): The vegetations are 3 to 4 mm in size, composed of degenerating valve tissue; func-tional disability is minimal; ventricular surface of the mitral valve is commonly involved; aortic valve involvement is rare; entire valve apparatus can be involved.

SUBACUTE BACTERIAL ENDOCARDITIS (SABE)

Clinical Features

- Persistent fever
- Progressive pallor
- Tachycardia
- Clubbing
- Petechiae in dorsum of hands
- *Osler's node* [Tender papule about the size of pin head to pea and is seen in the pulp of fingers, toes and palms (due to embolism or arteritis)]
- Splinter hemorrhage (linear longitudinal hemorrhage under the nail)
- *Janeway's spot* (nontender maculopapular lesion in palm)
- Pansystolic murmur (due to pre-existent mitral regurgitations), i.e. there may be change in the pre-existent murmur or appearance of a new diastolic murmur
- Mild, tender splenomegaly
- Tender renal angle
- Ophthalmoscopy—Roth spots.

Investigations

Blood

- Anemia
- Leukocytosis
- Raised ESR
- Mild hyperbilirubinemia
- Repeated blood culture (4-6 blood cultures are taken at ½ hour interval under aseptic technique; both aerobic and anaerobic cultures are done).

Urine

- Microscopic hematuria
- Slight proteinuria
- Echocardiography: Demonstration of parent disease and vegetations.

CAUSES OF HEMOPTYSIS IN RHD

- Pulmonary apoplexy due to rupture of thin-walled, dilated bronchopulmonary veins usually as a consequence of a sudden rise in left atrial pressure.
- Blood stained sputum associated with episodes of paroxysmal nocturnal dyspnea due to pulmonary congestion.
- Pink, frothy sputum of pulmonary edema.
- Blood stained sputum as a result of recurrent bronchitis and bronchiectasis.
- Pulmonary infarction, a late complication of mitral stenosis associated with heart failure.

DUKE'S CRITERIA FOR INFECTIVE ENDOCARDITIS

Major Criteria

- Positive blood culture:
  - Typical organisms in two separate blood cultures
  - Persistently positive blood culture: > 3 positive cultures 12 hours apart
- Endocardium involved
  - Positive echocardiogram (vegetation, abscess or dehiscence of prosthetic valve) or
  - New valvular regurgitation (change in murmur not sufficient).

Minor Criteria

- Predisposition (cardiac lesion, IV drug abuse)
- Fever > 38° C
- Vascular or immunologic sign
- Positive blood culture that do not meet major criteria
- Positive echocardiogram that do not meet major criteria.

Definitive Diagnosis based on

- Two major criteria or
- One major and 3 minor criteria or
- All 5 minor, criteria.

CRITERIA FOR ENDING ABSOLUTE BEDREST AND REDUCING DOSE OF SUPPRESSION THERAPY

- Normal temperature
- Absence of joint symptoms and signs
- Absence of increased sleeping pulse rate
- Absence of signs of cardiac insufficiency
- Stabilization of murmurs and heart sounds
- Reduction in heart size
- ESR less than 25 mm
- Negative CRP
- Return of PR interval to normal.

REBOUND PHENOMENA

When suppressive therapy is tapered or discontinued, clinical and laboratory findings may reappear. Rebound is more common with steroids. Two hypotheses are considered for rebound phenomena:

- Rheumatic inflammatory process has not run its full course and premature withdrawal of drugs allow resumption of natural disease process.
- Suppressive therapy prevents dispersion of rheumatic inflammatory process and the accumulated residual inflammation appears in the form of rebound.

ECG FINDINGS IN RHD

Mitral stenosis	P mitrale (bifid) due to enlarged LA Prolonged PR interval (RV hypertrophy) Cardiac arrhythmia
Mitral regurgitation	Left axis deviation P mitrale Prolonged PR interval LV hypertrophy
Aortic stenosis	LV hypertrophy 1st degree AV block, LBBB
Aortic regurgitation	LV hypertrophy, volume overload

CHAPTER 16

RESPIRATORY SYSTEM

PLEURAL EFFUSION

HISTORY

CHIEF COMPLAINTS

- Cough/fever
- Breathlessness
- Chest pain.

HISTORY OF PRESENT ILLNESS

History of Disease

Cough

- Onset: How it started
- Duration: Acute (< 2 weeks); Chronic (> 2 weeks)
- Aggravating or relieving factors
- Diurnal variation
- Noisy breathing: Stridor; wheezing
- Dry or productive
- Color of sputum
- Amount of sputum
- Odor
- Blood in sputum
- Associated symptoms: Ear ache; ringing in ears.

Breathlessness

- Onset
- Progression
- Increases on any particular position like lying down
- Nature of difficulty: Faster than usual (tachypnea); harder than normal (dyspnea)

Chest Pain

- Localized to which side
- Type of pain
- Radiation
- Increases on respiration and cough.

Fever

- Onset and progression
- Associated with chills, night sweats
- Evening rise in temperature

- Does it touch baseline and responds to medications.

History of Complications

- Sinus formation.
- To assess severity:
  - Inability to feed
  - Lethargic/unconscious
  - Convulsions
  - Persistent vomiting
  - Cyanosis.

History of Differential Diagnosis

- Tuberculosis: Evening rise in temperature, Anorexia, weight loss, night sweats, contact with tuberculosis patient
- Trauma to chest
- Bone pains/weight loss/bleeding manifestations (neoplasms)
- Liver abscess: History of dysentery, High fever with chills, right upper abdominal pain
- Fever with rash (measles/SLE)
- Edema over feet/puffiness of face/breathlessness on exertion/pallor/hematuria
  - S/o CCF/hypoproteinemia/anemia/ nephritic syndrome (all causes of transudates)
- Failure to thrive/poor dietary history/skin and hair changes—Kwashiorkor
- Skin boils/rapid progression/deterioration (Staphylococcus infection)
- Chest pain localised to one side (empyema)
- Sounds during breathing:
  - Stridor:Laryngotracheobronchitis, epiglottitis, foreign body
  - Wheeze: Bronchiolitis.
- Drooling of saliva: Epiglottitis
- History of foreign body aspiration/ episodes of choking
- Day care center/ exposure to passive smoke/ crowding/ premature birth (bronchiolitis)
- Known HIV infection
- Recurrent episodes with:
  - Atopy/ eczema/ rhinitis / night cough / family history of asthma (reactive airway disease, asthma)
  - Temporal relation to feeding or posture (gastroesophageal reflex disease)
  - History of malabsorption (cystic fibrosis)
  - Multiple multifocal infections (immunodeficiencies)
  - Feeding diaphoresis (acyanotic CHD).

IMMUNIZATION HISTORY

- BCG Test

FAMILY HISTORY

- Tuberculosis
- Bronchial asthma
- Atopic dermatitis
- Cystic fibrosis.

OCCUPATIONAL HISTORY

- Not important in paediatric history-taking. Numerous chemicals, moulds, organic dust and animal proteins can cause asthma and allergic alveolitis.

GENERAL PHYSICAL EXAMINATION

- Respiratory distress
  - any irregularity in rate, depth and rhythm of respiration
  - Inability to speak without frequent pauses resulting in short, jerky, breathless sentences.
  - Movement of alae nasi and accessory muscle involvement

- ♦ Depression of intercostals spaces and subcostal retraction.
- ❖ Anthropometry
- ❖ Cyanosis, clubbing, edema
- ❖ Jugular veins
- ❖ Other signs of respiratory distress: head bobbing, pulsus paradoxus
- ❖ Lymphadenopathy
- ❖ Position of trachea
- ❖ Skin examination
- ❖ Spine examination
- ❖ Stigmata of tuberculosis
  - ♦ Phylectenular conjunctivitis
  - ♦ Scars and sinuses
  - ♦ Thickened spermatic cord
  - ♦ Erythema nodosum.
- ❖ BCG mark
- ❖ Examine nose and see for patency of both nostrils by occluding each side and listening for airflow through other nostril
- ❖ Examine maxillary and frontal sinuses for tenderness in older children to rule out chronic sinusitis
- ❖ Examination of oral cavity: Posterior pharyngeal wall; tonsils
- ❖ Ear examination: Look for wax, discharge and tympanic membrane
- ❖ Eye examination: Discharge from eyes.

SYSTEMIC EXAMINATION

RESPIRATORY SYSTEM EXAMINATION

Inspection

- Shape and symmetry of the chest
- Movements of the chest
- Apical impulse
- Respiration:

  Rate (count for 1 full minute)

  Pattern of Breathing:
  - ❖ Rapid and deep: Metabolic acidosis.
  - ❖ Irregular (CNS lesions, usually not associated with chest indrawing).
  - ❖ Paradoxical: Severity, diaphragmatic paralysis

  Respiratory Effort:
  - ❖ Intercostal recession
  - ❖ Accessory muscles of respiration are working or not
  - ❖ Flaring of alae nasi
  - ❖ Paradoxical movement: Inward movement of chest wall during inspiration is paradoxical breathing, while both chest wall and abdominal wall outward during normal inspiration.
- Fullness or depression
  - ❖ Unilateral or bilateral
  - ❖ Localized or generalized
- Skin
- Back examination—Scoliosis, kyphosis, drooping of the shoulder, winging of the scapula, gibbus, position of inferior angle of both scapula, symmetry of interscapular areas (spinoscapular distance).

Palpation

- Temperature
- Tenderness
- Corroboration of the findings of inspection: Examine the spinal deformity
- Position of the trachea and the apex beat (i.e. position of the mediastinum): Place second and fourth fingers on two heads of sternocleidomastoid muscle and gently pass the third finger over the trachea to look for position of trachea.
- Movements of the chest (measure both in full inspiration and in full expiration): Place both

palms on thorax at level of nipples, gently apposing the thumbs in midline. During inspiration thumbs separate and this gives measure of chest expansion and symmetry.
- Tactile vocal fremitus: Ask the child to say ninety-nine repeatedly and feel for vibrations with ulnar aspect of both hands placed on either side of chest.
  - Decreased (effusion, pneumothorax, collapse)
  - Increased (consolidation)
- Friction rub: Pleuritis.

Percussion

- Stony dullness on ipsilateral side of chest (pleural effusion)
- Hyperresonant: Pneumothorax
- Impaired / dull: Consolidation, pleural thickening.

Auscultation

- Breath sounds: Diminshed vesicular breath sound on ipsilateral side
- Adventitious sounds (rhonchi, crepitations and pleural rub)
- Vocal resonance (diminished, whispering pectoriloquy, aegophony).

Examination of Neck

- Jugular venous pressure.

CVS EXAMINATION

- Search for pericardial effusion (as a complication of anasarca) and signs of cor pulmonale.

GI SYSTEM EXAMINATION

- Hepatosplenomegaly
- Ascites and hydrocele: In patients with hydrothorax.

DIFFERENTIAL DIAGNOSIS

PNEUMONIA

- Cough with fast breathing
- Lower chest wall indrawing
- Fever
- Coarse crackles on auscultation
- Nasal flaring
- Grunting
- Head nodding.

PNEUMONIC CONSOLIDATION

- Acute onset with high fever, rusty sputum, chest pain and respiratory distress.
- No mediastinal shift
- Resonant on percussion
- Bronchial breath sounds on auscultation.

PNEUMOTHORAX

- Sudden onset
- Hyperresonance on percussion on ipsilateral side of the chest
- Shift in mediastinum to opposite side.

EFFUSION/EMPYEMA

- Stony dullness to percussion
- Air entry absent
- Shift in mediastinum to opposite side.

HYDROPNEUMOTHORAX

- Horizontal fluid level on chest X-ray
- Succussion splash
- Shifting dullness.

LUNG COLLAPSE

- Crowding of ribs, drooping of the shoulder and retraction of intercostals spaces; flat chest

- Shift of mediastinum to same side
- Impaired resonance on percussion; never stony dull
- Diminished breath sound.

PERICARDIAL EFFUSION

Considered only in left sided pleural effusion.

- JVP–Engorged and may be pulsatile. Kussmaul's sign present
- Pulsus paradoxus
- Muffled heart sounds
- Apex beat (if possible to localize) is medial to outer border of cardiac dullness.

LIVER ABSCESS

Considered only in right sided pleural effusion:

- Patient looks toxic; fever with chills
- Severe upper abdominal pain with right sided intercostal tenderness
- Upper border of liver dullness shifts upward.

FOREIGN BODY

- History of sudden onset of choking or wheezing
- Wheeze may be unilateral
- Air trapping with hyperresonance and mediastinal shift
- Signs of lung collapse: Reduced air entry and impaired percussion note
- No response to bronchodilators.

ASTHMA

- History of recurrent wheeze, some unrelated to coughs and colds
- Diurnal variation, seasonal variation
- Hyperinflation of the chest
- Prolonged expiration
- Reduced air entry (if very severe, airway obstruction)
- Good response to bronchodilators.

BRONCHIOLITIS

- First episode of wheeze in a child aged < 2 years
- Wheeze episode at time of seasonal bronchiolitis
- Hyperinflation of the chest
- Prolonged expiration
- Reduced air entry (if very severe, airway obstruction)
- Poor/no response to bronchodilators.

RETROPHARYNGEAL ABSCESS

- Soft tissue swelling
- Difficulty in swallowing
- Fever.

DIPHTHERIA

- Bull neck appearance due to enlarged cervical nodes and Edema
- Red throat
- Oral examination reveals grey pharyngeal membrane
- Blood-stained nasal discharge
- No history of DPT vaccination.

CARDIAC FAILURE

- Raised jugular venous pressure and enlarged palpable liver
- Apex beat displaced to the left
- Gallop rhythm
- Heart murmur
- Basal fine crackles
- Difficulty in feeding or breastfeeding.

CONGENITAL ANOMALY

- Stridor present since birth.

INVESTIGATIONS

- Complete blood count with ESR

- Chest X-ray (PA view):
  - Opacity with a curved upper border which is concave medially
  - Obliteration of costophrenic angle (earliest site of fluid collection)
  - Displacement of mediastinum to opposite side
  - Lateral view is done to differentiate it from lobar consolidation.
- Pleural tap for:
  - Confirmation of diagnosis
  - Examination of the nature of fluid: Transudate or exudate
  - Smear examination: Gram's stain, Ziel-Nelson stain
  - Culture (culture of *M. tuberculosis* in Lowenstein-Jensen media)
  - BACTEC gives result within 7 to 10 days:
- Ultrasound chest:
  - Differentiates pleural effusion from consolidation.
  - To localize effusion before aspiration or pleural biopsy.
- Sputum examination—Done on two consecutive days:
  - For demonstration of acid fast bacilli
  - To diagnose the etiology of pneumonia (if effusion develops from pneumonia).
- Mantoux test:
  - Positive in cases of tuberculosis.
- Fine needle aspiration cytology (FNAC) or excision biopsy of lymph nodes (axillary or cervical).

Confirmation of Diagnosis

- Chest X-ray: PA and lateral view, PLUS
- Aspiration of pleural fluid (absolute proof).

TREATMENT

An empyema is treated with parenteral antibiotics and prompt chest tube drainage.

- Antibiotics:
  - Empiric therapy is with:
    - Ceftriaxone (good gram-negative coverage) and
    - Cloxacillin (good Staphylococcus coverage) and
    - Gentamycin (good anerobic coverage) until a definitive organism is identified on pleural fluid cultures and sensitivities are obtained.
- Include vancomycin for Methicillin resistant *Staphylococcus aureus.*
- Pleural fluids or sputum specimens that are obtained should be cultured for *M. tuberculosis* as well.
- Antitubercular drug therapy: $2(HRZ)_3 + 4(HR)_3$ (If tuberculosis is etiology)
- Adequate drainage of pus by:
  - *Closed tube thoracostomy* at the most dependent part of empyema (chest tube insertion is avoided, if tuberculosis is etiology due to sinus formation):
    - Tube thoracostomy fails if:
      - Pus is too thick
      - Bronchopleural fistula develops
      - Pus is loculated.

  A chest drain should be inserted for early empyema. Late presenting empyema should be treated by decortication, if the patient is fit. The fibrous wall of empyema cavity is stripped off the parietal and visceral pleura in decortication.
- Fibrinolytic therapy.

Indication: Stage 2 of empyema (see discussion)

Dose:

- Streptokinase 15,000 units/kg in 50 ml of normal saline daily for 3-5 days
- Urokinase 40,000 units in 40 ml of normal saline twice daily for 6 doses
- Complication: Anaphylaxis, hemorrhage.

Procedure

The fibrinolytic substance is diluted in 100 ml saline and instilled via the chest tube. The tube is then clamped for 1-4 hours. The instillation is usually repeated once daily, and is continued for several days. After 1 to 4 hours, the catheters are unclamped and as much fluid as possible aspirated. The net amount of fluid is recorded.

- Open drainage with rib resection is done if the patient is unfit for decortication.
- Nutritional management.

DISCUSSION

DIAGNOSIS OF EMPYEMA IN ABSENCE OF PUS ASPIRATION

- Pleural fluid pH < 7.2
- Pleural fluid LDH > 1000 IU/L
- Pleural fluid glucose < 40 mg/L.

PLEURAL EFFUSION WITH MIDDLE TRACHEA

- Mild pleural effusion
- Loculated or encysted pleural effusion
- Bilateral pleural effusion
- Pleural effusion associated with old apical fibrosis (ipsilateral).

BRONCHIAL BREATHING

Tubular

- High-pitched
- Seen in:
  - Pneumonic consolidation
  - Collapsed lung or lobe when large draining bronchus is patent
  - Above the level of pleural effusion (in partially collapsed lung with patent bronchus).

Cavernous

- Low-pitched
- Seen in: Thick-walled cavity with a communicating bronchus

Amphoric

- Low-pitched, with a high tone and a metallic quality
- Seen in:
  - Large superficial smooth-walled cavity
  - Bronchopleural fistula
  - Tension pneumothorax.

VOCAL RESONANCE (FIG. 16.1)

Ask the child to say ninety-nine repeatedly and hear for the voice sound with the chest piece of the stethoscope. Types:

- *Bronchophony:* Voice sounds appear to be heard near the earpiece of stethoscope and words are unclear, e.g. consolidation, cavity communicating with a bronchus, above the level of pleural effusion. It is normally heard in proximity to trachea and larynx.
- *Aegophony:* When the intensity of spoken voice is increased and there is nasal quality, the auditory quality is called egophony. It has quality of sound produced by bleating of goat. Heard above the level of pleural effusion and pneumothorax.
- *Whispering pectoriloquy:* If bronchophony is extreme even a whisper can be heard, clearly through stethoscope as if uttered directly into the examiner's ear and is called as whispering pectoriloquy. It is heard in consolidation and Large cavity communicating with bronchus.

POSITION OF MEDIASTINUM

Center

- Pneumonia

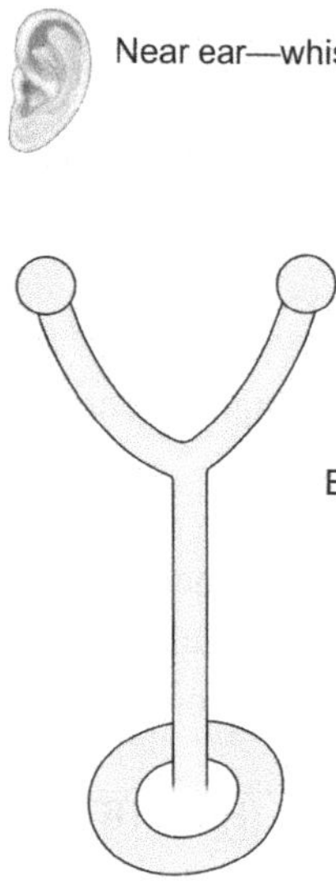

Fig. 16.1: Vocal resonance

- Emphysema
- Bronchiectasis
- Bronchial asthma.

Opposite Side

- Pneumothorax
- Pleural effusion
- Space occupying lesion (tumor).

Same Side

- Collapse
- Fibrosis
- Tactile vocal fremitus.

TACTILE VOCAL FRAMITUS

Increased

- Consolidation
- Superficial cavity

Decreased

- Pneumothorax
- Pleural effusion
- Lung collapse
- Bronchial obstruction.

FRICTION RUB

- Originates due to rubbing of the two inflamed and roughened surfaces of the pleura.
- It is a dry, crackly, grating low-pitched sound and is heard in both expiration and inspiration.
- Common site of pleural friction is the lower part of the axilla.
- Friction rub should be distinguished from crackles by the following points (Table 16.1.)

Table 16.1: Difference between friction rub and crackles

Friction rub	*Crackles*
• Superficial, scratchy sound	Deeper sound
• Associated with pleuritic pain	No pain
• Intensify with pressing stethoscope	No effect over the chest
• Does not alter with cough	Disappear or intensify following coughing

DULL NOTE ON PERCUSSION

Stony Dullness

- Pleural effusion
- Massive collapse consolidation.

Impaired Note

- Bronchopneumonia
- Collapse
- Thickened pleura
- Fibrosis
- Abscess.

DIFFERENCE BETWEEN TRANSUDATE AND EXUDATE

Pleural Exudate

- Protein > 2.5 gm%
- LDH > 200 IU

- Ratio of pleural fluid protein to serum protein > 0.5
- Ratio of pleural fluid LDH to serum LDH > 0.6.

Pleural Transudate

- Protein < 2.5 gm%
- LDH < 200 IU
- Ratio of pleural fluid protein to serum protein <0.5
- Ratio of pleural fluid LDH to serum LDH < 0.6.

DIFFERENCE BETWEEN EMPYEMA AND PARAPNEMONIC EFFUSION

Empyema

- pH < 7.2
- Pleural fluid sugar < 40
- LDH > 1000 IU/L.

Parapnemonic Effusion

- pH > 7.2
- Pleural fluid sugar > 60
- LDH < 1000 IU/L.

CAUSES OF PLEURAL EFFUSION

Transudates

- Congestive cardiac failure
- Anemia
- Nephrotic syndrome
- Hypoproteinemia.

Exudates

- Tuberculosis
- Lung abscess
- Bronchiectasis
- Pneumonia
- Neoplasm
- Trauma.

In tuberculosis, exudate is much more common (because of direct affection of pleura), however transudate is also present in the form of an allergic manifestation.

PATHOLOGICAL STAGES IN THE DEVELOPMENT OF PNEUMONIA

- Stage of congestion—Fine crackles heard
- Stage of red hepatization—Tubular type of bronchial breathing heard
- Stage of gray hepatization—Tubular type of bronchial breathing heard
- Stage of resolution—Coarse crackles heard.

CLASSIFICATION OF EMPYEMA (AMERICAN THORACIC SOCIETY)

Stage 1. Exudative with swelling of the pleural membranes.

Stage 2. Fibrinopurulent with heavy fibrin deposits.

Stage 3. Organization with ingrowth of fibroblasts and deposition of collagen.

CAUSES OF RECURRENT PNEUMONIA

- Foreign body
- Sequestration of lung
- Bronchiectasis
- Neoplasia (benign or malignant).

SPECIAL CHARACTERISTICS OF VARIOUS PNEUMONIAE

Pneumococcal pneumonia

- Production of rusty sputum is characteristic and the patient may be icteric.

- It usually involves a lobe and pleuritic reaction is common.

Staphylococcal pneumonia

- This is common in cystic fibrosis and influenza.
- Multiple, thin-walled staphylococcal abscesses are common (pneumatoceles).
- Pneumothorax is a complication.
- It occurs in extremes of age and in immunosuppressed patients.

Klebsiella pneumonia

- Massive consolidation and excavation of upper lobe with expectoration of chocolate colored sputum (brick red currant jelly).
- Lobes characteristically increase in size and it simulates tuberculosis.
- Pneumatoceles are common.

Legionella pneumonia

- This is transmitted through infected water from cisterns, vapor or ventilation systems.
- Patient is toxic with hemoptysis; CNS or renal problems, myoglobinuria, may be present.
- Diagnosis by serology or immunofluorescence.

Viral pneumonia (Atypical pneumonia)

- Prodromal symptoms precede the onset of pneumonia by one week.
- Despite extensive radiological findings, respiratory signs and symptoms are minimal. Hemoptysis and parapneumonic effusions are rare.
- Common viruses causing pneumonia are Varicella, H. simplex, CMV, measles, influenza, adenovirus and RSV.

Mycoplasma pneumonia

- Presents with dry cough, erythema multiforme, arthralgia, myalgia.
- Predilection to lower lobe.
- Cold agglutinins positive.

Pneumonia due to Chlamydia

- Patient has pneumonia, systemic illness, hepatosplenomegaly.
- Patchy consolidation is common.
- Diagnosed by serology.

Nosocomial pneumonia

- Pneumonia developing in a patient who has been hospitalized for > 48 hours.
- Infection by *Staph. aureus*, Pseudomonas and anaerobes are common.

Table 16.2: IMNCI classification of cough or difficult breathing

Signs and symptoms		*Classification*	*Therapy*
• No signs of pneumonia OR very severe disease		No pneumonia Cough or cold	If coughing more than 30 days-refer for assessment Soothe the throat and relieve cough with safe remedy Advice mother when to return immediately Follow-up in 2 days
• Fast breathing *RR/min* 60 or more 50 or more 40 or more	 *Age* <2 months 2-12 months 12-60 months	Pneumonia	Cotrimoxazole OR Amoxycillin Soothe the throat and relieve cough with safe remedy Advice mother when to return immediately Follow-up in 2 days
• Any general danger sign Lower Chest indrawing Stridor in calm child		Severe pneumonia or very severe disease	Give first dose of appropriate antibiotic Refer urgently to hospital

CAUSES OF UNRESOLVED PNEUMONIAE

- Incorrect microbiologic diagnosis
- Inadequate dose or wrong choice of antibiotics
- Endobronchial obstruction (poor local host defences)
- Immunocompromised states (disease or drugs)
- Malignancy.

INDICATIONS FOR CHEST TUBE INSERTION

- Grossly purulent pleural fluid
- pH level less than 7.2
- WBC count greater than 50,000 cells/μl (or polymorphonuclear leukocyte count of 1,000 IU/dl)
- Glucose level less than 40 mg/dl
- Lactate dehydrogenase level greater than 1,000 IU/ml
- Positive pleural fluid culture
- Decubitus chest X-ray fluid thickness >1 cm
- LDH pleural fluid serum ratio >0.6
- Proteins pleural fluid serum ratio >0.5
- A pleural fluid marker currently being studied is tumor necrosis factor (TNF)–alpha. In patients who have pleural effusions, a TNF-alpha level higher than 80 pg/mL is suggestive of an empyema or complicated parapneumonic effusion.

INDICATIONS FOR CHEST TUBE REMOVAL

- Clinical improvement with resolution of fever and leukocytosis is desirable. However, if alternate source of fever is apparent (i.e. persistent pneumonia), it is not necessary that the white blood cell count be normal and the patient afebrile.
- Radiographic evaluation of drainage of pleural fluid.
- Not more than 20 ml of net drain output over a 24-hour period.

PNEUMOTHORAX

History and examination are almost similar to pleural effusion with stress on following points:

SYMPTOMS

- Respiratory distress
- Pain in the chest
- Fever.

GENERAL PHYSICAL EXAMINATION

- Decubitus—propped-up position
- Respiration—abdominothoracic, less movement on side of pneumothorax
- Cyanosis
- Febrile.

SYSTEMIC EXAMINATION

RESPIRATORY SYSTEM EXAMINATION

Inspection

- Full intercostal spaces
- Diminished ipsilateral movement
- Shift of apical impulse.

Palpation

- Diminished movement on ipsilateral side
- Trachea and apex beat is shifted towards opposite side

- Vocal fremitus is diminished (or absent)
- Normal resonant note on percussion over opposite side of the chest
- Subcutaneous emphysema (pneumomediastinum).

Auscultation

- Breath sounds diminished
- Vocal resonance diminished.

INVESTIGATIONS

- Chest X-ray—both inspiratory and expiratory films are taken.
  - Increased radiolucency with absence of lung markings.
  - Collapsed lung is seen as a homogeneous opacity with sharp outline.
  - Shifting of mediastinum towards opposite side.
  - Costophrenic angles are clear.
- Blood—lymphocytosis with high ESR point towards tuberculosis.
- Mantoux test.
- Sputum for AFB is done for consecutive three days.

TREATMENT

- *Small pneumothorax (less symptoms)*: Air is absorbed spontaneously within few days and no treatment is required. Small pneumothorax needs close observation.
- *Large pneumothorax or tension pneumothorax*: O_2 inhalation and propped-up position. Thoracostomy tube is inserted into the pleural cavity in the second intercostals space along the midclavicular line (preferable) or in the fourth or fifth intercostals space behind the anterior axillary fold (more comfortable and cosmetic for a female patient). If no bubbling is seen for 24 hours or the patient is relieved of dyspnea or the chest X-ray shows complete re-expansion of lung, the tube is removed. The whole process takes approximately 3 to 4 days.
- *Recurrent spontaneous pneumothorax:* Chemical pleurodesis is done by kaolin, talcom, minocycline, 50% glucose solution, iodized oil.
- Antituberculosis chemotherapy, whenever indicated.
- Antibiotics to prevent secondary infection.
- *Surgery*: For open pneumothorax.
- Thoracoscopy and cauterization of the breach in the pleura or excision of the bulla.
- Pleurectomy (in recurrent type when pleurodesis fails).
- Decortication and closure of bronchopleural fistula, lobectomy or thoracoplasty.
- The rate of reabsorption of air is about 1.25% of the total radiographic area per day and thus a 50% pneumothorax (occupying 50% of hemithorax) may take 4 to 6 weeks to resolve totally.

Immediate Management of Tension Pneumothorax

- O_2 inhalation and propped-up position.
- Do not wait for the chest X-ray and immediately insert a wide-bore needle into the pleural space through the second intercostals space at midclavicular line. If large amount of gas escapes from the needle, the diagnosis is confirmed and the patient is relieved. The needle should be left in place until a water-seal drainage system can be arranged at the earliest opportunity. If tension penumothorax is dealt in this way, circulatory collapse can be prevented.
- Treatment of shock and circulatory collapse, if present.

Patency of Water-Seal Drainage

- Bubbling occurs, during expiration or coughing
- Water column ascends during inspiration.

Types of pneumothorax

- **Traumatic**
  - Chest trauma, pleural or lung biopsy, pericardiocentesis, bronchoscopy
- **Spontaneous**
  - Develops without antecedent trauma
  - *Closed*
    - Due to rupture of emphysematous bulla or subpleural tuberculous focus.
    - Dyspnea not very severe
    - Infection of pleural space does not occur
    - Mediastinal shift present
  - *Open*
    - Free communication between pleural space and the bronchus (bronchopleural fistula).
    - Infection of the pleural space (pyopneumothorax)
    - Due to tuberculous cavity/ lung abscess/ apical sub-pleural bleb/ penetrating wound.
    - Dyspnea present
    - Mediastinal shift present
  - *Tension*
    - Check-valve allows air to enter into the pleural cavity during inspiration but prevents escape during expiration.
    - Severe dyspnea with mediastinal shift

- Tube should be changed *weekly* (always remove after clamping it) and water should be changed every 48 hours.

DISCUSSION

PNEUMOTHORAX IN RELATION TO ATMOSPHERIC PRESSURE

- *Closed type:* Intrapleural pressure < Atmospheric pressure.
- *Open type:* Intrapleural pressure = Atmospheric pressure.
- *Tension:* Intrapleural pressure > Atmospheric pressure.

CHAPTER 17

Gastrointestinal System

Hepatosplenomegaly

HISTORY

CHIEF COMPLAINTS

- Progressive paleness/Yellowness of body
- Swelling over body
- Fever
- Bleeding.

HISTORY OF PRESENT ILLNESS

History of Disease

The history should be elicited keeping in mind following clinical points:

- Lump in the abdomen
- Abdominal distension
- Fever
- Jaundice
- Pallor
- Edema
- Bleeding manifestations
- Swelling in the neck
- Feeding difficulties
- Convulsions
- Developmental delay
- Reduced vision and speech.

Fever

- Onset: Sudden, insidious
- Associated with chills and rigor
- Associated with sweating
- Documented or not
- Intermittent, remittent, continuous
- History of convulsions associated with fever
- History of immunization.

Diarrhea

- Acute onset or persistent
- Frequency of stools
- Accompanied by blood or mucus
- Presence of tenesmus (painful urgency is seen in invasive diarrhea)
- Presence of foul smelling, bulky stool difficult to flush (malabsorption, cystic fibrosis)
- Associated with abdominal pain or vomiting
- Ingestion of unusual food (food poisoning)
- Urine output (assess severity of dehydration)
- Use of antibiotics.

Vomiting

- Frequency
- Time of occurrence
- Projectile or non-projectile
- Content of vomitus
- Antecedent symptoms:
  - Abdominal pain, diarrhea (GIT problem)
  - Headache (intracranial space occupying lesion, meningitis)
  - Cough (posttussive vomiting)
  - Urinary symptoms (fever and vomiting may be due to urinary tract infection)
  - Ear symptoms (vertigo)
  - Abdominal distension (surgical cause).
- Urine output
- Jaundice
- Association with history of drug intake.

Jaundice

- Present from birth and progressively increasing (biliary atresia)
- Anemia (hemolytic cause)
- Color of stool (clay colored suggests obstructive cause), urine (dark urine suggests cholestasis), sclera
- Anorexia and vomiting (hepatitis)
- Itching (obstructive cause)
- Abdominal pain (gallstones)
- Drug ingestion (antitubercular)
- Source of water, drug injection, blood transfusion, contact with jaundice patient (infective hepatitis)
- Playing in rat infested area (leptospirosis).

Hematemesis

- Epigastric pain (acid peptic disease)
- Bleeding diathesis
- Drug ingestion (aspirin, steroids)
- Jaundice (liver disease)
- Swallowed blood in vomitus.

Abdominal Pain

- Site of pain, intensity, type of pain, mode of onset
- Aggravating or relieving factors
- Radiation
- Associated symptoms (dysuria, vomiting, diarrhea)
- Associated diarrhea (enterocolitis)
- Recent introduction of any new food (food allergy)
- History of rashes (Henoch-schönlein purpura).

History of Complications

- Edema feet, pain abdomen, difficulty in respiration, feeding difficulties, failure to thrive (congestive cardiac failure)
- Bleeding—Petechiae (< 2 mm), purpura (2-10 mm), ecchymosis (>10 mm) (thrombocytopenia) [liver cell failure]
- Pallor (anemia), fever (infection) [to look for hypersplenism]
- Delayed milestones, myoclonic seizures, incoordination, reduced vision and hearing (storage disorders).

FAMILY HISTORY

- *Consanguinity*: Important in hemolytic anemia, Wilson's disease and inborn errors of metabolism.

GENERAL PHYSICAL EXAMINATION

- Vitals
- Anthropometry
- Facies (hemolytic facies, butterfly rash in SLE)
- Pallor (cirrhosis/thalassemia)
- Clubbing/cyanosis/edema feet
- Lymphadenopathy (lymphoma/leukemia/ infectious mononucleosis)

- ❖ Jaundice (cirrhosis/thalassemia)
- ❖ Petechial hemorrhages
- ❖ Leg ulcers (congenital hemolytic anemia)
- ❖ Sternal tenderness (acute leukemia)
- ❖ Anterior fontanelle – Delayed closure seen in Toxoplasmosis (hydrocephalus)
- ❖ Eyes:
  - ❒ Cataract (Intrauterine infections, galactosemia)
  - ❒ K-F ring (Wilson's disease)
  - ❒ Chorioretinitis (Intrauterine infections)
  - ❒ Iridocyclitis (Juveline rheumatoid arthritis)
  - ❒ Phlycten (tuberculosis).
- ❖ Signs of liver cell failure:
  - ❒ Fetor hepaticus
  - ❒ Parotid enlargement
  - ❒ Spider nevi.
- ❖ Signs of portal hypertension:
  - ❒ Ascites
  - ❒ Splenomegaly
  - ❒ Dilated veins over abdomen
  - ❒ Caput medusae
  - ❒ Esophageal varices.
- ❖ Signs of vitamin A deficiency:
- ❖ Conjunctival/Corneal xerosis
- ❖ Bitot's spots.
- ❖ Signs of vitamin B deficiency:
  - ❒ Angular stomatitis
  - ❒ Cheilosis.
- ❖ Signs of vitamin D deficiency – Rickets.
- ❖ Signs of vitamin E deficiency – Petechiae, purpura.

SYSTEMIC EXAMINATION

ABDOMEN EXAMINATION

Abdomen is divided into 9 quadrants by 2 vertical and 2 horizontal lines.

Vertical lines: Two vertical lines are drawn passing through the tips of both the ninth costal cartilages above and the femoral arteries below.

Horizontal lines: First horizontal line passes through lowest points of both the costal margins while the second horizontal line passes through both the iliac tubercles.

9 quadrants of abdomen from above downwards are:

i. Right hypochondrium, epigastric and left hypochondrium;
ii. Right lumbar, umbilical and left lumbar;
iii. Right iliac, suprapubic and left iliac.

Inspection

- *Skin and subcutaneous tissue:*
  - ❖ Any visible abdominal lump
  - ❖ If superficial veins are engorged—their location.
- *Umbilicus*—everted (ascites): Displaced upwards or downwards by ascites or swelling.
- *Contour of abdomen:*
  - ❖ Movements—visible
  - ❖ Peristaltic or any pulsatile movement
  - ❖ Look for liver biopsy mark, ascitic tap mark, bone marrow biopsy mark.

Palpation

- Temperature
- Tenderness or hyperesthesia
- Consistency of feel (normal elastic feel, muscle guard or rigidity)
- Localized lump
- Fluid thrill with girth of the abdomen at the level of the umbilicus
- If superficial veins are engorged—their direction of blood flow; empty the vein of blood by placing two fingers side by side over the vein.

Move one finger away while keeping the other fixed.

Now, release the finger one by one to see the direction through which the blood fills the vein. If direction of flow of blood is towards the umbilicus, it suggests inferior vena cava obstruction while the direction of blood flow away from the umbilicus suggests portal hypertension.

- Superficial and deep palpation to look for any tenderness: Tenderness is pain elicited by the palpating hand when pressure is applied to the abdomen wall. It is a sign that the peritoneum under the abdominal wall or the underlying organ is inflamed.
- Rebound tenderness is pain elicited when pressure applied to the abdomen wall by the palpating hand is suddenly released. It is a sign that the underlying peritoneum is inflamed.

Description of Splenomegaly

- Enlarged….. cm below the left costal margin along its long axis and has crossed the umbilicus towards the right iliac fossa
- Nontender (tenderness is seen in splenic infarction, especially in a very big spleen)
- Presence of notch in the anterior border
- Consistency: Firm, soft
- Moves freely with respiration
- Surface: Smooth, nodular
- Margin: Sharp, rounded
- Fingers cannot be insinuated between the spleen and the left costal arch
- Neither bimanually palpable nor ballottable
- No colonic resonance over the mass
- No splenic rub (present in case of splenic infarction)
- Auscultate for any bruit.

Description of Hepatomegaly

- Enlarged…. cm below the right costal margin at right MCL
- Upper border of liver dullness is at right 5th ICS at right MCL
- Moving with respiration
- Nontender
- Surface: Smooth, granular, nodular
- Consistency: Soft, firm, hard
- Margins: Sharp, rounded
- Left lobe is not palpable
- No pulsation/rub/bruit.

Percussion

- During abdomen percussion, always proceed from a tympanitic or resonant site towards a dull site. The middle finger should be positioned, so that it receives the strike parallel to the anticipated border and not perpendicular to it.
- To delineate the liver borders, start percussing along the mid-clavicular line at the 4th intercostal space. The percussion note will change from resonant to dull at the 5th intercostal space where the upper border of the liver normally lies. This dullness will continue till the lower border of liver which is just below the costal margin in a normal subject.

Puddle Sign

If the fluid in the peritoneal cavity is minimal, make patient prone so that, he bears weight over his knees and elbows and the abdomen is off the couch. When the patient assumes this posture, the fluid gravitates down around the centre and percussion over the umbilicus will give a dull note.

Fluid thrill

Fluid thrill is demonstrable only if a large volume of ascitic fluid is present.

1. Lay the subject supine and place one hand flat against his flank on one side.
2. Ask an assistant to place the ulnar aspect of his hand firmly in the midline of the abdomen.

3. Now, tap the opposite flank of the abdomen with your other hand. If ascitic fluid is present, the impulse generated by the tap will be transmitted to your hand on the flank. The hand on the abdomen is to prevent transmission of the impulse through the subcutaneous fat of the abdominal wall.

Shifting Dullness

1. Expose the abdomen and ask the child to lie supine. Keep the plexor finger perpendicular to the mid-line at a point between the xiphisternum and umbilicus. Percussing here, normally elicits a resonant note.
2. Percuss downwards from this point towards the umbilicus up to suprapubic region. The note should remain resonant. A dullness suggests an underlying full urinary bladder. Ask the child to void so that the bladder becomes empty.
3. After the percussion note at the umbilicus is resonant, keep the plexor finger at the umbilicus in the direction of the midline.
4. Start percussing from the umbilicus and go laterally towards the right or the left flank.
5. If the note remains resonant throughout up to the flanks, this indicates absence of significant fluid in the peritoneal cavity. A dull note in the dependent flanks suggests presence of fluid because of gravitation.
6. If the flanks are dull, turn the patient towards the opposite side without removing your plexor finger. Wait for some time to let the fluid shift to the other flank because of gravitv. Percuss again over the same area. A resonant note now confirms that the fluid has shifted to the dependent area.

Auscultation

Auscultation is generally done over the abdomen to hear the bowel sounds. They are exaggerated in intestinal obstruction. The abdomen will be silent in patients of ileus or peritonitis.

A renal bruit should be heard in patients with renal artery stenosis like hypertension or arteritis.

CARDIOVASCULAR SYSTEM

- Effect of anemia on CVS with special reference to hemic murmur
- Look for features of heart failure.

RESPIRATORY SYSTEM

- Occasional rhonchi and crepitations due to respiratory tract infection
- Fundus examination is must.

DIAGNOSIS

Mild/moderate/severe hepatomegaly; with/without splenomegaly (mild/moderate/severe); with/without ascites; with/without signs of liver cell failure; with/without icterus; with/without pallor; with/without signs of PEM Grade———— by IAP Classification;
Most probable etiology being ————

DIFFERENTIAL DIAGNOSIS

PAINFUL HEPATOMEGALY

- *Hepatitis*
  - Lethargy, anorexia, and malaise
  - Elevation of ALT (SGPT) levels
  - Physical examination, shows icterus and tender hepatomegaly.
- *Congestive cardiac failure*
  - Fatigue, effort intolerance, anorexia, abdominal pain, dyspnea, and cough
  - Elevated jugular venous pressure, liver enlargement, tachypnea and tachycardia
  - Orthopnea, crepitations and rhonchi are generally present

- ❖ Edema is seen in dependent portions of the body
- ❖ Cardiomegaly and gallop rhythm.

- *Pyogenic/amebic liver abscess*
  - ❖ Fever, chills, night sweats, malaise, fatigue, nausea, abdominal pain
  - ❖ Right upper quadrant tenderness, Hepatomegaly and jaundice
  - ❖ Ultrasound or CT scan can confirm diagnosis.
- *Hepatoblastoma*
  - ❖ Presents as large, asymptomatic abdominal mass
  - ❖ Weight loss, anorexia, vomiting, and abdominal pain may be present.
  - ❖ Metastatic spread involves regional lymph nodes and the lungs.
  - ❖ α-fetoprotein (AFP), is used for diagnosis and monitoring.

HEPATOMEGALY

1. Infective:
   - *Hepatitis* (see above)
   - *Typhoid*:
     - ❖ High-grade fever
     - ❖ Generalized myalgia, abdominal pain, hepatosplenomegaly and anorexia.
     - ❖ In children, diarrhea is present in initial stages, followed by constipation.
     - ❖ Positive widal test or blood culture can help.
   - *Tuberculosis:*
     - ❖ Gradual onset with vague ill health, high fever with sweats and loss of weight
     - ❖ Cough, breathlessness and anorexia
     - ❖ Tachycardia, paucity of signs in chest
     - ❖ Mild to moderate hepatosplenomegaly.
   - *Amebic/pyogenic liver abscess* (see above)
   - *Hydatid cyst:*
     - ❖ Mass effect leading to pain, obstruction of adjacent organs
     - ❖ Nodular liver enlargement
     - ❖ History of contact with animals
     - ❖ Less commonly, secondary bacterial infection, distal spread of daughter cysts.
2. Hematological:
   - *Associated with anemia*
   - *Sickle-cell disease*
     - ❖ Most children have functional asplenia
     - ❖ Recurrent bacterial infection (*Streptococcus pneumoniae*; *Haemophilus influenzae* type B)
     - ❖ Red cell aplasia (parvovirus B19 infection)
     - ❖ Acute chest syndrome, glomerulonephritis, and stroke are commonly seen.
     - ❖ Dactylitis, Priapism.
3. Metabolic: (see text)
   - *Glycogen storage disease (III, VI and IX)*
   - *Tyrosinemia*
   - *Galactosemia*
   - *Mucopolysaccharidosis.*
4. Malignancy:
   - *Hepatoblastoma* (see above)
5. Drug-induced hepatitis:
   - Isoniazid
   - Sulfonamides
   - Nitrofurantoin
   - Dapsone
   - Methyldopa.
6. Fatty liver: Kwashiorkor (firm liver with normal transaminase levels, diagnosis by biopsy).
7. Cirrhosis.
8. Congestive cardiac failure (see above).

MILD SPLENOMEGALY

- *Infective endocarditis*
  - Prolonged fever, myalgia, arthralgia, headache, chills, nausea and vomiting.
  - New or changing heart murmurs.
  - Splenomegaly and petechiae.
  - Neurologic complications like embolic strokes, cerebral abscesses, mycotic aneurysms, and hemorrhage.
  - Skin manifestations: Osler nodes (tender, pea-sized intradermal nodules in pads of fingers and toes), Janeway lesions (painless small erythematous or hemorrhagic lesions on palms and soles), and splinter hemorrhages (linear lesions beneath the nails). These lesions represent vasculitis due to circulating antigen-antibody complexes.
- *Typhoid* (see above)
- *Septicemia*
  - Alterations in temperature regulation (hyperthermia or hypothermia), tachycardia, and tachypnea.
  - Decreased cardiac output: Hypotension, delayed capillary refill, diminished peripheral and central pulses, cool extremities, and decreased urine output.
  - Alterations in mental status: Confusion, agitation, lethargy, anxiety or coma.
  - Lactic acidosis occurs as shock progresses.
- *Early stages of hemolytic anemia/leukemia*

MODERATE–MASSIVE SPLENOMEGALY

1. Infective:
   - *Chronic malaria*
     - Symptoms vary: Fever, headache, drowsiness, anorexia, vomiting, diarrhea, pallor, cyanosis, splenomegaly, hepatomegaly, anemia, thrombocytopenia, a normal or low leukocyte count, or combination of these.
     - Cerebral malaria is characterized by a depressed level of consciousness, seizures, irregular respirations, hypoxia, hypotension, tachycardia, dehydration, hypoglycemia, metabolic acidosis, and hyperkalemia.
   - *Kala-azar*
     - High fever, marked splenomegaly, hepatomegaly and severe cachexia.
     - Gross wasting, pancytopenia and jaundice, edema, and ascites may be present.
     - Anemia may be severe enough to precipitate heart failure.
     - Bleeding episodes, especially epistaxis, are frequent.
2. Hematological:
   - *Hemolytic anemia*
   - *Thalassemia major/intermedia*
     - Normal at birth and manifest during second 6 month of life
     - Persistent and progressive pallor
     - Splenohepatomegaly
     - Jaundice
     - Facio skeletal changes
     - Skin changes
     - Leg ulcer
     - Growth retardation.
3. Metabolic disease: *Gaucher's disease* (see text)
4. Malignancy:
   - *Hodgkin's disease*
     - Commonly cervical group is involved first then gradual painless lymphadenopathy
     - Discrete, rubbery or firm, non-tender lymphadenopathy

- ❖ Fever, night sweats, loss of weight
- ❖ Hepatosplenomegaly.
- *Chronic myeloid leukemia*

5. Congestive:
   - *Portal hypertension*
     - ❖ Most commonly: Bleeding esophageal varices
     - ❖ Jaundice and stigmata of cirrhosis such as palmar erythema and vascular telangiectasias
     - ❖ Ascites present in intrahepatic causes of portal hypertension
     - ❖ Splenomegaly, may be seen first.
6. Idiopathic.

HEPATOSPLENOMEGALY WITH ASCITES

- Abdominal or disseminated TB (see above)
- Cirrhosis with portal hypertension (see above)
- Congestive cardiac failure (see above)
- Malignancy.

HEPATOSPLENOMEGALY WITH PALLOR

1. Infective
   - *Malaria*
   - *Disseminated tuberculosis*
   - *Infective endocarditis*
   - *Kala-azar.*
2. Hematological
   - *Thalassemia*
   - *Sickle-cell anemia*
   - *Hereditary spherocytosis.*
     - ❖ Anemia, jaundice, fatigue, and exercise intolerance.
     - ❖ Extramedullary hematopoiesis.
     - ❖ Splenomegaly and pigmentary (bilirubin) gallstones may form as early as age 4-5 years.
     - ❖ Aplastic crisis, primarily as a result of parvovirus infection.
3. Metabolic
   - *Wilsons' disease*
     - ❖ Asymptomatic hepatomegaly (with or without splenomegaly)
     - ❖ Hepatic dysfunction: Cirrhosis, portal hypertension, ascites, edema, variceal bleeding.
     - ❖ Neurologic disorders: Intention tremor, dysarthria, dystonia, lack of motor coordi-nation, deterioration in school performance, or behavioral changes.
     - ❖ Kayser-Fleischer rings uncommon with liver disease but always present with neurologic symptoms.
     - ❖ Psychiatric manifestations: Depression, anxiety, or psychosis.
   - *Gaucher's disease*
4. Malignancy
   - *Leukemia*
     - ❖ Fever may be very high
     - ❖ Discrete, non-tender adenopathy
     - ❖ Moderate splenomegaly with hepatomegaly
     - ❖ *Anemia:* Pallor, fatigue, tachycardia, dyspnea and occasional cardiovascular decompensation
     - ❖ *Leukopenia:* Low to marked temperature elevation with infections
     - ❖ *Thrombocytopenia:* Petechiae, mucosal bleeding and epistaxis
     - ❖ Presence of sternal tenderness, bone pains.
   - *Lymphoma*
5. Cirrhosis with portal hypertension (see above)
6. Collagen-vascular disease
   - *Systemic lupus erythematous*
   - *Juveline rheumatoid arthritis*
     - ❖ Hemolytic anemia is the first possibility. It is rather a splenohepatomegaly

- Family history, early age of onset, repeated transfusions and hemolytic facies point towards congenital hemolytic anemia.

HEPATOSPLENOMEGALY WITH ICTERUS

1. Infective:
   - *Hepatitis* (see above)
   - *Disseminated TB* (icterus is more due to anti TB drugs)
     - High rise of temperature with drenching sweats, loss of weight, progressive anemia, cough.
     - Matted, painless lymphadenopathy but may be associated with cold abscess.
     - Paucity of signs in the chest. Often few crepitations are heard late in the disease.
     - Mild hepatomegaly with mild, tender splenomegaly
     - Choroidal tubercles seen in the retina by ophthalmoscopy.
   - *Malaria* (see above)
2. Hematological:
   - *Thalassemia* (jaundice mild due to hepatobiliary system becoming adjusted to continous low-grade hemolysis)
   - *Hereditary spherocytosis* (see above)
3. Metabolic:
   - *Galactosemia* (see text)
   - α-1 *antitrypsin* deficiency
     - Chronic pulmonary symptoms, including dyspnea, wheezing, cough, and emphysema
     - Growth failure, increased antero-posterior diameter of chest and clubbing
     - Emphysema depresses diaphragm, making the liver and spleen palpable
     - α_1-antitrypsin levels decreased (normal serum levels are 180-280 mg/dl)
     - Chest CT: Hyperexpansion in the lower lung zones, with bronchiectasis.
4. Malignancy:
   - *Leukemia* (see above)
   - *Lymphoma* (see above)
5. Cirrhosis
6. Drugs:
   - *Anti-tubercular drugs*
   - *Anticonvulsants*.

HEPATOSPLENOMEGALY WITH BLEEDING MANIFESTATIONS

1. Infective
   - *Viral hemorrhagic fever like dengue, septicemia*
   - *Intrauterine infections* (see text).
2. Hematological
   - *Chronic ITP* (splenomegaly unlikely in acute ITP)
   - *Thalassemia* (petechiae secondary to hypersplenism) (see above)
   - *Henoch-Schönlein purpura*
     - Rash, characterized as palpable purpuras
       Local angioedema (due to damage to cutaneous vessels)
     - Arthritis, usually localized to the knees and ankles.
     - Colicky abdominal pain (damage to the vasculature of the gastrointestinal tract)
     - Renal involvement manifest with hematuria, proteinuria, nephritis or acute renal failure.
3. Malignancy:
   - *Leukemia* (see above)
   - *Lymphoma* (see above).

4. Cirrhosis with hypersplenism (see above)
5. Metabolic
   - *Gaucher's Disease*
     - Neuroregression (due to accumulation of glycosphingolipids in CNS)
     - Hepatosplenomegaly (due to accumulation of glycosphingolipids in visceral cells)
     - Skeletal abnormalities
     - Bleeding manifestations due to thrombocytopenia
     - Chronic fatigue due to anemia
     - Bone pain or pathologic fractures (in 20%).
   - *Niemann-Pick Disease*
     - History of prolonged neonatal jaundice
     - Neuroregression
     - Hepatosplenomegaly
     - Moderate lymphadenopathy.

HEPATOSPLENOMEGALY WITH LYMPHADENOPATHY

1. Infective
   - *Disseminated* TB (see above)
   - *HIV*
     - History of receiving blood transfusion or presence of HIV in parents
     - Persistent generalized lymphadenopathy, chronic diarrhea, weight loss and oral candidiasis.
     - Rapid downhill course
     - Biopsy of lymph nodes shows reactive hyperplasia
   - *Toxoplasmosis (see text)*
   - *Kala-azar (see above).*
2. Hematological: *Thalassemia* (see above)
3. Malignancy
   - *Leukemia* (see above)
   - *Lymphoma* (see above)
   - *Histocytosis.*
4. Drugs
   - *Phenytoin*
   - *Dapsone.*
5. Collagen vascular disorder: *SLE, JRA.*

METABOLIC DISORDERS

Glycogen Storage Disease

Type I (glucose-6-phosphatase or translocase deficiency, von gierke disease):

- Neonate with hypoglycemia, lactic acidosis, hepatomegaly and hypoglycemic seizures.
- Doll-like facies with fat cheeks, thin extremities, short stature, protuberant abdomen due to massive hepatomegaly; kidneys enlarged, whereas the spleen and heart are normal.

Type III (debrancher deficiency, limit dextrinosis):

- Indistinguishable from type I GSD because hepatomegaly, hypoglycemia, hyperlipidemia, and growth retardation are common.
- Splenomegaly may be present, but the kidneys are not enlarged.
- Definite diagnosis requires enzyme assay in liver, muscle, or mutation analysis.

Type IV (branching enzyme deficiency, amylopectinosis, or andersen disease)

- The most common and classic form.
- Cirrhosis manifests as hepatosplenomegaly, failure to thrive and progresses to portal hypertension, ascites, esophageal varices, and liver failure that usually leads to death by 5 years of age.
- *Diagnosis:* Demonstration of the deficient branching enzyme activity in liver, muscle, cultured skin fibroblasts, or leukocytes.

Tyrosinemia

Tyrosinemia Type I

- Fever, irritability, vomiting, hemorrhage, hepatomegaly, jaundice, elevated levels of serum transaminases, and hypoglycemia are common.
- Odor resembling boiled cabbage, due to increased methionine metabolites.
- Episodes of acute peripheral neuropathy resembling acute porphyria characterized by severe pain in legs, associated with hypertonic posturing of the head and trunk, vomiting, paralytic ileus, and, occasionally, self-induced injuries of the tongue or buccal mucosa.
- Renal involvement is manifested as a Fanconi-like syndrome with normal anion gap metabolic acidosis,hyperphosphaturia, hypophosphatemia, and vitamin D-resistant rickets.
- Diagnosis-elevated levels of succinylacetone in urine or blood. Succinylacetone, which is not detected by the current screening methods, is the preferable initial metabolite tested.

Tyrosinemia Type II

- Ocular manifestations of excessive tearing, redness, pain, and photophobia often occur before skin lesions. Corneal lesions are presumed to be due to tyrosine deposition.
- Skin lesions, include painful, nonpruritic hyperkeratotic plaques on the soles, palms, and fingertips.
- Mental retardation occurs in 50% of patients.
- Diagnosis is established by assay of plasma tyrosine concentration.

Alcaptonuria

- Ochronosis and arthritis, occurs in adulthood.
- The only sign of the disorder in children is a blackening of the urine on standing. This is caused by oxidation and polymerization of the homogentisic acid.
- The diagnosis is confirmed by finding massive excretion of homogentisic acid in urine.

Galactosemia

Milk and dairy products contain lactose, the major dietary source of galactose.

Galactosemia denotes the elevated level of galactose in the blood: galactose-1-phosphate uridyl transferase, galactokinase, and uridine diphosphate galactose-4-epimerase. The term *galactosemia,* generally designates the transferase deficiency.

Galactose-1-phosphate Uridyl Transferase Deficiency (Galactosemia)

- Suspected in newborn or young infants with: Jaundice, hepatomegaly, vomiting, hypoglycemia, convulsions, lethargy, irritability, feeding difficulties, poor weight gain, aminoaciduria, cataracts, liver cirrhosis, ascites, splenomegaly, or mental retardation.
- Symptoms improve when milk is temporarily withdrawn and replaced by intravenous or lactose-free nutrition.
- Diagnosis: Reducing substance in urine specimens collected while the patient is receiving human milk, cow's milk, or any other formula containing lactose.

Mucopolysaccharidoses

The most common subtype is MPS-III, followed by MPS-I and MPS-II.

Mucopolysaccharidosis I (Hurler Syndrome)

- Normal at birth, but inguinal hernias are often present.
- Diagnosed at 6 and 24 months of age with hepatosplenomegaly, coarse facial features, corneal clouding, large tongue, prominent forehead, joint stiffness, short stature, and skeletal dysplasia.
- Premature death, usually by 10 yr of age.

Mucopolysaccharidosis II (Hunter's Disease)

- MPS II is similar to Hurler disease except for the lack of corneal clouding and slower progression.
- Coarse facial features, short stature, dysostosis multiplex, joint stiffness, and mental retardation manifest between 2 and 4 yr of age.

Mucopolysaccharidosis III (Sanflippo's Disease)

Onset between 2 and 6 yr in a normal child. Features include delayed development, hyperactivity with aggressive behavior, coarse hair, hirsutism, sleep disorders, and mild hepatosplenomegaly.

Diagnosis of MPS

- Radiographs of chest, spine, pelvis, and hands are useful to detect early signs of dysostosis multiplex.
- Semiquantitative spot tests for increased urinary GAG excretion are useful for initial evaluation.
- Quantitative analysis of single GAG by various methods, or of oligosaccharides by tandem mass spectrometry, reveals type-specific profiles.
- Morquio disease (MPS type IV) is often missed in urinary assays but can reliably be diagnosed in serum using monoclonal antibodies to keratan sulfate.
- Serum, leukocytes, or cultured fibroblasts are used as the tissue source for measuring lysosomal enzymes.

Gaucher's Disease

- Neuroregression (due to accumulation of glycosphingolipids in CNS)
- Hepatosplenomegaly (due to accumulation of glycosphingolipids in visceral cells)
- Skeletal abnormalities
- Bleeding manifestations due to thrombocytopenia
- Chronic fatigue due to anemia
- Bone pain or pathologic fractures (in 20%).

Niemann-Pick Disease

- History of prolonged neonatal jaundice
- Neuroregression
- Hepatosplenomegaly
- Moderate lymphadenopathy.

INTRAUTERINE INFECTIONS

Common signs and symptoms: Intrauterine growth restriction, microcephaly or hydrocephalus, intracranial calcifications, chorioretinitis, cataracts, myocarditis, pneumonia, hepatosplenomegaly, direct hyperbilirubinemia, anemia, thrombocytopenia, hydrops fetalis, and skin manifestations, including petechiae, purpura, and vesicles. Late sequelae include sensorineural hearing loss, visual disturbances, seizures, and neuro-developmental abnormalities.

Toxoplasmosis

Acquired Toxoplasmosis

Infection acquired postnatally

- Combination of fever, stiff neck, myalgia, arthralgia, maculopapular rash that spares the palms and soles.
- Lymphadenopathy, hepatomegaly, hepatitis, reactive lymphocytosis, meningitis, encephalitis, pneumonia, polymyositis, pericarditis, pericardial effusion, and myocarditis.

Congenital Toxoplasmosis

- Lymphadenopathy is the most common symptom in infected mothers.
- Triad of chorioretinitis, hydrocephalus, and cerebral calcifications.
- Manifestations vary from hydrops fetalis and perinatal death to small size for gestational age,

prem aturity, peripheral retinal scars, persistent jaundice, mild thrombocytopenia, CSF pleocytosis.
- Neurologic signs: Convulsions, hydrocephalus.

Cytomegalovirus

- Intrauterine growth restriction, prematurity, hepatosplenomegaly, jaundice, blueberry muffin-like rash, thrombocytopenia, purpura, microcephaly, intracranial calcifications.
- Other neurologic problems include chorioretinitis, sensorineural hearing loss, and mild increases in cerebrospinal fluid protein.

Rubella

- Prodrome of fever, sore throat, red eyes, headache, malaise, anorexia, and lymphadenopathy.
- Suboccipital, postauricular, and anterior cervical lymph nodes are most prominent.
- In children, the 1st manifestation is usually the rash, which begins on the face and neck as small, irregular pink macules, and it spreads to involve the torso and extremities, where it tends to occur as discrete macules (measles like rash).
- The rash fades from the face as it extends to the rest of the body. Rash lasts for 3 days, and resolves without desquamation.

INVESTIGATIONS

β Thalassemia

- Peripheral blood smear
  - Anisocytosis (variation in size), poikilocytosis (variation in shape), microcytic hypochromic anemia, target cells, tear-drop cells, cigar-shaped cells, basophilic stippling.
  - Reticulocytosis.
- Hemoglobin concentration and bilirubin
  - Hemoglobin (low)
  - Serum bilirubin is raised (unconjugated).
- Radiology
  - X-ray of skull—*Hair on end appearance* (separation of two tables of skull with perpendicular trabeculae in between)
  - X-ray of small bones of hands—*Mosaic patterns* (widening of medullary space with thinning of cortex and criss–cross trabeculae in between).
  - Hemoglobin electrophoresis is diagnostic —Show presence of HbF (>2% of total Hb) and variable amount of HbA_2 and HbA (HbA_2 is increased more in thalassaemia minor than in major).
- Alkaline denaturation test—HbF is resistant to alkaline denaturation (i.e. positive test).
- Osmotic fragility test—Increased resistance of red cells to osmotic lysis (osmotic fragility is increased in hereditary spherocytosis).
- Ferrokinetics—Serum iron concentration is increased and TIBC usually remains normal.
- Bone marrow—Hypercellular with erythroid hyperplasia with increased erythroblasts and sideroblasts.
- Antenatal diagnosis
  - Measurement of globin chain synthesis
  - Analysis of fetal DNA by gene mapping techniques after extraction from fibroblasts of chorion.
- Carrier detection—Hemoglobin decreased, microcytic hypochromic anemia, increased HbA_2, NESTROF test, DNA studies.

Hereditary Spherocytosis

- Peripheral smear showing spherocytes
- Increased osmotic fragility of erythrocytes
- Increased reticulocyte count, increased serum bilirubin
- Urine-urobilinogen present, no bile pigment (acholuric jaundice)

- Negative direct antiglobin test
- Study of other members of family—osmotic fragility, excess urobilinogens, reticulocyte count.

Autoimmune Acquired Hemolytic Anemia

- Blood picture shows reticulocytosis, spherocytosis
- Positive direct antiglobin test (Coombs' test).

Portal Hypertension and Cirrhosis

- Liver function test
- Occult blood in stool
- Ultrasound—to look for dilated portal vein, ascites, increased echotexture in cirrhosis
- Barium study—filling defects (varices)
- Endoscopy
- Liver biopsy—cirrhosis of various cause
- Transplenic portal venography
- CT scan—abdomen
- Ceruloplasmin levels
- Urinary copper excretion
- Immunofluorescence and immunocytochemical studies of intracytoplasmic globules seen in periportal hepatocytes in alpha-1 Antitrypsin deficiency.

Storage Disorders

Gaucher's Disease

- Liver or bone marrow biopsy shows Gaucher's cells
- Beta glucosidase deficiency in WBC.

Niemann-Pick's Disease

- Liver or bone marrow biopsy shows foam cells
- Sphingomyelinase enzyme deficiency in WBC.

Malaria

Peripheral smear for malarial parasite and occasionally parasites in bone marrow and splenic puncture material.

Tropical Splenomegaly

- Fluorescent antibody titer for malaria
- Immunoglobulin levels—Rise in IgM fraction
- Bone marrow study—Hyperplastic bone marrow
- Liver biopsy shows varying degrees of hepatic sinusoidal lymphocytosis and Kupffer cell hypertrophy.

Chronic Myeloid Leukemia

- High total WBC
- Myelocyte in peripheral smear
- Philadelphia chromosome in adult variety of CML.

DISCUSSION

DEFINITIONS

Diarrhea: Increase in frequency, fluidity or volume of bowel movements relative to usual habit of individual. For infants and children this would result in stool output greater than 10g/kg/24 hour or more than adult limit of 200g/24 hour.

Chronic diarrhea: Diarrhea lasting longer than 2 weeks (Table 17.1).

Cyclic vomiting: Syndrome with numerous episodes of vomiting (approx 9 episodes/month) interspread with well intervals.

Toddler's diarrhea: Pattern of intermittent loose stools between 1 and 3 years of age due to frequent drinking and snacks.

Loss of electrolytes in stool:

- Sodium: 20-25 mEq/L
- Potassium: 50-70 mEq/L
- Chloride: 20-25 mEq/L.

Table 17.1: Difference between osmotic and secretory diarrhea

	Osmotic diarrhea	Secretory diarrhea
Volume of stool	< 200 ml/day	> 200 ml/day
Response to fasting	Diarrhea stops	Diarrhoea continues
Stool Na+	< 70 mEq/L	> 70 mEq/L
Reducing substances	Positive	Negative
Stool pH	< 5	> 6

DIFFERENTIAL DIAGNOSIS OF JAUNDICE

Hemolytic Jaundice

- History: Blood transfusion, drug abuse, abdominal pain during acute episode
- Examination: Pallor, Splenomegaly
- Investigations:
  - Serum bilirubin—Mild increase
  - SGOT/SGPT—Usually normal
  - Alkaline phosphatase—Usually normal
  - Urine bilirubin—Absent
  - Urine urobilinogen—Present
  - Stool stercobilinogen—Present
  - Reticulocyte count—Increased.

Hepatocellular Jaundice

- History: Pruritis, abdominal pain, weight loss
- Examination: Tenderness over liver, ascites.
- Investigations:
  - Serum bilirubin—Increased
  - SGOT/SGPT—Increased
  - Alkaline phosphatase—Increased
  - Urine bilirubin—Present
  - Urine urobilinogen—Present
  - Stool stercobilinogen—Present
  - Reticulocyte count—Normal.

Obstructive Jaundice

- History: Contact with jaundice patient, anti-tubercular therapy, vomiting, right hypochondric pain.
- Examination: Pallor, scratch mark, ascites
- Investigations:
  - Serum bilirubin—Moderate increase
  - SGOT/SGPT—Moderate increase
  - Alkaline phosphatase—Marked increased
  - Urine bilirubin—Present
  - Urine urobilinogen—Absent
  - Stool stercobilinogen—Absent
  - Reticulocyte count—Normal.

SEROLOGIC PATTERN IN HEPATITIS B

Positive markers	*Interpretation*
HBsAg, IgM anti HBc	Acute hepatitis B infection
IgM anti HBc	Acute hepatitis B infection
HBsAg, IgM anti HBc, HBeAg	Chronic hepatitis B with active viral replication
Anti HBs, IgG anti HBc	Recovery from hepatitis B (immunity)
Anti HBs	Vaccination
IgG Anti HBc	False positive infection or infection in remote past

ANICTERIC HEPATITIS

Jaundice is not clinically evident; symptoms are few though the liver becomes enlarged and tender. These patients usually suffer from chronic liver disease (chronic active hepatitis, etc.) later in life.

TRANSUDATE VS EXUDATIVE ASCITIC FLUID

Transudate (Cirrhosis)

- < 2.5 g% protein
- Specific gravity of < 1.016.

Exudate (Peritonitis)

- > 2.5 g% protein
- Specific gravity of > 1.016.

ROLE OF SERUM ASCITES ALBUMIN GRADIENT (SAAG) (TABLE 17.2)

- Rather than total protein content of ascites, SAG is used to characterize ascites.
- It correlates directly with portal pressure.
- Gradient > 1.1 g/dl (high-gradient) suggests uncomplicated cirrhotic ascites and differentiates ascites due to portal hypertension from ascites not due to portal hypertension in > 95 % of cases.
- Gradient < 1.1 g/dl (low-gradient) suggests ascites is not due to portal hypertension with > 95 % accuracy.

Table 17.2: Classification of ascites based on SAAG

High albumin gradient (more than 1.1 gm/dl)	*Low albumin gradient (more than 1.1 gm/dl)*
Cirrhosis	Tuberculous peritonitis
Fulminant hepatic failure	Nephrotic syndrome
Hepatitis	Pancreatic ascites
Budd-Chiari syndrome	Serositis in connective tissue diseases
Cardiac ascites	Postoperative lymphatic leak
Myxedema	Peritoneal carcinomatosis
	Portal vein thrombosis

MANAGEMENT OF ASCITES

SAAG decides the mode of therapy.

Low Albumin Gradient Ascites

These patients do not respond to salt restriction and diuretics, as they do not have portal hypertension. Treatment of the cause cures ascites.

High Albumin Gradient Ascites

Salt-restricted diet and Diuretics.

COMPLICATIONS OF ASCITES

- Mechanical complication: Respiratory distress, hernia, pressure over inferior vena cava—edema feet
- Collapse of lower lobe of lung—right sided pleural effusion, waddling gait
- Subacute bacterial peritonitis
- Hepatorenal syndrome.

CAUSES OF DISPROPORTIONATE EDEMA (ASCITES) VS PROPORTIONATE EDEMA

Disproportionate Edema (Ascites)

- Hepatic causes
- Peritoneal tuberculosis
- Chylous ascites
- Constricitive pericarditis
- Malignancy-like lymphomas.

Proportionate Edema

- Renal causes
- Cardiac causes leading to CCF
- Protein energy malnutrition
- Hypoproteinemia
- Anemia.

REFRACTORY ASCITES

It is defined as fluid overload unresponsive to salt restriction and high-dose diuretic.

Management

- Therapeutic paracentesis: Large volume fluid tap upto 100 ml/kg
- Peritoneal venous shunt (Le Veen shunt)
- Orthotropic liver transplantation.

CAUSE OF RAISED ESR IN HYPOPROTEINEMIA

Normally fibrinogen inhibits roulette formation and in the absence of fibrinogen—there is raised ESR because of increased roulette formation.

CAUSES OF CHRONIC LIVER DISEASE

- Hepatitis—Chronic active/passive hepatitis due to hepatitis B virus
- Wilson's disease
- Indian childhood cirrhosis
- Alpha—1 antitrypsin deficiency
- Cystic fibrosis
- Collagen vascular disease
- Glycogen storage disease.

FEATURES OF HEPATOCELLULAR FAILURE

- General failure of health.
- Jaundice.
- Skin changes
  - Spider nevi
  - Palmar erythema
  - Diffuse pigmentation
  - White nails
  - Clubbing (common in biliary cirrhosis)
  - Loss of axillary and pubic hair
  - 'Paper money' skin (usually on upper arms).
- Endocrine changes
  - Gynecomastia
  - Testicular atrophy.
- Bleeding manifestation—Petechiae, ecchymosis (due to hypoprothrombinemia and low platelet count).
- Fever (due to endotoxemia with production of cytokines).
- Fetor hepaticus (sweetish-fecal smell of the breath and urine due to methyl L mercaptan derived from methionine).
- Hepatic encephalopathy (disturbed consciousness, personality changes, intellectual deterioration with asterixis).
- Ascites and bipedal edema.
- Circulatory changes.
- Hyperkinetic circulation
  - Capillary pulsation
  - Bounding pulse (high pulse pressure with low diastolic BP).
  - Tachycardia.
  - Hyperdynamic apex
  - Ejection systolic murmur at the apex.
- Cyanosis and clubbing—Due to pulmonary arteriovenous shunts.

TREATABLE CAUSES OF NEONATAL CHOLESTASIS

- Sepsis
- Endocrinopathy: Hypothyroidism, panhypopituitarism
- Metabolic: Galactosemia, tyrosinemia
- Choledochal cyst
- Biliary atresia.

FUNDUS CHANGES IN INTRAUTERINE INFECTIONS

- Chorioretinitis (toxoplasma and CMV)
  - Chorioretinitis with microcephaly and hepatosplenomegaly—suggestive of CMV
  - Chorioretinitis without other manifestations—suggestive of toxoplasma.
- Cataract (rubella)
- Optic atrophy
- Salt and pepper appearance (rubella).

PERITONITIS

Peritoneal fluid containing > 250 WBC's and > 50% polymorphs;
OR > 250 WBC's with signs and symptoms
OR > 500 WBC's without signs and symptoms.

Primary Peritonitis

- No cause readily detected
- Does not require surgical treatment
- Proteins in ascitic fluid < 1 gm%
- No relation between serum and fluid LDH
- Sugar not less than 50 gm%
- Usually only a single type of organism detected.

Secondary Peritonitis

- Secondary to surgical condition/perforation
- Usually requires surgery
- Proteins in ascitic fluid > 1.1 gm%
- Ascitic fluid LDH > serum LDH
- Sugar < 50 gm%
- Multiple types of bacteria may be detected.

VIRAL AGENTS OF GASTROENTERITIS

- Rotavirus
- Astrovirus
- Enteric adenovirus
- Norwalk virus (MC cause of gastroenteritis outbreaks in older children and adults).

CRITERIA FOR DIAGNOSIS OF SLE

MDP SOARHINA (Name of African Prince)

- **M**alar rash
- **D**iscoid rash
- **P**hotosensivity
- **S**erositis
- **O**ral ulcers
- **A**rthritis: Nonerosive arthritis involving two or more peripheral joints
- **R**enal disorder: Persistent proteinuria > 3+ or cellular casts
- **H**ematologic disorder: Hemolytic anemia or leucopenia or lymphopenia or thrombocytopenia
- **I**mmunologic disorder: Positive LE cell or Anti DNA antibody or Anti Sm
- **N**eurologic disorder: Seizures or psychosis
- **A**ntinuclear antibody.

GRADING OF SPLENOMEGALY

Mild splenomegaly: Spleen is few centrimeters.

Moderate splenomegaly: Spleen measures several centimeters but does not cross midline.

Severe splenomegaly: Spleen crosses midline in direction of right iliac fossa.

DIFFERENCE BETWEEN SPLEEN AND RENAL LUMP

Spleen

- Notch on medial border
- Not bimanually palpable or ballotable
- Fingers cannot be insinuated between lump and costal margin
- Moves with respiration.

Kidney

- No notch
- Bimanually palpable and ballotable
- Fingers can be insinuated between lump and costal margin
- Restricted movement with respiration.

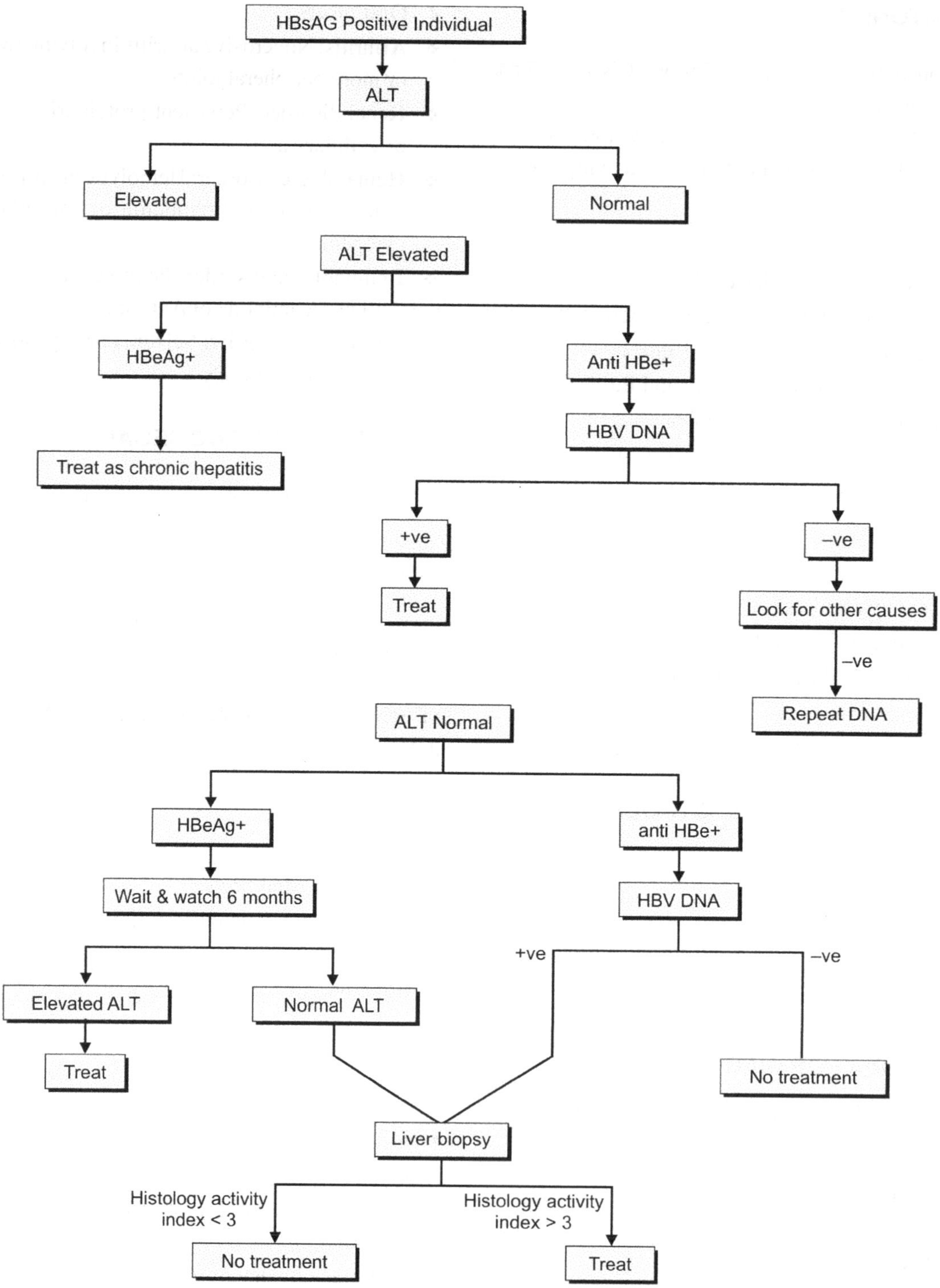

Fig. 17.1: Approach to chronic hepatitis

LIVER FUNCTION TESTS

Markers of Hepatic Damage

- *Alanine aminotransferase (ALT)*—More liver specific but less sensitive than AST
- *Aspartate aminotransferase (AST)*—Not liver specific but sensitive indicator of hepatic damage. Its level is proportional to degree of hepatocellular damage.
- *Lactate dehydrogenase (LDH)*—Insensitive and nonspecific.

Markers of Cholestasis

- Bilirubin
- Alkaline phosphatase
- Gamma glutamyl transferase.

Markers of Reduced Synthetic Function

- Albumin
- Clotting factors
- Cholinesterase.

Indicators of Function

- Lignocaine metabolites.

Indicators of Hepatic Blood Flow

- Indocyanine green clearance
- Bromosulphthalein clearance.

TYPHIDOT VS WIDAL TEST

Typhidot test is a ELISA test that detects IgM and IgG antibodies against the outer membrane protein (OMP) of the *Salmonella typhi*. The typhidot test becomes positive within 2-3 days of infection. It is highly sensitive and specific test, rapid, easy to perform, more reliable test for typhoid fever as compared to widal test.

The **Widal test** is a serological test for Enteric fever or Undulant fever. In case of *Salmonella* it is a demonstration of agglutinating antibodies against antigens O-somatic and H-flagellar in the blood. For brucellosis, only O-somatic antigen is used. It's not a very accurate method, since presence of other bacteria (e.g. *Salmonella enteritidis*, *Salmonella typhimurium*); past history of typhoid fever, typhoid vaccination can cause a false-positive result. As with all serological tests, the rise in antibody levels needed to make the diagnosis takes 7-14 days, which limits their use.

CHAPTER 18

CENTRAL NERVOUS SYSTEM

TUBERCULOUS MENINGITIS (TBM)

HISTORY

CHIEF COMPLAINTS

- Fever
- Altered sensorium
- Seizures
- Decreased movement of any part of body.

HISTORY OF PRESENT ILLNESS

History of Disease

Convulsions

- Partial/generalized/partial with secondary generalization
- Nature of seizures—Tonic-clonic/tonic/clonic
- Associated with uprolling of eyeballs, frothing from mouth, incontinence of urine/stools
- Associated with any aura/automatism
- Associated with loss of consciousness
- Duration of the seizure
- Number of seizures
- Postictal state (drowsiness, consciousness, delirium, hemiplegia, etc.)
- If multiple seizures, the state of consciousness in the interval between 2 successive convulsions.
- Is patient on any drugs to control seizures and his compliance.

Altered Sensorium

- Inability to recognize parents
- Passing urine and stool in bed
- Abnormal behavior: Aggression, biting, pulling clothes, irrelevant talking.

Associated History

- Vomiting, headache, convulsions, focal neurological deficits (increased intracranial tension)
- Cranial nerve palsies: Vision, hearing, speech, drooling of saliva and pooling of secretions
- Sensory deficits: Numbness, tingling, loss of balance especially in dark, pain/burning
- Any bleeding manifestations
- Intake of antitubercular therapy.

History of Complications

- Inability to move a limb (hemiplegia)
- Involuntary movements
- Contractures
- Bed sores
- Activities of daily living—"DEATH", i.e. dressing, eating, ambulating, toileting, hygiene.

History of Risk Factors

- Fever with rash (measles)
- Recurrent diarrhea/respiratory infections/loss of weight (HIV)
- Contact with tuberculosis patient
- Immunosuppressive drug intake
- History of any other vaccination (postvaccinial encephalopathy pertussis)
- Head trauma
- Ear discharge (pyogenic meningitis, cerebral abscess)

PAST HISTORY

- Tuberculosis
- Similar episodes in past.

DIETARY HISTORY

- Food intake during 24 hours prior to the onset of illness
- Calculate the approximate calorie and protein intake per day prior to illness
- Compare the calorie and protein intake of child with that of normal child
- Diet includes fruits and is rich in fiber or not.

FAMILY HISTORY

- History of seizures in any member of family.

SOCIOECONOMIC HISTORY

- Number of members in family
- Age, occupation, education and income of parents and other siblings
- Housing conditions—whether living in a kaccha house/pacca house/slum
- Number of rooms in house
- Source of drinking water; water disposal; storage of water supply
- Sewage disposal/defecation habit
- Details of schooling.

IMMUNIZATION HISTORY

- BCG vaccine/measles vaccine.

GENERAL PHYSICAL EXAMINATION

- General appearance: Comatose, emaciated and lying in decerebrate posture
- Vitals: Temperature/pulse/respiration/BP
- Anthropometry: Malnutrition in TBM
- Posture: Decorticate, decerebrate
- Pallor/cyanosis/clubbing/icterus/lymphadenopathy/edema feet
- Anterior fontanel: bulging or not
- BCG mark
- Signs of vitamin A deficiency
  - Conjunctival/Corneal xerosis
  - Bitot's spots.
- Signs of vitamin B deficiency
  - Angular stomatitis
  - Cheilosis.
- Signs of vitamin D deficiency—rickets
- Signs of vitamin E deficiency—petechiae, purpura
- Allergic manifestation of TB—phylycten/erythema nodosum/tache cerebrale
- Bedsores
- Skull/spine/scars/sinus

- ❖ Presence/absence/patency of shunt (VP shunt) if present.
- ❖ Signs favoring differential diagnosis:
  - ❒ Ear discharge, pulmonary infections, skin infections, CSF rhinorrhea (pyogenic meningitis)
  - ❒ Bleeding from any site (leukemic infiltration)
  - ❒ Bruit over skull (AV malformation).

SYSTEMIC EXAMINATION

NERVOUS SYSTEM

- **Higher mental functions**
  - ❖ Consciousness
  - ❖ Orientation—time, space and person
  - ❖ Intelligence and judgment
  - ❖ Memory
  - ❖ Speech.
- **Cranial nerves:** Always search for optic atrophy and VIIth nerve palsy
  - ❖ *Olfactory:* Test the smell sensation with common bedside objects like soap, toothpaste, etc.
  - ❖ *Optic*
    - ❒ Acuity of vision
    - ❒ Field of vision
    - ❒ Color vision
    - ❒ Ophthalmoscopy.
  - ❖ *Oculomotor, trochlear and abducent*
    - ❒ Ptosis
    - ❒ Squint
    - ❒ Extraocular movements
    - ❒ Nystagmus
    - ❒ Pupil—size, shape, reaction (light reflex, consensual light reflex and accommodation reflex).
  - ❖ *Trigeminal*
    - ❒ Motor function (masseter, pterygoids and temporalis)
    - ❒ Sensory function (sensation over the face)
    - ❒ Corneal reflex.
  - ❖ *Facial*
    - ❒ Palpebral fissure, frowning, eye closure, nasolabial folds, angle of the mouth
    - ❒ Ask the patient to show his teeth, epiphora, salivation, etc.
    - ❒ Taste sensation of anterior 2/3rd of the tongue.
  - ❖ *Vestibulocochlear*
    - ❒ Positional nystagmus
    - ❒ Hearing—Watch test, Rinne's test, Weber's test.

Rinne's Test

Method

Place a vibrating tuning fork (512 or 256 Hz) initially on the mastoid process until sound is no longer heard, the fork is then immediately placed just outside the ear. Normally, the sound is audible at the ear.

Description	*Interpretation*
In normal ear, air conduction is better than bone conduction	Positive Rinne
In conductive hearing loss, bone conduction is better than air	Negative Rinne
In sensorineural hearing loss, bone conduction and air conduction are both equally depreciated, maintaining their relative difference (there may be false negative Rinne)	Positive Rinne

Weber's Test

Method

A vibrating tuning fork (either 256 or 512 Hz) is placed in the middle of the forehead. The patient is asked to in which ear the sound is heard louder. In a normal patient, the sound is heard equally loud in both ears (no lateralization). However a patient with symmetrical hearing loss will have the same findings. Thus, there is diagnostic utility only in asymmetric hearing losses.

Conductive Hearing Loss

A patient with a unilateral conductive hearing loss would hear the tuning fork loudest in the affected ear.

Sensorineural Hearing Loss

A patient with a unilateral sensorineural hearing loss would hear the sound louder in the unaffected ear.

- *Glossopharyngeal and vagus*
  - Soft palate—movements
  - Pharyngeal reflex
  - Taste sensation of posterior 1/3rd of the tongue.
- *Spinal accessory*
  - Power of sternocleidomastoids
  - Power of trapezius.
- *Hypoglossal*
  - Deviation of tongue
  - Atrophy and fasciculation of tongue.

Motor Functions

- Nutrition—Attitude of limbs/Atrophy
- Bulk—Shape, size and symmetry of muscle
- Tone
  - Inspection: Observe the posture
  - Palpation: Palpate for feel of muscle
  - Passive movement at joint.
- Power (For detailed power examination see chapter on Duchenne Muscular Dystrophy)
  Grading of Muscular Weakness
  - Grade 0: Complete paralysis
  - Grade 1: Flicker of contraction only (visible or palpable)
  - Grade 2: Movements with elimination of gravity
  - Grade 3: Movement against gravity but not against resistance
  - Grade 4: Movement possible against gravity plus resistance but weaker than normal.
  - Grade 5: Normal power

    Often, '+' or '–' symbols are used to improve the sensitivity of the grading.
- Involuntary movements.

Reflexes

- *Superficial*
  - Abdominal (T7 to T 12): Abdominal wall is stroked from lateral to medial side. This elicits contraction of muscles of anterior abdominal wall.
  - Cremasteric (L1)—lost bilaterally: This is elicited by stroking a line along the medial thigh and watching the movement of testis. A normal reflex elicits elevation of the ipsilateral testis.
  - Plantar response (S1, S2)—extensor flexor in both the lower limbs: Lateral aspect of sole is stroked with a blunt pointed object. The stimulus should be gentle but firm. Normal response is plantar flexion of great toe, which is considered as absent (negative) *Babinski's sign*. Dorsiflexion (positive sign) of great toe suggests upper motor neuron lesion. This is accompanied by fanning out of other toes (this is not necessary).

Gordon's sign: Squeezing of calf muscles causing fanning of great toe.

Oppenheim's sign: Scratching the inner side of leg causes fanning of great toe.

Chaddock's sign: Irritation of external malleolar skin causes fanning of great toe.

- *Deep:*
  - Biceps jerk (C5, C6)
  - Triceps jerk (C7, C8)
  - Supinator jerk (C6)
  - Knee jerk (L2, L3, L4)
  - Ankle jerk (S1)
  - Clonus (ankle and patellar).
- *Visceral:*
  - Bladder: Catheterized or not
  - Bowel: Incontinent or not.

Grading of Deep Tendon Reflexes

0 Absent
1+ Sluggish or present only with rein-forcement
2+ Readily elicited
3+ Brisk without evidence of clonus
4+ Associated with clonus.

Sensory Functions

- Spinothalmic—light touch, pain and temperature
- Dorsal column
  - Joint sense
  - Vibration sense
  - Touch localization.
- Cortical sensation—two point localization (discrimination of two closely placed stimuli as separate), Stereognosis (Identification of object by touch and manipulation alone), Graphesthesia (Identification of letter or number written on skin surface).

Touch is assessed by stimulating the skin with cotton wisp.

Pain is tested by using new pin.

Temperature is tested by using a metal object (i.e. tuning fork) that has been immersed in cold and warm water.

Vibration is tested by using a 128 Hz tuning fork applied to distal phalanx of great toe just below nail bed. By placing finger on opposite side of joint being tested, examiner compares the patients threshold of vibration perception with his own.

Joint position (propioception) testing is done by grasping the great toe between your index finger and thumb. Grasp the side of digit so that movement is not felt as pressure up or down. Move the toe up and down 3-4 times and finally rest either up or down. Ask the child position of toe. Repeat for alternative position.

Romberg's sign: Ask child to stand erect with his feet close together, arms by the side and eyes open. The child with a posterior column dysfunction sways.

Cortical sensation is mediated by parietal lobes, testing cortical sensation is meaningful only when primary sensation is intact. With the patients eye closed, examiner lightly touches one or both hands and asks the patient to identify the stimuli. With a parietal lobe lesion, the patient may be unable to identify the stimulus on contralateral side when both hands are touched.

Sensory Scoring for Light Touch and Pinprick

0: Absent
1: Impaired or hyperesthesia
2: Intact

A score of zero is given if the patient cannot differentiate between the point of a sharp pin and the dull edge.

Cerebellar Functions

Truncal and Gait ataxia: Cerebellar lesion is associated with broad based gait.

Intention tremors: Oscillating tremors that accelerates on approaching the target. Ask the child to extend and abduct his arm to 90° and touch the tip of his nose (finger to nose test) OR Ask him to touch your finger with his finger (finger to finger test). In cerebellar disease, tremors are seen when child finger start approaching the nose or your finger.

Dyssynergia (Inco-ordination): This is elicited by heel- shin test.

Dysmetria and Past pointing: Overshooting a target while attempting to reach an object. Generally tested by finger to nose or finger to finger test.

Dysdiadochokinesia: Inability to perform rapid alternating movements like simultaneously pronation and supination of hand.

Dysarthria: Staccato, slurred or scanning speech.

Pendular Knee Jerk

Nystagmus: Nystagmus is seen when child is asked to look in a particular direction (gaze evoked).

Signs of Meningeal Irritation

Neck Rigidity

Place your hand under the supine child's head and gently try to flex the neck. Undue resistance implies irritation of cranial nerve roots from meningeal inflammation. A conscious child should be asked to flex the neck and touch the chin to chest.

Kernig's Sign

With child supine, flex the hip and knee on one side, then extend the knee with the hip still flexed. With meningeal inflammation, there is pain in posterior thigh muscle and knee extension becomes difficult. With severe meningeal inflammation, the opposite knee may also flex during the test.

Brudzinski Sign

To elicit Brudzinski sign, place your hand behind the child's head and place the other hand on child's chest. Then, flex the child's head while hand on chest restrains the child and prevents the child from rising. Flexion of child's hips and knees constitutes a positive sign.

Cranium and Spine

Examine skull for microcephaly, macrocephaly, encephalocele and cracked pot sign in children with raised intracranial tension.

Look for spinal deformities like vertebral defects, dermal sinus, hypertrichosis, kyphosis, scoliosis.

Trophic changes: Bed sores

Autonomic functions: Loss of sweating below the level of umbilicus.

Fundus Examination

RESPIRATORY SYSTEM

- Any crepitations, consolidation or pleural effusion.

GI AND GENITOURINARY SYSTEM

- Any organomegaly or ascites
- *Percuss the bladder* and see the colour of the urine present in the tube or urosac (chalky or turbid urine is seen in Urinary tract infections, orange colored urine suggests intake of rifampicin).

CARDIOVASCULAR SYSTEM

- Look for hemic murmur due to anemia.

LYMPHORETICULAR SYSTEM

- Lymphadenopathy.

DIAGNOSIS

Chronic meningoencephalitis; with/without raised intracranial tension; with/without cranial nerve palsies; with/without hemiparesis most probable cause being an infarct in opposite middle cerebral artery probably in internal capsule region (commonest), Probable etiology being Tuberculous meningitis.

DIFFERENTIAL DIAGNOSIS

PYOGENIC MENINGITIS

- Acute onset
- Focus of infection present: Pyoderma/ear discharge/bronchopneumonia
- Focal neurological deficits, cranial nerve palsies, hydrocephalus rare
- CSF turbid, glucose decreased, proteins increased, Neutrophils seen on cytology, Gram staining and culture positive
- Prognosis—better, i.e. if it is picked up early
- Rapid and better response to treatment and less morbidity.

VIRAL ENCEPHALITIS

- Seasonal clustering
- Short history of fever
- Associated rash, rhinopharyngitis, diarrhea
- Lack of meningeal signs
- Focal neurological deficits usually absent
- CSF clear, glucose normal, proteins slightly increase, lymphocytic pleocytosis
- Viral serology positive.

ASEPTIC MENINGITIS

- History of viral illness, mumps
- Headache, vomiting
- Neck rigidity positive
- Sensorium relatively spared
- Focal deficits absent
- CSF similar to viral encephalitis.

FUNGAL MENINGITIS

- Seen in immunocompromised children
- Presentation similar to Tuberculous meningitis
- CSF- India ink preparation (cryptococci)
- Gram's stain-Candida
- Fungal culture positive.

INVESTIGATIONS

To confirm the diagnosis of Tuberculous meningitis:

LUMBAR PUNCTURE (AFTER FUNDUS EXAMINATION TO R/O RAISED ICT)

In CSF one should look for:

- Opening pressure (high in acute meningitis)
- Gross appearance of the CSF (clear or turbid)
- Biochemistry, sugar, proteins
- Cytology including total cell counts and differential counts, should be done within 30 minutes of doing a lumbar puncture
- Giemsa staining is essential to determine DLC as a chamber evaluation of cells.
- Other tests:
  - *Culture in LJ medium:* 7-10 weeks of incubation is necessary for detection of organisms. Yield of culture varies from 30-70%.
  - *BACTEC for tuberculosis:* Average time required for detection is 9-14 days. It detects growth of AFB radiometrically by measuring the release of CO_2.
  - *PCR for TB:* Sensivity is 4-80% and specificity is 80-100%. A negative PCR never eliminates possibility of TB and positive is not confirmatory.
  - ELISA for detection of antibodies.
  - *Adenosine deaminase assay (ADA):* ADA is enzyme produced by T lymphocytes. Results are available in 24 hours and have sensivity and specificity of diagnosing TBM is 70% and 92% respectively.
  - *Tuberculostearic acid assay:* Detects tuberculostearic acid (component of mycobacterial cell wall). Sensivity is 95% and specificity is 91-99%.

- *Bromide partition test:* Involves determination of ratio of concentration of bromide between serum and CSF after loading dose of bromide is given. The ratio decreases with disruption of blood brain barrier in TBM.

To look for supportive evidence of tuberculosis

- Total leukocyte count (lymphocytosis)
- ESR—Increased in TB
- Chest X-ray—To locate primary lesion
- Gastric lavage for acid fast bacilli
- FNAC of lymph nodes if lymphadenopathy is present
- Mantoux test > 10 mm
- Ultrasound abdomen—Retroperitoneal lymphadenopathy.

To look for complications

- USG skull—with open fontanel and signs of raised ICT
- CT scan brain—to rule out presence of hydrocephalus and tuberculoma
- BERA—to r/o deafness
- Ophthalmologic examination to look for blindness.

Baseline Tests before Starting Treatment

- Liver function tests
- Renal function tests.

TREATMENT

Specific Antitubercular Treatment

Plan

2 $(HRZS)_3$ + 7 $(HRE)_3$ + Steroid for 6 weeks (RNTCP protocol)

Dosage:

Drugs	*Daily therapy*	*Thrice weekly therapy*
Isoniazid	5 mg/kg	10 mg/kg
Rifampicin	10 mg/kg	10 mg/kg
Pyrazinamide	25 mg/kg	35 mg/kg
Ethambutol	15 mg/kg	30 mg/kg
Streptomycin	15 mg/kg	15 mg/kg

- *Corticosteroids:* To decrease complications Dexamethasone: 0.15 mg/kg/dose intravenously thrice a day for 3-5 days and when patient starts accepting orally start Predinisolone.
  Prednisolone (2 mg/kg/day) to be given for 1 month and then to be tapered over 15 days.
- *To decrease the raised ICT:* Mannitol (20%)-5-8 ml/kg/dose thrice a day for 2 days then. Acetazolamide or glycerol may be given orally or through infant feeding tube in chronic cases if raised intracranial tension persists.

Treatment of Complications

- *Treatment of hydrocephalus:* If moderate to severe: VP shunt surgery
- *Treatment of seizures:*
  - Diazepam 0.3 mg/kg slowly
  - Phenytoin 15 mg/kg loading dose followed by 5 mg/kg/day in 2 divided doses.

General Care

- *Care of unconscious/bed-ridden patient:*
  - Change position 2 hourly
  - Apply talc to pressure points
  - Administer methylcellulose eye drops frequently and keep eyes closed by eye pads.
  - Bladder and bowel care
  - Maintain oral hygiene
  - Regular physiotherapy to prevent contractures.

- *Nutritional care:*
  - High-protein and calorie diet through Ryle's tube to prevent malnutrition.

DISCUSSION

DEFINITIONS

- *Chronic pyogenic meningitis* is persistence of symptoms and signs of meningitis for more than 4 weeks associated with CSF pleocytosis.
- *Partially treated pyogenic meningitis* is a case of meningitis which has been treated with inappropriate selection of the drugs or in inadequate doses/duration resulting in an altered clinical picture and non-clearance of CSF.
- *Recurrent pyogenic meningitis* is defined as separate episodes of meningitis at least 1 week or more apart during which time the patient's clinical profile is essentially normal.
- *Situation related epilepsy:* Convulsions occurring within 7 days of causative insult, e.g. birth asphyxia leading to epilepsy.
- *Primary focus:* Inflamed area at the point of entry of tubercle bacilli.
- *Primary complex:* Primary focus, draining lymphatic and inflamed regional lymph nodes are collectively called primary complex.
- *Puhl's lesion:* Site of isolated lesion of chronic pulmonary tuberculosis. It is situated at apex of lung because blood flow and diffusion is sluggish.
- *Assman's focus:* Infraclavicular lesion of chronic pulmonary tuberculosis.

Table 18.1: CSF picture in meningitis caused by different etiological agents

Normal	*Pyogenic*	*Viral*	*Mycobacterial*	*Fungal*
Gross appearance	Turbid	Clear to turbid	Clear Cobweb coagulum forms	Turbid
Sugar (>2/3rd of blood sugar)	< 40	Normal	<50	30-40
Protein (<40 mg %)	100-500	Normal or slight increase	Up to 300, may be increased >500	100 (20-500)
Total cells (<10/mm^3, no polys)	Up to several 1000	Up to 100	25-100 (rarely>500)	Up to 50
Predominant cell type	Neutrophils	Lymphocytes generally	Lymphocytes	Lymphocytes generally

INCREASED INTRACRANIAL TENSION

Symptoms

- Headache (early morning headache which increases by coughing and straining).
- Vomiting (sometimes projectile; no nausea; unrelated to food).
- Convulsions (usually generalized; focal due to space occupying lesion).
- Altered consciousness to coma.
- Rarely, dizziness; visual problems like deterioration of visual acuity and peripheral constriction of visual field.

Signs

- Bradycardia; but if the intracranial pressure continues to increase the pulse becomes very rapid.
- Blood pressure—There may be hypertension.
- Slow and deep respiration; later on it becomes rapid and shallow, and lastly Cheyne-Stokes breathing appears.
- Papilledema.
- False localization signs:
  - Unilateral or bilateral VIth nerve palsy
  - Bilateral Babinski's sign
  - Bilateral grasp reflex.

- Bulging anterior fontanelle in infants.
- A chronically increased intracranial tension may produce features of 'hypopituitarism', e.g. loss of body hairs, hypothyroidism, hypoadrenalism, etc.

Investigations

- X-ray skull:
  - Silver-beaten appearance
  - Sutural diastasis.
  - Erosion of clinoid process
  - Deepened sella turcica
  - Enlargement of internal auditory meatus.
- CT or MRI scan—Diagnoses raised intracranial tension with etiology.
- Lumbar puncture is contraindicated in raised intracranial tension with papilloedema because of the risk of development of cerebellar pressure cone syndrome.

WHEN TO SUSPECT TBM

- Any chronically ill, febrile child with meningeal signs
- Disseminated, miliary tuberculosis even without frank CNS manifestations
- Infants with non-specific CNS features such as irritability and strong history of contact
- Febrile child with hydrocephalus
- Febrile child with focal deficits.

If in a case of tuberculous meningitis; hepatosplenomegaly is significant then consider possibility of disseminated tuberculosis.

CAUSES OF VOMITING IN TUBERCULOUS MENINGITIS

- Drug induced hepatitis (associated with hepatomegaly and elevated liver transaminases)
- Raised intracranial tension due to hydrocephalus (associated with spasticity, garbled speech, brisk deep tendon reflexes and papilledema on funduscopy).
- Gastritis due to steroids (associated with epigastric pain)
- Metabolic decompensation due to carbonic anhydrase inhibitor. (Carbonic anhydrase inhibitor like acetazolamide leads to metabolic acidosis which can lead to vomiting. Vomiting leads to metabolic alkalosis due to loss of hydrogen ions in vomitus).

POOR PROGNOSTIC FACTORS IN TBM

- Age < 2 years
- Malnutrition
- HIV infection
- Altered sensorium/seizures
- Inadequate treatment
- Residual neurological deficit
- Complications like hydrocephalus, infarct.

POOR PROGNOSTIC FACTORS IN PYOGENIC MENINGITIS

- Age < 6 months
- 10^6 colony forming units of bacteria/ml in CSF
- Seizures occurring more than 7 days into therapy
- Coma or focal neurologic signs.

COMPLICATIONS IN TBM

- Hydrocephalus
- Motor/cranial nerve deficits
- Mental retardation
- Seizures
- Behavioral problems
- Endocrine problems
- Visual complications and optic atrophy
- Complications of treatment:
  - Lumbar puncture—headache
  - Drugs—hepatitis/peripheral neuritis
  - Shunt complications.

CAUSES OF SEIZURES IN TBM

- Raised intracranial tension
- Electrolyte imbalance
- Infarction
- Febrile convulsions
- Tuberculoma
- Vasculitis
- Syndrome of inappropriate diuretic hormone
- Isoniazid therapy.

CAUSES OF HEMIPLEGIA IN TBM

- Vasculitis
- Basal exudates in sylvian fissure entrapping middle cerebral artery
- Lacunar infarcts in internal capsule
- Tuberculoma
- Calcification
- Edema.

STAGES IN TBM

- *Prodromal stage or stage of invasion*: Nonspecific symptoms such as irritability, excessive cry, apathy, behavior disturbances.
- *Stage of meningitis*: Signs of meningeal irritation, raised ICT, altered sensorium, convulsions.
- *Stage of coma or diffuse or focal cerebral involvement*: Deep coma, fixed and dilated pupils, decerebrate and decorticate rigidity.

PRINCIPLES OF CHEMOTHERAPY

- *Drugs acting in acid medium:* Pyrazinamide—acts on intracellular organisms
- *Drugs acting in alkaline medium:* Streptomycin—acts on extracellular organisms
- *Drugs acting on intracellular, extracellular organisms in both acid and alkaline medium:* INH; Rifampicin—acts on persisters also
- *Drugs crossing blood-brain barrier:* Isoniazid, rifampicin and pyrazinamide;streptomycin crosses the blood-brain barrier poorly.

It takes 3 weeks for sputum conversion if regimens containing rifampicin are used and 3 months for regimens without rifampicin.

Table 18.2: Testing spinal tracts

Ascending	
Lateral spinothalamic	Superficial pain Temperature
Anterior spinothalamic	Superficial touch Deep pressure
Posterior column	Vibration Deep pressure Position Stereognosis Point location Two-point discrimination
Anterior and dorsal spinocerebellar	Proprioceptive
Descending	
Lateral and anterior	Rapid rhythm with alternating movement
Pyramidal	Voluntary movement Deep tendon reflexes Plantar reflex
Medial and lateral reticulospinal	Posture, gait, Romberg's

RNTCP FLOW CHART FOR DIAGNOSIS OF TUBERCULOSIS

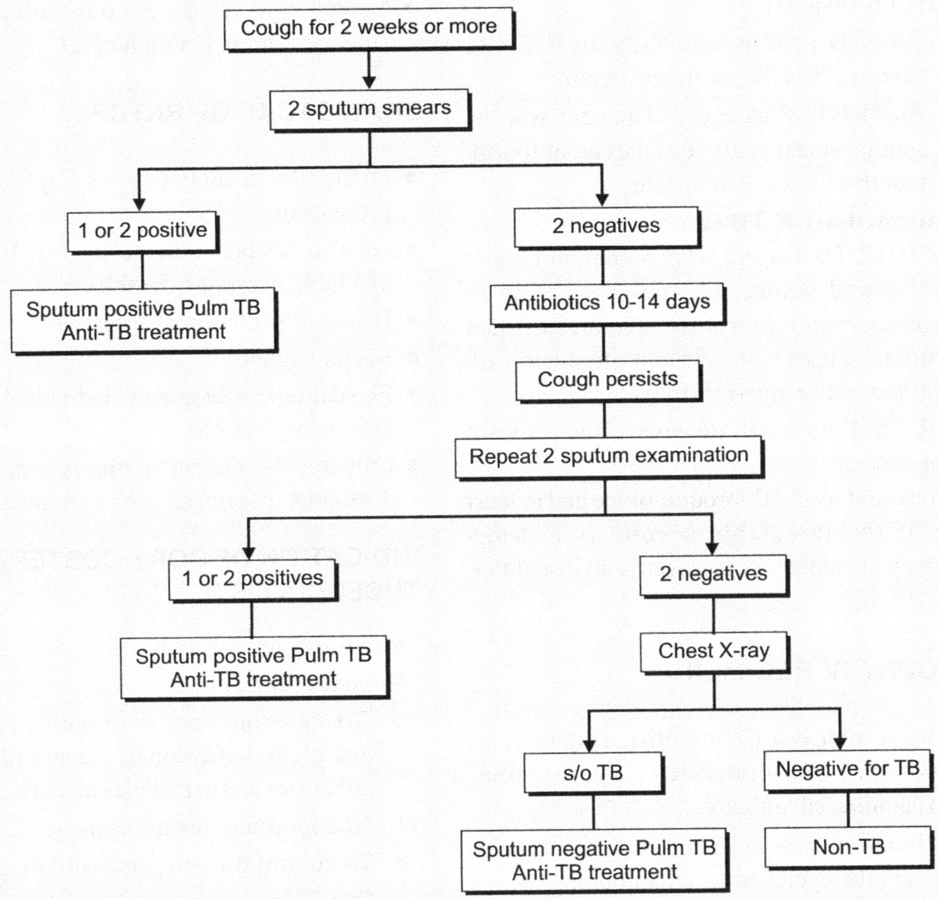

RNTCP CATEGORIES OF TREATMENT

Category of treatment	*Type of patient*	*Regimen*
Category I	New sputum smear-positive Seriously ill New sputum smear-negative Seriously ill New extra-pulmonary	$2(HRZE)_3 + 4(HR)_3$
Category II	Sputum smear-positive relapse Sputum smear-positive failure Sputum smear-positive treatment after DEFAULT	$2(HRZES)_3$ $+ (HRZE)_3$ $+ 5(HRE)_3$
Category III	New sputum smear-negative, not seriously ill New extra-pulmonary, not seriously ill	$2(HRZ)_3 + 4(HR)_3$
Category IV	Multi drug resistant tuberculosis	6(9)Km Ofx Eto Cs ZE/18Ofx Eto Cs E

MULTIDRUG RESISTANT TUBERCULOSIS

- **MDR TB suspect:**
  - ❖ Any TB patient who fails an RNTCP category I or III treatment regimens.
  - ❖ Any RNTCP category II patient who is sputum smear positive at the end of fourth month of treatment or later.
- **Confirmed MDR TB case:**
  Any MDR TB suspect who is sputum culture positive and whose tuberculosis is due to *Mycobacterium tuberculosis* that are resistant in vitro to at least isoniazid and rifampcin with or without other anti-TB drugs.
- **XDR TB** [Extreme (Extensive) Drug resistant tuberculosis]:
  TB resistant to any fluoroquinolone and at least one of the injectable second line drugs (kanamycin, amikacin, capreomycin) in addition to MDR TB.

CATEGORY IV REGIMEN

- Intensive phase-6 (9) months: Kanamycin, oflaxacin, ethionamide, cycloserine, pyrizinamide, ethambutol.
- Continuation phase-18 months: Oflaxacin, ethionamide, cycloserine, ethambutol.
- Minimum duration of intensive phase is 6 months.
- After 6 months start continuation phase (if culture at 4th month negative).
- Maximum duration of Intensive phase-9 months.
- Continuation phase of 18 months.
- 4 sputa collected and examined by smear and culture (30 day apart) from 3rd to 7th month of treatment and at 3 monthly interval from 9th month onward till completion of treatment.
- If any of the culture in last 3 quarter becomes positive it will be followed by monthly cultures in the following 3 months.
- Culture converted—2 consecutive negative cultures at least 1 month apart.
- Smear converted—2 consecutive negative smears at least 1 month apart.

DRAWBACKS OF RNTCP

- Difficulty in diagnosis—symptoms, sputum production.
- Gastric lavage, tuberculin test, FNAC—not available at primary health center.
- Direct observation of treatment.
- Social stigma.
- Fixed drug combination—individual dose calculation not possible.
- Category I—patient sputum smear positive at 3 months, continues with continuation phase.

INDICATION OF CORTICOSTEROIDS IN TUBERCULOSIS

- ❖ Miliary tuberculosis
- ❖ Neurotuberculosis
- ❖ TB in serous sacs (peritonitis, pericarditis and pleural effusion to prevent fibrosis and adhesions and to facilitate absorption of fluid)
- ❖ Genitourinary tuberculosis
- ❖ To control drug hypersensitivity reaction
- ❖ Rarely for regression of lymph nodes during chemotherapy
- ❖ Lymph node tuberculosis causing airway obstruction.

Dose: 1-2 mg /kg /day up to 4 mg/kg for 4–8 weeks (maximum dose 60 mg/day).

DIAGNOSTIC CRITERIA OF CONGENITAL TUBERCULOSIS

Infant must have proven tuberculous lesion and at least one of the following:

- Lesions in 1st week of life
- A primary hepatic complex or caseating hepatic granuloma

- Tuberculous infection of the placenta or the maternal genital tract
- Exclusion of possibility of postnatal transmission.

BABY BORN TO MOTHER WITH TB (DIAGNOSED IN THIRD TRIMESTER OR DURING DELIVERY)

- Breastfeeding to be continued
- BCG at birth
- If chest X-ray is normal, then 6HR
- If chest X-ray is abnormal, then 2HRZ + 4 HR
- Congenital tuberculosis 2 HRZ + 7HR.

DIFFERENCE BETWEEN TUBERCULAR AND ATYPICAL MYCOBACTERIAL LYMPHADENITIS

Mycobacterial lymphadenitis	*Atypical mycobacterial lymphadenitis*
Site: Posterior triangle, Supraclavicular	Site: Submandibular, Preauricular
Multiple and bilateral	Solitary, unilateral
Constitutional symptoms present	Constitional symptoms absent
Sinuses/fistula common	Sinuses rare
Contact history positive	Contact history negative
Chest X-ray findings may be present	Chest X-ray normal
Mantoux positive	Mantoux negative

CAUSES OF NEGATIVE MANTOUX IN TUBERCULOSIS

- Malnutrition, Tuberculous meningitis, miliary tuberculosis
- Viral infections: Measles, mumps, chickenpox
- Immunosuppresion: HIV infection, immunosuppressive drugs, malignancies
- Chronic renal failure
- Young infants
- Stress due to surgery, burns, etc.

CRITERIA FOR DIAGNOSIS OF PAPILLEDEMA

- Elevation of the optic disk
- Venules: Enlargement, dilatation, tortuosity, absence of pulsations
- Deflection of vessels over edge and elevated optic disk
- Blurred disk (temporal)
- Reddish optic disk
- Flame shaped hemorrhages near optic disk
- Few exudates
- Folds and edema of retina
- Usually bilateral
- Advanced cases—blurring and constriction of visual fields.

FUNDUS EXAMINATION IN PAPILLEDEMA AND OPTIC NEURITIS

Papilledema	*Optic neuritis*
• Bilateral (often)	Unilateral
• Vision-normal	Diminished
• No pain	Pain present
• Venous pulsations absent	Present

MODIFIED GLASGOW COMA SCALE FOR INFANTS AND CHILDREN

Child	*Infant*	*Score*
Eye Opening (E)		
Spontaneous	Spontaneous	4
To verbal command	To verbal command	3
In response to pain	In response to pain	2
No response	No response	1
Best Motor Response		
Obeys command	Moves purposefully	6

Contd...

Localizes painful stimulus	Withdraws to touch	5
Withdraws to painful stimulus	Withdraws to painful stimulus	4
Flexion in response to pain	Flexion in response to pain (Decorticate posture)	3
Extension in response to pain	Extension in response to pain (Decerebrate posture)	2
No response	No response	1
Verbal Response		
Oriented, appropriate	Coos and babbles	5
Confused conversation	Irritable cries	4
Inappropriate words	Cries to pain	3.
Incomprehensible sounds	Moans to pain	2
No response	No response	1

Maximum GCS Score at

- < 6 months is 9
- 6 months—1 year is 11
- 1 year is 12
- 5 years is 13
- > 5 years is 14.

Minimum GCS score at any time is 3. Even a dead child will have GCS 3.

DOLL'S EYE MOVEMENT

It is a vestibulo-ocular reflex acting through pons and medulla. It is not possible to demonstrate in conscious child due to their ability to fix at objects.

Response: When head is tilted to one side, eyes move to the opposite direction.

Appearance of Doll's eye: Deep coma with intact brainstem.

Disappearance of Doll's eye: Brainstem lesion.

STAGES OF COMA

- *Stage I or stupor:* Patient can be aroused briefly and shows verbal or motor response to stimuli.
- *Stage II or light coma:* Patient cannot be aroused easily, except with painful stimuli.
- *Stage III or deep coma:* No response to painful stimuli. Patient is either in decorticate or decerebrate posture.
- *Stage IV or brain death:* Loss of cerebral functions. Pupillary reflexes are absent, no spontaneous respiratory effort. However, local spinal reflexes may be lost.

HEMIPLEGIA

HISTORY

CHIEF COMPLAINTS

- Weakness of one-half of body
- Deviation of face to opposite side.

HISTORY OF PRESENT ILLNESS

History of Disease

Weakness

- Note the specific date and time of onset of paralysis
- Sudden/acute/chronic onset
- Precipitating factor (exertion/fever/convulsions)
- Progression—progressive/static/improving (complete recovery indicates cerebral embolism)
- Degree of paralysis
  - Is child able to walk
  - If unable to walk, does the child move legs in the bed
  - Does he lift arm to comb hair, lift objects.
- Site—upper limb/lower Limb or both.
- Weakness—proximal/distal.
- Sensory involvement.
- Cranial nerve involvement.

- Speech/gait abnormality.
- Involuntary movements (Extrapyramidal involvement/abnormal behavior).
- Any sphincter disturbance (autonomic system involvement).
- *Recovery:* Disappeared rapidly, slowly regressed over a period of time or persisting indefinitely.

History of Complications

- Bed sores
- Limb shortening
- Contractures
- Behavioral problems
- Activities of daily living—"DEATH", i.e. dressing, eating, ambulating, toileting, hygiene
- Todd's palsy: Following epileptiform convulsion there may be development of paralysis (commonly monoplegia, rarely hemiplegia) due to exhaustion of cerebral neurons. Todd's palsy usually recovers within 24 hours.

History of Risk Factors

- Focal seizures prior to hemiplegia (Todd's paralysis, stroke)
- Recurrent attacks of hemiplegia on same or opposite side (Alternating hemiplegia)
- Vaccination in recent past (Rabies)
- Early morning headache, projectile vomiting, focal seizures (Intracranial space occupying lesion)
- Mental retardation (degenerative and metabolic disorders)
- Recent exanthemas (Varicella)
- *Hematological causes:*
  - ❖ Paleness of body
  - ❖ Pain in abdomen/hand/foot (Sickle cell dactylitis)
  - ❖ Bleeding from any site/joint swelling (Coagulopathies)
  - ❖ Fever/bone pains/weight loss (leukemia)
  - ❖ Diarrhea/vomiting/decreased urine output/ blood in urine (Hemolytic uremic syndrome)
  - ❖ Repeated blood transfusion (Thalassemia major, sickle cell anemia).
- *Cardiac causes:*
  - ❖ Congestive cardiac failure (edema feet/ anorexia/suck-rest-suck cycle/failure to thrive)
  - ❖ Fever with chills/petechial hemorrhages/ Hematuria (infective endocarditis)
  - ❖ Blueness of body/cyanotic spells (cyanotic heart disease)
  - ❖ Breathlessness/chest pain/syncopal attacks/ joint pain (rheumatic heart disease).
- *Collagen vascular diseases/metabolic causes:*
  - ❖ Fever/facial rash/joint pain/exacerbation of symptoms on sun exposure (SLE)
  - ❖ Similar family history (hyperlipidemia/ homocystinuria).
- *Infections causes:*
  - ❖ Contact with tuberculosis
  - ❖ Rashes (herpes simplex/chickenpox)
  - ❖ Fever/altered sensorium/convulsions (meningitis)
  - ❖ Ear discharge with signs of raised intracranial tension (brain abscess).
- *Drug intake*: Cytotoxic drugs or cranial irradiation.
- *Trauma:* This is one of the important causes.

ANTENATAL AND PERINATAL HISTORY

- Preterm/breech
- Delayed cry at birth: Birth asphyxia

- Decreased activity/poor feeding/abdominal distension (septicemia)
- Rash, fever, petechial hemorrhages, prolonged jaundice, cataract (intrauterine infections)
- Exchange transfusion (embolism).

PAST HISTORY

- Similar type of attacks or monoplegia in the past which recovered completely (indicates Transient ischemic attacks)
- Head injury (subdural hematoma)
- Hypertension (cerebral thrombosis or hemorrhage)
- Rheumatic fever (valvular heart disease and cerebral embolism)
- Epilepsy (Todd's palsy)
- Tuberculosis (tuberculoma, tuberculous arteritis or tuberculous meningitis)
- Fever (meningitis, cerebral abscess, encephalitis, leukemia or lymphoma)
- Recent weight loss (brain tumor, tuberculosis).

FAMILY HISTORY

- Hypertension
- Diabetes mellitus
- Similar illness among other members of the family
- Epilepsy or migraine.

SOCIAL HISTORY

- Living conditions, upbringing
- Parent child relationship, peer group relationship
- Economic and cultural background
- Educational achievements.

OCCUPATIONAL HISTORY

- Relevant in days of child labor in poor and underprivileged.

GENERAL PHYSICAL EXAMINATION

- Consciousness of patient
- Pulse/BP/temperature/lymphadenopathy/edema/clubbing/cyanosis
- *Head:* Bulging anteior fontanelle, separated sutures (subdural hematoma, Intracranial space occupying lesion), bruit (AV malformation)
- *Face:* Butterfly rash (SLE)
- *Eyes:* Retinal hemorrhage (subdural hemorrhage), Roths spots (Subacute bacterial endocarditis), lens dislocation (homocystinuria)
- *Ears:* Ear discharge (Acute suppurative otitis media).
- *Oral cavity:* Cyanosis (cyanotic CHD), pallor (leukemia)
- *Skin:* Petechiae (bacterial endocarditis, leukemia), rash (measles, chickenpox), Xanthoma (hyperlipoproteinemia)
- *Signs of vasomotor instability:* Tachycerebrale, palmar erythema
- *Bones and joints:* Arthritis (SLE, Rheumatoid arthritis), Dactylitis (sickle cell anemia), joint effusions (hemophilia, collagen vascular diseases)
- Handedness (to establish dominant hemisphere), cortical thumb
- Facial asymmetry
- *Decubitus posture*
  - Upper limb (ipsilateral side): Flexed, adducted and semipronated
  - Lower limb (ipsilateral side): Extended, adducted and plantiflexed
  - Contralateral side: Within normal limit.
- *Neurocutaneous markers:*
  - Facial naevus
  - Adenoma sebaceum (Multiple erythematous papules on the lower half

of face-cheeks, nasolabial folds, sides of the nose and chin)
- Café-au-lait spots [Pigmented macules (>1 cm) on the trunk]
- Subungual fibromas (ulcerative lesions at base or corners of nails)
- Neurofibromas
- Ash-leaf spots (Hypopigmented macules generally 1 to 3 cm in size, multiple and discrete)
- Axillary freckling
- Shagreen patch (leathery plaques of subepidermal fibrosis, usually situated on the trunk).

SYSTEMIC EXAMINATION

NERVOUS SYSTEM EXAMINATION

Higher Mental Functions

- Consciousness
- Orientation—time, space and person
- Intelligence and judgment
- Memory
- Speech.

Cranial Nerves Examination

- *Olfactory*: Test the smell sensation with common bedside objects like soap, toothpaste, etc.
- *Optic*
  - Acuity of vision
  - Field of vision
  - Color vision
  - Ophthalmoscopy.
- *Oculomotor, trochlear and abducent*
  - Ptosis
  - Squint
  - Extraocular muscles movement
  - Nystagmus
  - Pupil—size, shape, reaction (light reflex, consensual light reflex and accommodation reflex).
- *Trigeminal*
  - Motor function (masseter, pterygoids and temporalis)
  - Sensory function (sensation over the face)
  - Corneal reflex.
- *Facial*
  - Palpebral fissure, frowning, eye closure, nasolabial folds, angle of the mouth
  - Ask the patient to show his teeth, epiphora, salivation, etc.
  - Upper half of face escaped or not
  - Taste sensation of anterior 2/3rd of the tongue.
- *Vestibulocochlear*
  - Hearing—Watch test, Rinne's test, Weber's test (for details see CNS examination in TBM).
  - Positional nystagmus.
- *Glossopharyngeal and vagus*
  - Soft palate—movements
  - Pharyngeal reflex
  - Taste sensation of posterior 1/3rd of the tongue.
- *Spinal accessory*
  - Power of sternocleidomastoids
  - Power of trapezius.
- *Hypoglossal*
  - Deviation of tongue
  - Atrophy or fasciculation of tongue.

Motor Functions

Compare Right with the Left

- Nutrition—Attitude of limbs/atrophy
- Bulk—Shape, size and symmetry of muscle
- Tone

- *Inspection*—Observe the posture
- *Palpation*—Palpate for feel of muscle
- Passive movement at Joint.

- Power.

Grading of Muscular Weakness

- Grade 0: Complete paralysis
- Grade 1: Flicker of contraction only (visible or palpable)
- Grade 2: Movements with elimination of gravity
- Grade 3: Movement against gravity but not against resistance
- Grade 4: Movement possible against gravity plus resistance but weaker than normal.
- Grade 5: Normal power.

Often, '+' or '–' symbols are used to improve the sensitivity of the grading.

- Compare hand size and thumb size
- Measure length of limb to detect shortening of limb
- Any dystonia or spasticity of limbs
- Involuntary movements.

Reflexes

- *Superficial:* Look for abdominal, cremastric and plantar response (Compare right with the left)
- *Deep:*

	Right	*Left*
Biceps jerk	+/–	+/–
Triceps jerk	+/–	+/–
Supinator jerk	+/–	+/–
Knee jerk	+/–	+/–
Ankle jerk	+/–	+/–
Clonus (ankle and patellar)	+/–	+/–

- *Visceral:* Bladder, bowel and swallowing reflexes.

Sensory Functions

Compare right with the left (for details see CNS examination in TBM)

- Spinothalmic—light touch, pain and temperature
- Dorsal column:
  - Joint sense
  - Vibration sense
  - Touch localization.
- Cortical sensation:
  - Two point localization (discrimination of two closely placed stimuli as separate)
  - Stereognosis (identification of object by touch and manipulation alone)
  - Graphesthesia (identification of letter or number written on skin surface).

Cerebellar functions: Normal (for detailed cerebellar examination see chapter on TBM).

Signs of meningeal irritation: Neck rigidity, Kernigs sign, Brudzinski sign.

Cranium and Spine

Trophic changes: Bed sore over sacrum

Autonomic functions: Normal.

Fundus Examination

Gait

- Describe gait
- Tiptoe walking
- Posture of upper limb
- Dystonia of upper limb or chorea.

CARDIOVASCULAR EXAMINATION

- Always search for a mitral diastolic murmur, especially in a patient with cerebral embolism
- Rheumatic heart disease—Cerebral embolism
- Hypertensive heart disease—Cerebral thrombosis and hemorrhage
- Congenital cyanotic heart disease—May give rise to cerebral abscess
- Bruit over the eyeballs/anterior fontanelle (for arteriovenous malformation).

RESPIRATORY SYSTEM EXAMINATION

Look for crepitations and rhonchi due to aspiration pneumonitis.

DIAGNOSIS

Acute/subacute; progressive/nonprogressive; Right/Left; hemiparesis/hemiplegia of congenital/acquired origin; with/without cranial nerve palsies/focal deficits with lesion at level of internal capsule/MCA territory with probable vascular etiology, probably occlusive/or hemorrhagic probably due to .... D/D

DIFFERENTIAL DIAGNOSIS

1. **Acute hemiplegia**
   - Spontaneous/catastrophic (in minutes)
     - Hemorrhage/embolism/trauma.
   - Acute (in 1-2 days)
     - Pyogenic meningitis/encephalitis/thrombosis/electrolyte imbalance/toxins.
   - Subacute/insidious (in days—weeks)
     - Infections—tuberculosis malignancies—brain tumor/partially treated pyogenic meningitis/neuroregression.
2. **Chronic nonprogressive hemiplegia**
   - Hemiplegic cerebral palsy
3. **Chronic progressive hemiplegia**
   - Intracranial space occupying lesions
     - Brain tumor, brain abscess, AV malformations.
   - Demyelinating diseases

     ALD, late onset globoid leukodystrophy
4. **Paroxysmal**
   - Epilepsy/migraine/periodic paralysis

INVESTIGATIONS

- Complete blood count with ESR, PT, PTTK, Fibrin degradation products
- Blood sugar, lipid profile, urea
- ECG to diagnose chamber enlargement in heart, arrhythmia
- Chest X-ray
- Echocardiography
- Carotid angiography and CSF study are not routinely done (carotid angiography may precipitate thrombosis in another territory of brain). Lumbar puncture is diagnostic in subarachnoid hemorrhage.
- Doppler flow studies in carotids
- CT scan of the brain—No information is obtained within first 48 hours; isodense for first 48 hours, hypodense with contrast enhancement thereafter (in case of infarction, i.e. thrombosis or embolism). CT scan is helpful for localization and extension of infarction with or without cerebral edema. CT scan can differentiate infarction (hypo-dense) from hemorrhage (hyperdense). MRI scan may be done.
- Prothrombotic workup
  - Protein C, S levels
  - Antithrombin III levels
  - Antiphospholipid levels
  - Blood, urine homocysteine levels
  - Peripheral smear for sickle cells.
- Serum lactate, pyruvate levels.

TREATMENT

- Neurosurgical intervention is required for the following causes:
  - Trauma
  - Tumour
  - Abscess.
- For CNS infection
  - Antibiotics (bacterial infection)
  - Antitubercular therapy (Tuberculous meningitis)
  - Acyclovir (herpes encephalitis).

- For vascular causes
  - Ischemic (aspirin prophylaxis)
  - Embolic (anticoagulants)
  - Hemorrhagic (correct underlying coagulation abnormalities).
- Patient should lie with frequently changing postures; insert Ryle's tube, put a self-retaining catheter and take care of the airway.
- Treat cerebral edema by:
  - 20% mannitol
  - Oral glycerol
  - Injection dexamethasone (if not hypertensive)
  - Injection frusemide.
- Treatment of diabetes mellitus, hypertension (maintain the BP), valvular heart disease
- Antiplatelet drugs (in thrombosis)—Low-dose aspirin or dipyridamole or ticlopidine for long-term prophylaxis. Pentoxifylline (changes viscosity of blood) may be beneficial in cerebral infarction if used within 12 hours of onset of stroke.
- Role of cerebral vasodilators are contradictory (5% CO_2 with 95% O_2, cyclandelate, nicotinic acid, papaverine, aminophylline, etc.) due to steal phenomenon.
- Anticoagulant therapy may the given (heparin) in an evolving stroke if cerebral hemorrhage is ruled out by early CT scan. Anticoagulant therapy is not of value in the treatment of completed stroke.
- Physiotherapy—Started as soon as the patient recovers from the neural shock stage. Changes of posture in bed must be done to avoid bed sores. Physiotherapy is advised to prevent joint contractures and to promote recovery of strength.
- Speech and occupational therapy.

DISCUSSION

The term **Acute Infantile Hemiplegia** is used only till onset within 4 years of age, because the growth of brain is till 4 years of age.

DEFINITIONS

Plegia means paralysis and '*paresis*' means weakness or partial paralysis.

Hemiplegia: Paralysis of one-half of the body (especially of face, arm and leg).

Hemiplegia cruciata: Paralysis of ipsilateral lower limb and contralateral upper limb. It occurs due to arm fibers crossing before leg fibers at the lower part of medulla.

Paraplegia: Paralysis of both the lower limbs.

Diplegia: Bilateral hemiplegia of cortical origin where the lower limbs are more affected than the upper limbs.

Double hemiplegia: Both halves of body involved with upper limbs more affected than lower limbs.

Triplegia: Diplegia with superimposed hemiplegia.

Quadriplegia: Paralysis of all the four limbs.

Monoplegia

- Paralysis of one limb
- Brachial monoplegia: Paralysis of one upper extremity
- Crural monoplegia: Paralysis of one lower extremity.

Crossed hemiplegia: Paralysis of ipsilateral cranial nerves (LMN type) with contralateral hemiplegia.

Stroke: A stroke or CVA is defined as a 'focal neurological deficit of abrupt onset due to a pathological process in the blood vessels'. The term *apoplexy* (transient cessation of cerebral circulation) is still sometimes used for severe strokes, especially when the patient is unconscious.

LOCALIZATION OF LESION IN HEMIPLEGIA

See figure 18.1

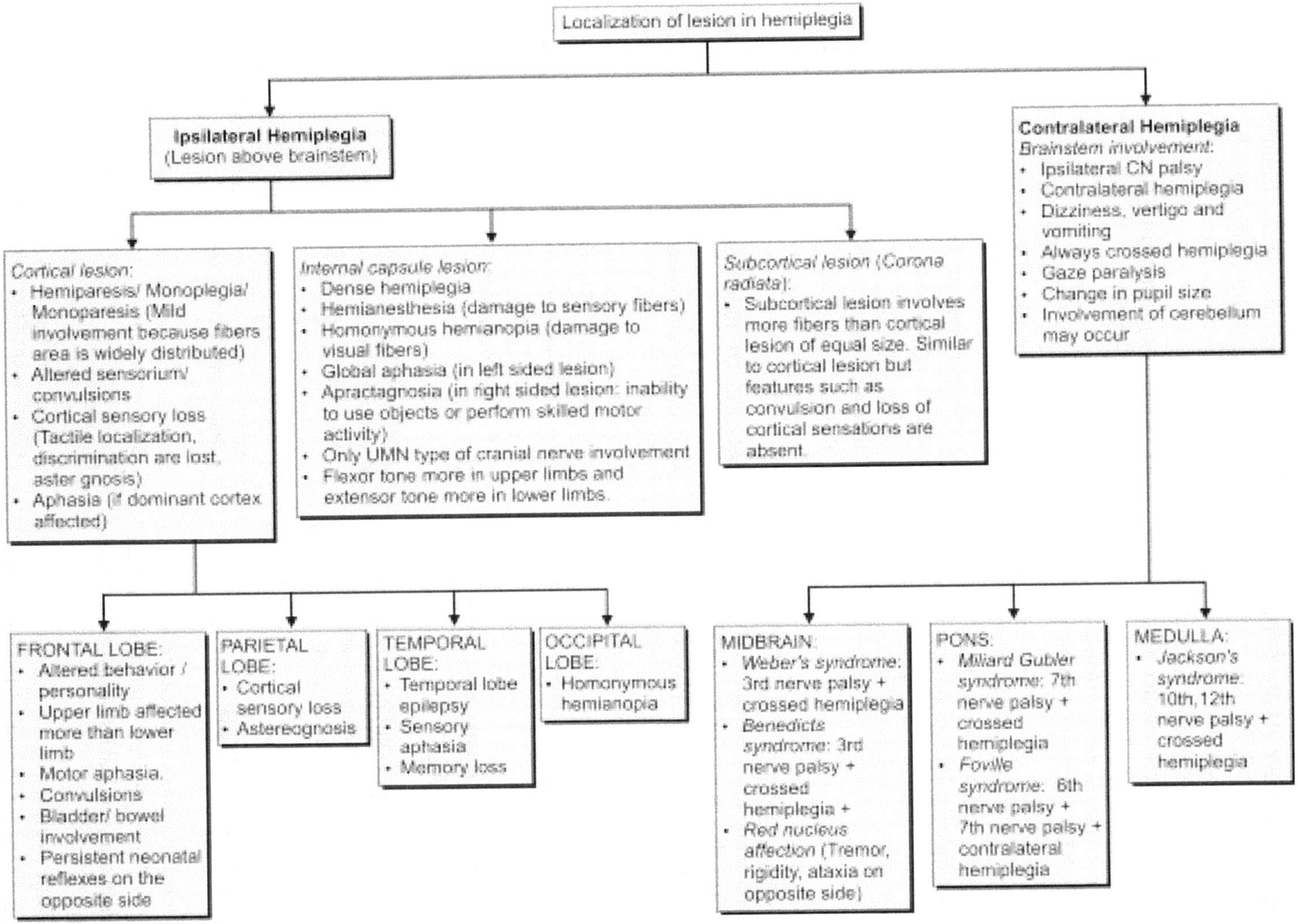

Fig. 18.1: Localization of lesion in hemiplegia

VIITH NERVE PALSY (UMN TYPE)

- All cranial nerve nuclei are bilaterally supplied by pyramidal fibers except the lower part of the VIIth cranial nerve nuclei which supplies pyramidal fibers only from the opposite side. So the lower face is easily affected (i.e. UMN type of VIIth nerve palsy) in patient of hemiplegia.
- UMN type of VIIth cranial nerve palsy is always associated with same sided hemiplegia while hemiplegia, if at all present with LMN type of VIIth cranial nerve palsy, is always crossed.

Site of Lesion

- VIIth cranial nerve palsy (UMN type) with ipsilateral hemiplegia—Lesion is above the pons (opposite side)
- VIIth cranial nerve palsy (LMN type) with contralateral hemiplegia (lesion is at VIIth cranial nerve nucleus)—Lesion is at pons on the side of VIIth nerve palsy
- No facial nerve involvement (incomplete hemiplegia)—Lesion is below the level of pons.

DIFFERENCE BETWEEN 9TH AND 10TH CRANIAL NERVE PALSY

Gag reflex is absent in both 9th and 10th cranial nerve palsy. If the child wretches on attempted gag reflex then the sensory arc is intact—9th cranial nerve is intact.

SUPERFICIAL REFLEXES

- Red nucleus inhibits superficial reflexes
- Causes of exaggerated superficial reflex: Chorea, extrapyramidal lesion, psychoneurosis, hysteria
- Aseptic meningitis
- No organisms are identified by routine CSF analysis, despite a high neutrophil and lymphocyte count.
- Causes include viruses (mumps, measles), fungi, brucellosis, atypical TB, sarcoidosis, partially treated pyogenic meningitis.

ALTERNATING HEMIPLEGIA OF CHILDHOOD

- Onset before 18 months of age
- Repeated attacks of hemiplegia involving either side of body
- Other paroxysmal disturbances like dystonic attacks, nystagmus, dyspnea
- Disappearance of symptoms on going to sleep, with recurrence 10-20 minutes after awakening
- Evidence of developmental delay and mental retardation.

CAUSES OF RECURRENT HEMIPLEGIA

- Cardiovascular system: Multiple emboli from heart
- Prothrombotic conditions
  - Protein C, S deficiency
  - Antithrombin III deficiency
  - Antiphospholipid antibody
  - Increased homocysteine levels.
- Metabolic
  - MELAS
  - Leighs encephalopathy.
- Moya moya disease
- Alternating hemiplegia of childhood.

Table 18.3: Stages of hemiplegia

1. Stage of neural shock (may extend up to 2-3 weeks) • Patient may be in coma • Hypotonia • Absence of deep tendon reflexes.
2. Stage of recovery • Recovery is in the following order • Face (earliest) • Lower limb (extensors recover first) • Upper limb (flexors recover first) • Dorsiflexion of foot (minimal recovery) • Fine movements of finger.
3. Stage of residual paralysis • Some amount of deficit persists.

BLOOD SUPPLY OF BRAIN

Blood supply of brain

- Anterior cerebral artery
  - Frontal and parietal lobes
  - Part of internal capsule
  - Paracentral lobule, i.e. the center for movements of the lower limbs plus the center
  - For micturition and defecation.
- Middle cerebral artery
  - Motor, sensory and speech areas
- Posterior cerebral artery
  - Visual cortex, occipital lobe and part of the temporal lobe
  - Part of the posterior limb of internal capsule

PARAPLEGIA

HISTORY

CHIEF COMPLAINTS

- Weakness of both the lower limb
- Hesitancy of micturition and loss of bowel control
- Cough with evening rise of temperature.

HISTORY OF PRESENT ILLNESS

History of Disease

Motor Symptoms

- Note the specific date of onset of paralysis
- Sudden (acute transverse myelitis, spinal injury) or gradual (caries spine)
- Precipitating factors: Spinal injury/vaccination (commonly antirabies vaccine and rarely hepatitis B vaccine)
- Evolution: Whether both the limbs are affected simultaneously or one after the other
- Progression:
  - Increasing in severity and extent: Cord compression
  - Improving: Inflammatory, acute transverse myelitis
  - Static, slowly progressing: Degenerative lesion (Friedreich's ataxia).
- *Degree and duration of paralysis:*
  - Is patient able to stand with or without support
  - Able to walk with or without support
  - Noticed any abnormality while walking.
- *Neonates:* Paucity of movement, persistent fisting
- *Older children:* Difficulty in climbing stairs, dressing, rising from floor
- Involuntary movements
- Cranial nerve involvement—visual loss, facial asymmetry, dysarthria, etc.

Sensory Symptoms

- Loss of sensation
- Girdle—like sensation or sense of constriction (find out the level)
- Paraesthesia, numbness or tingling
- Any hyperaesthesia (find out the level)
- Root pain (distribution and precipitating factors)
- Sensation of pins and needles in the lower extremities.

Autonomic Symptoms

- Sweating, loss of temperature control

- Bowel, bladder complaints—retention, incontinence, constipation.

History of Complications

- Bed sores
- Limb shortening
- Contractures
- Foot deformities: Pes cavus, hammer toes
- Abnormal gait:Scissoring, waddling, toe walking
- Activities of daily living: "DEATH", i.e. dressing, eating, ambulating, toileting, hygiene
- Cognitive decline.

History of Risk Factors

- Trauma to spine
- Prolonged fever, back pain (tuberculosis)
- Fever, rash, diarrhea and upper respiratory tract infection (acute transverse myelitis)
- Weight loss, bony pains (malignancy)
- Recent exanthem or vaccination
- Drug intake or toxin exposure
- HIV risk factors
- Any chronic systemic illness.

FAMILY HISTORY

- Hypertension (as a routine)
- Paraplegia in other members of the family (if present may indicate hereditary spastic paraplegia or paraplegia with hereditary ataxia)
- Tuberculosis
- History of consanguinity.

SOCIAL HISTORY

- Living conditions, upbringing
- Parent child relationship, peer group relationship
- Economic and cultural background
- Educational achievements.

OCCUPATIONAL HISTORY

- Relevant in days of child labor in poor and underprivileged.

GENERAL PHYSICAL EXAMINATION

- Conscious and co-operative
- Decubitus—lying without any movement of the lower limbs and with extension of all joints (lower limb). Upper limbs are within normal limit
- Lymph nodes—not palpable (tuberculosis, lymphoma or malignancy)
- Respiration—search for respiratory depression in Gullian Barre syndrome
- Blood pressure
- Temperature (tuberculosis, acute transverse myelitis, urinary tract infection)
- Edema—look for sacral edema
- Spine—kyphoscoliosis, gibbus, local tenderness
- Skin—absence of neurofibroma or Café-au-lait spot or any rash
- Pes cavus
- Decubitus ulcers
- Dribbling of urine.

SYSTEMIC EXAMINATION

NERVOUS SYSTEM EXAMINATION

Higher mental functions

Cranial nerve examination: Optic, facial and 9, 10, 12 cranial nerve examination.

Motor functions: Both the upper limbs are within normal in all respect

- Nutrition: Attitude of limbs/Atrophy

- Bulk: Shape, size and symmetry of muscle
- Tone
  - Inspection: Observe the posture
  - Palpation: Palpate for feel of muscle
  - Passive movement at joint
- Power
- Involuntary movements.

Reflexes

Superficial

- Abdominal
- Cremasteric—lost bilaterally
- Plantar response—extensor in both the lower limbs

Deep	Right	Left
Biceps jerk	Normal	Normal
Triceps jerk	Normal	Normal
Supinator jerk	Normal	Normal
Knee jerk	Brisk	Brisk
Ankle jerk	Brisk	Brisk
Clonus (ankle and patellar)	Present	Present

Visceral

- *Bladder:* Catheterized
- *Bowel:* Incontinence present or not
- Swallowing.

Sensory functions

Both the upper limbs are normal

- Spinothalmic—light touch, pain and temperature
- Dorsal column
  - Joint sense
  - Vibration sense
  - Touch localization.
- Cortical sensation—two point localization (discrimination of two closely placed stimuli as separate), Stereognosis (Identification of object by touch and manipulation alone), Graphesthesia (Identification of letter or number written on skin surface)
- Zone of hyperesthesia.

Signs of Meningeal Irritation

Neck Rigidity

Place your hand under the supine child's head and gently try to flex the neck. Undue resistance implies irritation of cranial nerve roots from meningeal inflammation. A conscious child should be asked to flex the neck and touch the chin to chest.

Kernig's Sign

With child supine, flex the hip and knee on one side, then extend the knee with the hip still flexed. With meningeal inflammation, there is pain in posterior thigh muscle and knee extension becomes difficult. With severe meningeal inflammation, the opposite knee may also flex during the test.

Brudzinski Sign

To elicit Brudzinski sign, place your hand behind the child's head and place the other hand on child's chest. Then, flex the child's head while hand on chest restrains the child and prevents the child from rising. Flexion of child's hips and knees constitutes a positive sign.

- **Cranium and spine** (Do not forget to examine spine in all patients with paraplegia)
- **Cerebellar functions:** Normal
- **Trophic changes:** Bed sores
- **Autonomic functions:** Loss of sweating below the level of umbilicus
- **Fundus examination**.

RESPIRATORY SYSTEM

- Tuberculosis: Crepitations at the apex, consolidation or pleural effusion

- Lymphoma: Superior venae cava syndrome or pleural effusion.

GI TRACT AND GENITOURINARY SYSTEM

- Organomegaly or ascites (Tuberculosis, lymphoma)
- Percuss the bladder and see the color of the urine present in urobag (chalky or turbid urine is seen in UTI, orange colored urine is due to rifampicin).

CARDIOVASCULAR SYSTEM

- Routine CVS examination.

LYMPHORETICULAR SYSTEM

- Sternal tenderness, lymphadenopathy.

DIAGNOSIS

This is a case of spastic/flaccid paraparesis (or paraplegia) due to compressive/uncompressive myelopathy caused by—— (e.g. caries spine) and the lesion is at the level of —— segment of the spinal cord.

If compressive myelopathy further classify it as Extramedullary or Intramedullary. Extramedullary lesions are further classified as extradural and intradural.

DIFFERENTIAL DIAGNOSIS

COMPRESSIVE MYELOPATHY

Cervical:

- Trauma
- Congenital anomalies (Klippel Fiel syndrome, Atlanto axial dislocation)
- Syringomyelia.

Thoracic:

- Pott's spine
- Subdural abscess
- Meningioma.

Lumbar:

- Lesions of intervertebral disk
- Spinabifida
- Neoplastic (ependymoma).

NONCOMPRESSIVE MYELOPATHY

Acute (Usually up to 4 weeks):

- Viral (Poliomyelitis, Enterovirus 70)
- Immunological (Acute transverse myelitis)
- Toxic
- Demyelinating diseases.

Subacute (4-8 Weeks):

- Lathyrism
- Tropical spastic paraplegia
- Infectious.

Chronic (> 8 Weeks):

- Infections (Tuberculosis)
- Toxic myelopathies
- Radiation myelopathy.

Pott's Spine

- Deformity/swelling/tenderness in the vertebra
- Root pain present
- Upper border of sensory loss present
- Girdle-like sensation or sense of constriction at the level of lesion (posterior column involvement)
- Zone of hyperesthesia is present 1 segment above the level of girdle-like sensation (compression of posterior nerve roots)
- Loss of deep reflexes, if the particular segment is involved. The reflexes will be brisk below the involved segment
- Lack of sweating below the level
- X-ray of the spine, CT scan or MRI confirms the diagnosis.

Acute Transverse Myelitis

- Fever may be present before onset of AFP, but rarely during onset.
- Paralysis is symmetrical in lower limbs
- Profound anesthesia to all forms of sensation (sensory involvement)
- Hypotonia and absent DTRs
- Early bladder involvement
- Though behaves like compressive variety, usually there is absence of root pain, spinal tenderness or spinal deformity. Girdle constriction at the level of lesion with zone of hyperesthesia just above may be obtained.
- Plantar response is extensor and there is partial or complete sensory loss with definite upper level (In acute infective polyneuropathy where these two features are: flexor plantar response and no demonstrable sensory loss respectively).
- No cranial nerve involvement/No signs of encephalitis.

Traumatic Neuritis

- Onset of AFP in lower limb occurs 1 hour to 5 days after injection in gluteal region.
- Fever may be present before onset of paralysis as injection is given for preexisting febrile illness.
- Accompanied by pain in gluteal region or affected leg atrophy may appear 40 to 60 days after.
- Knee jerk is present, ankle jerk is absent or diminished. Child walks with a foot drop.

Guillain-Barré Syndrome

- History of fever 2-3 weeks prior to illness.
- Flaccid, symmetric paralysis with absence or diminished DTRs.
- Commonly, paralysis of GBS is ascending, affecting lower limbs first followed by trunk, then upper limbs.
- Bilateral cranial nerve involvement is common. Facial nerve is most common followed by difficulty in swallowing secondary to 9th and 10th cranial nerve involvement.
- Sensory involvement is frequently present
- Hypoesthesia or anesthesia in glove and stocking distribution.
- CSF findings: In poliomyelitis CSF shows 20-300 WBCs and protein is normal or minimally elevated while in GBS, WBCs usually < 10 and proteins are up to 200 mg.
- Nerve conduction velocity: Normal in poliomyelitis, but is reduced in GBS.
- Electromyography: Abnormal in polio with signs of denervation and giant action potential, while in GBS it is normal or slightly abnormal.

INVESTIGATIONS

- Complete blood count, blood sugar and urea
- Urine routine and culture sensitivity test
- Mantoux test—Positive in tuberculosis
- Chest X-ray—To exclude tuberculosis
- X-ray of the spine (anteroposterior and lateral view)—Helps in the diagnosis of caries spine, metastasis, fracture and detection of the site of spinal lesion.
- Lymph node biopsy
- CSF examination:
  - Cytology
  - Protein
  - Sugar
  - PCR for *Mycobacterium tuberculosis*, isolation of virus.
- MRI scan: Spinal cord and brain:
  - Rule out compression
  - Localisation of lesion
  - Demyelination
  - Intramedullary tumors.

- Antinuclear antibody
- Serum B_{12} levels
- Serology for HIV/ enteroviruses
- Electromyogram/nerve conduction velocity/ muscle biopsy, if required.

TREATMENT

- Nutritious diet
- Care of the bladder, bowel and trophic ulcers:
  - *Bladder*—Put a self-retaining catheter under aseptic technique; change the catheter regularly at 2-3 weeks interval, bladder wash, to help in bladder control by application of clip to the drainage tube. Urine routine and culture sensivity as and when necessary, antibiotics in urinary tract infections.
  - *Bowel*—Constipation treated by laxatives
  - Trophic ulcers are cleaned by hydrogen peroxide, dressed; protect the other pressure points by adhesive plasters (attached to a distance from the pressure points).
- Muscle spasms are treated by diazepam, baclofen
- Treat underlying cause:
  - *In caries spine*—Traction in early stage. Later on 'plaster jacker' is applied for immobilization. Antitubercular chemotherapy (4 drugs regimen) is often continued for one year.
  - Treatment of carcinoma or lymphoma by radiotherapy/chemotherapy.
  - Acute transverse myelitis—ACTH or corticosteroid.
- Physiotherapy
- Surgery—Drainage of cold abscess, fusion of the vertebra, laminectomy for caries spine.

DISCUSSION

- ***Myelopathy*** denotes a pathologic involvement of the spinal cord
- Classified as compressive and non compressive
- Distinctive features between the two are Table 18.4:

Table 18.4: Differentiation between compressive and noncompressive myelopathy

	Compressive	*Noncompressive*
Onset and progression	Gradual and progressive	May be acute
Motor	• Unilateral to begin • Asymmetrical • Around the clock weakness (Elesberger phenomena)	• Usually bilateral • Symmetrical
Sensory	• Focal back pain present • Root pains present • Sacral sparing present • Dissociative anesthesia present • Girdle like sensation present • Sensory level present • Zone of hyperesthesia present	• Absent • Absent • Absent • Absent • Absent • Absent • Absent
Sphincter involvement	Late in extramedullary lesions early in intramedullary lesions	Late (early in acute transverse myelitis)
Vertebral deformity	Present	Absent
Spinal tenderness	Present	Absent
CSF cyto albumino dissociation	Present	Absent

When it is clear that spinal cord is involved by compressive lesion then differentiate whether the compressive lesion is Extramedullary or intramedullary (Table 18.5).

With extramedullary lesions, knife like pain is prominent, and there are early sacral sensory loss (lateral spinothalamic tract) and spastic weakness in the legs (corticospinal tract); this is due to superficial location of leg fibers in corticospinal tract.

Intramedullary lesions tend to produce poorly localized burning pain and spare sensation in perineal and sacral areas (sacral sparing) reflecting outermost localization of sacral and lumbar fibers.

Table 18.5: Differentiation between extramedullary and intramedullary lesions

	Extramedullary	*Intramedullary*
Symptom	Asymmetrical	Symmetrical
Cutaneous pain	Sharp, knife like	Burning ,poorly localized
Sensory deficit	• Marked sacral sensory loss • No dissociation of sensation	• Sacral sparing • Dissociative anesthesia (loss of pain, temp but preservation of vibration and propioception)
Motor	• Round the clock weakness in upper cervical lesion (Elesberg phenomenon) • Corticospinal tract sign early and Increased Reflexes	• Upper limb weakness is out of proportion to the lower limbs • Corticospinal tract sign late and Reflexes not increased
Sphincter	Late involvement	Early
CSF Changes	Frequent	Minimal

RELATIONSHIP OF BLADDER, HAND AND LEG FIBERS IN THE SPINAL CORD

The bladder fiber runs closest to the central canal in the spinal cord followed by hand fiber and the leg fiber runs laterally.

The order of involvement in different brain tumors with relation to the anatomy:

- *Intramedullary tumor (Table 18.5):* Bladder-Hand-Leg (as the tumor grows medial to lateral)
- *Extramedullary tumor(Table 18.5):* Leg-Hand-Bladder.

The extramedullary compression can be grouped into Extradural (generally malignant) and Intradural (generally benign) (Table 18.6). Long duration of symptoms favors an intradural origin.

Table 18.6 Differentiation between extradural and intradural lesions

	Extradural	*Intradural*
Root pains	Early and usually bilateral	Usually unilateral
Spinal ache	Prominent	Usually absent
Tenderness	Present	Usually absent
Signs of cord compression	Bilaterally symmetrical	Unilateral asymmetrical
CSF block	Late and less marked	Early and marked
CSF protein	Increased	Markedly increased

DETERMINATION OF SPINAL SEGMENTS IN RELATION TO VERTEBRA

The vertebral column grows more than the spinal cord hence the spinal segments are higher than the corresponding vertebral bodies.

- For lower cervical add one
- For T1-T6 add two
- For T7-T9 add three
- T10 overlies L1 and L2
- T11 overlies L3 and L4
- T12 overlies L5
- L1overlies sacral and coccygeal spinal segments
- Paraplegia results from lesions below T1

- Extensor plantar response: Lesion above L5
- At the site of lesion: LMN type of paralysis below that UMN type of paralysis.

UPPER MOTOR VS LOWER MOTOR NEURON LESIONS

Upper Motor Neuron

- Comprises of motor cortex and the corticospinal tracts
- Hypertonia
- Brisk reflexes
- Weakness in corticospinal distribution.

Lower Motor Neuron

- Comprises of the anterior horn cells, the motor nerve cells in the motor nuclei in brainstem, the motor nerve fibers, motor end plate and muscle fibers
- Diminished muscle tone
- Absent reflexes
- Muscle wasting and fasciculation's
- Weakness in distribution consistent with affected segment, nerve.

LOCALIZATION OF THE LEVEL OF COMPRESSION

- Distribution of root pain
- Upper border of sensory loss, i.e. examine from legs to thorax
- Girdle-like sensation or sense of constriction at the level of lesion (posterior column involvement)
- Zone of hyperesthesia is present 1 segment above the level of girdle like sensation (compression of posterior nerve roots)
- Abdominal reflex, i.e. if upper abdominal reflex is intact with loss of middle and lower one, the site of lesion is probably at T10 spinal segment.
- Atrophy of the muscles in a segmental distribution (involvement of anterior horn cells)
- Loss of deep reflexes, if the particular segment is involved. The reflexes will be brisk below the involved segment
- Analysis of *Beevor's sign* (do the rising test, in paralysis of lower part of rectus abdominis, umbilicus moves upwards and in paralysis of upper part of rectus, umbilicus goes downwards)
- Deformity/swelling/tenderness in the vertebra
- Lack of sweating below the level
- X-ray of the spine, CT scan or MRI.

Cervical Cord Lesions

- High cord lesions: Quadriplegia with respiratory paralysis
- Lesions at C4-5: Quadriplegia
- Lesions at C5-6: Loss of biceps and brachioradialis reflex with brisk triceps reflex
- Lesions at C7: Loss of triceps and wrist extensors resulting in paradoxical flexion (Unilateral-Jolly's sign; Bilateral-Thorborn's sign)
- Lesion at C8-T1: Loss of wrist and finger flexors
- Horner syndrome occurs ipsilaterally.

Thoracic Cord Lesions

- Identification of sensory level on the trunk
- Nipple at T4 and umbilicus at T10 important markers
- Lesion at T9-10: Paralysis of lower abdominal musculature spares the upper abdominal wall resulting in ***Beevors sign***
- Loss of superficial reflexes below the level of lesion.

Lumbosacral Cord Lesions

- Lesion at L1,2,3: Loss of hip flexion, adduction with loss of knee jerk
- Lesion at L4-S1: Loss of hip extension, plantar flexion, dorsiflexion, loss of knee flexion with loss of plantar and ankle reflex
- Lesion at S2: Affects intrinsic muscles of foot
- Lesion at S3,4: Loss of anal and bulbocavernous reflexes.

SENSORY IMPAIRMENT

- Inguinal area L1
- Pocket area L2
- Knee L3
- Medial aspect of leg L4
- Lateral aspect of leg, dorsum of foot with great toe L5
- Lateral aspect of foot S1
- Popliteal fossa S2
- Perianal area S2,3,4

Table 18.7: Differentiation between Conus medullaris and Cauda equina lesions

	Conus medullaris	*Cauda equina*
Onset	Sudden and Bilateral	Gradual and unilateral
Pain	Uncommon, Bilaterally symmetrical in perineum and thighs	Prominent; radicular
Sensory loss	Bilaterally symmetric in saddle area with dissociation of sensation	Unilateral asymmetric in saddle distribution, no dissociation
Motor deficit	Symmetric	Asymmetric, more marked
Reflex loss	Only achilles absent	Both knee and ankle may be absent
Bladder,bowel involvement	Early and marked	Late and less marked
Sexual functions	Impaired erection and ejaculations	Less affected
Decubitis	More common	Less common

DEEP TENDON REFLEXES

- Jaw jerk : Trigeminal
- Biceps : C5, 6
- Supinator : C6
- Triceps : C7
- Knee : L2, 3, 4
- Ankle : S1

RULE OF 3 (SENSORY DERMATOMES)

- C3 : Nape of Neck
- T3 : Axilla
- L3 : Knee
- S3 : Perianal area

CAUSES OF XANTHOCHROMIA IN CSF

- Old subarachnoid hemorrhage (due to pressure of old blood)
- Guillain-Barré syndrome (due to high protein)
- Froin's loculation syndrome (spinal subarachnoid block)
- Deep jaundice.

CAUSES OF ALBUMINO CYTOLOGICAL DISSOCIATION IN CSF

Increased protein in CSF without any rise in cell count

- Guillain-Barré syndrome

- Froin's loculation syndrome(Low pressure, xanthochromia, clot formation on standing, high protein content).
- Tuberculous arachnoiditis
- Anterior spinal artery occlusion
- Intraspinous tuberculoma.

CAUSES OF PARAPLEGIA IN SPINAL TUBERCULOSIS

- Nerve root compression due to Pott's spine
- Pressure effect of granulation tissue

PARAPLEGIA DUE TO CEREBRAL CAUSE

- Spastic diplegia
- Parasaggital tumor
- Anterior spinal artery thrombosis.

HYDROCEPHALUS

HISTORY

CHIEF COMPLAINTS

- Increase in size of head.

HISTORY OF PRESENT ILLNESS

History of Disease

- Increase in size of head
  - Congenital/acquired
  - Onset
  - Progression
  - Precipitating factor.
- Limb weakness:
  - Onset: Sudden/acute
  - Progression: Static/increasing
  - Weakness of upper or lower limb
  - Degree and duration of paralysis
  - Proximal or distal involvement
  - Evolution: Both limbs affected simultaneously or one after the other.
- Sensory symptoms
- Cranial nerve involvement
- Bowel/bladder complaints
- Involuntary movements
- Blindness/deafness
- Sunsetting of eyes
- Convulsions/unconsiousness (meningitis)
- Meningomyelocele with paraplegia
- Increased intracranial tension
  - Headache
  - Nausea, vomiting
  - Head banging, diplopia.
- Respiratory tract infection
  - Cough, fever
  - Difficulty in respiration
  - Activities of daily living- "DEATH", i.e. dressing, eating, ambulating, toileting, hygiene.

History of Risk Factors

- Maternal risk factors:
  - Drug intake (Vitamin A Toxicity)
  - Radiation exposure in 1st trimester
  - TORCH infection.
- Fetal risk factor:
  - Preterm child
  - Birth asphyxia.
- Contact with tuberculosis
- Trauma.

DEVELOPMENTAL HISTORY

In detail.

GENERAL PHYSICAL EXAMINATION

- Anthropometry:Increase in head circumference by more than 1 cm in every 2 weeks for the first 3 months of life makes clinician suspicious.
- Dysmorphic facies
- Pallor/cyanosis/icterus/lymphdenopathy/edema feet
- Skull:
  - Shape
  - Anterior fontanel/posterior fontanel
  - Sutural separation
  - Craniotabes.
- Transillumination test
- Bruit over head
- Eyes: Sunsetting/cataract
- Neurocutaneous markers
- Spine
- Presence and patency of shunt (VP shunt).

SYSTEMIC EXAMINATION

- Detailed CNS examination
- Examine neonatal reflexes.

DIAGNOSIS

.... year old child with enlargement of head with/without paraplegia, with/without raised intracranial tension, with developmental age of......; Diagnosis is hydrocephalus most probably due to .... (etiology of hydrocephalus).

DIFFERENTIAL DIAGNOSIS

Megaloencephaly

- Associated with severe mental retardation
- No signs of raised intracranial tension
- Ventricles not enlarged
- Causes: Hurler's syndrome, metachromatic leukodystrophy, Tay Sachs disease.

Chronic Subdural Hematoma

- Large head mostly in parietal region
- No prominent scalp veins or sunset sign.

Other Causes of Large Head

- Rickets
- Hydranencephaly
- Achondroplasia
- Hemolytic anemia.

INVESTIGATIONS

- Hemogram with ESR
- X-ray skull
  - Enlargement of calvarium
  - Sutural diastasis
  - Thinning of bone
  - Erosion of clinoid process
  - Deepened sella turcica.
- CT scan brain/MRI/Ultrasound brain
- CSF study (after fundus examination)
- Slit-lamp examination to r/o chorioretinitis.

TREATMENT

Depends on:
- Etiology
- Associated malformation
- Clinical course.

Arrested Hydrocephalus: No Treatment

Medical Management

To decrease the raised ICT:
- Mannitol (20%) : 5-8 ml/kg/dose every 6 hourly for 2 days, then,
- Acetazolamide (50-75 mg/kg/day) decreases CSF production or glycerol may be given orally or through RT in chronic cases, if raised intracranial tension persists.

Surgical Management

Indications

- Head size enlarging rapidly
- Congenital obstructive hydrocephalus
- Periventricular ooze, acquired hydrocephalus.

Shunt Operation

- Ventriculoatrial (commonly used)
- Ventriculoperitoneal (commonly used)
- Ventriculocaval (to jugular vein or superior vena cava)
- Lateral ventricle to cisterna magna
  - Different varieties of silastic valves are used and the commonly used one is 'Spitz-Holter' valve.
- Treatment of associated conditions like meningitis
- Nutritional management.

DISCUSSION

DEFINITION

Increased volume of CSF within the ventricles, resulting due to obstruction of the CSF circulation or there may be failure of CSF absorption by the arachnoid villi.

TYPES OF HYDROCEPHALUS

Congenital

Intrauterine Infections

- Rubella
- Cytomegalvirus
- Toxoplasmosis.

Malformations

- Aqueductal stenosis
- Dandy walker syndrome
- Arnold Chiari malformation.

Acquired

- Intracranial meningitis
- Tuberculous meningitis
- Intracranial hemorrhage
- Posterior fossa tumors.

Double compartment hydrocephalus (trapped 4th ventricle): Aqueductal stenosis associated with obliteration of 4th ventricle outlet.

Unilateral: Due to compression of opposite lateral ventricle and hemiparenchymal atrophy.

Hydrocephalus ex vacuo: Ventricular dilatation associated with cerebral atrophy and normal CSF pressure.

Normal pressure hydrocephalus: It is a misnomer, Initially there is increased pressure but ultimately CSF hemodynamics compromise (ventricles dilate) and it becomes normal or low pressure hydrocephalus. This is predominantly seen in old age with the triad of symptoms such as dementia, ataxia and urinary incontinence. Though it may result from head injury, subarachnoid hemorrhage or meningitis, many a time no cause is identified.

CIRCULATION OF CSF

Production

Eighty percent CSF comes from choroid plexus in lateral, 3rd and 4th ventricles. Rest from parenchyma, ependyma and capillary endothelium (See Fig. 18.2).

Rate of CSF Production

20 ml/hour or 400-500 ml/day. CSF is replaced 3 times/day.

Volume of CSF

50 ml in infant and 90 ml in children 4-13 years of age.

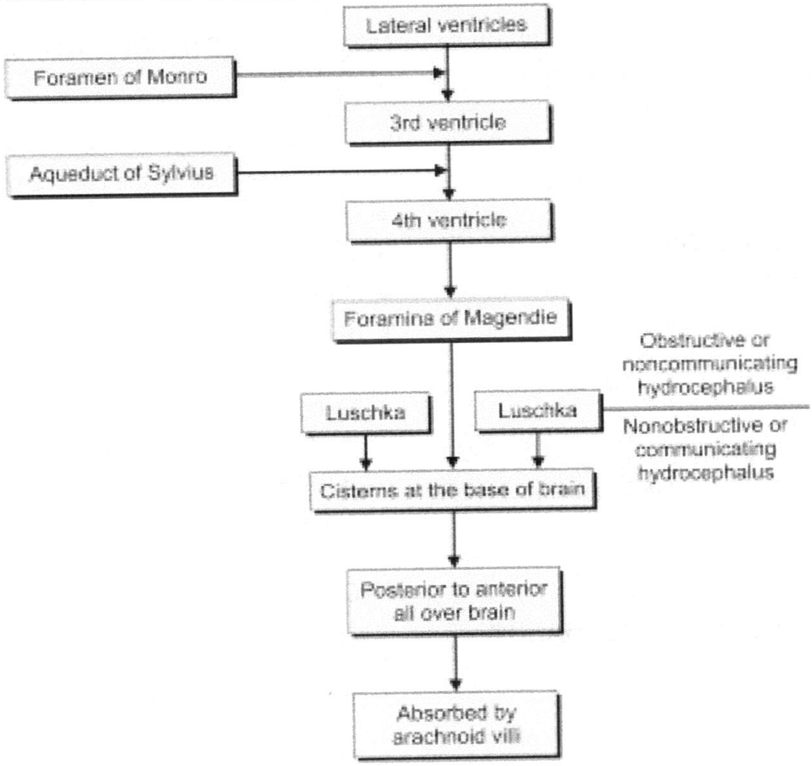

Fig. 18.2: Flow of CSF

FACTORS CAUSING HYDROCEPHALUS

- *Increased production of CSF:* Choroid plexus papilloma
- *Decreased absorption of CSF:* Obstruction of arachnoid villi or other peripheral subarachnoid pathways
- *Obstruction to flow of CSF:* Tumors/ inflammatory exudates/congenital failure of opening of foramina of Luschka and Magendie.

Diagnosis of Hydrocephalus

Signs and Symptoms

- Abnormal enlargement of head, especially the frontal area
- Sutural separation
- Bulging of the anterior fontanelle
- *Setting sun sign*: The eyes appear to be pushed down and thus the upper bulbar conjunctiva becomes visible
- Scalp veins are dilated and the skin over the scalp is thin and shiny
- *Macewen sign:* Skull is resonant on percussion
- High pitched cry
- Spastic limbs due to stretching of cortical fibers.

Examination and Investigations

- Serial recording of head circumference plus suggestive ultrasound helps in early diagnosis
- Head circumference increases more than 1cm every fortnight for 1st 3 months leads to suspicion of hydrocephalus

- CT scan and MRI brain helps evaluate ventricular size, cortical mantle, periventricular ooze and etiology of hydrocephalus
- X-ray skull: Separation of sutures, posterior clinoid process erosion, silver beaten appearance.

FEATURES OF LATE ONSET HYDROCEPHALUS

- Head size may not enlarge
- Sutural separation may not be present
- Mental retardation
- Presence of papilledema
- Spastic and ataxic child (legs are more involved)
- Urinary incontinence.

PHYSIOLOGICAL BUFFERS IN RESPONSE TO HYDROCEPHALUS

- Collapse of cerebral veins
- Shunting of CSF from ventricular compartment to spinal CSF compartment
- Skull enlargement
- Increased CSF absorption from arachnoid villi.

COMPLICATIONS OF CSF SHUNT SURGERY

Shunt should be kept for entire life. Revise shunt using a longer tube as the child grows.

- Shunt block
- Ventriculitis (by *Staphylococcus albus*)
- Shunt nephritis (acute glomerulonephritis)
- Bacterial colonization of shunt
- Fracture of tubing
- Abdominal complications:
  - Intestinal obstruction (volvulus)
  - Peritonitis.
- Ventricular collapse.

PROGNOSIS

- If untreated: 50% die, 50% survive
  - In survivors 50% have handicaps and 50% normal intelligence.
- Prognosis depends on cause of hydrocephalus
- Hydrocephalus with spina bifida has poor prognosis.

ACUTE FLACCID PARALYSIS

HISTORY

CHIEF COMPLAINTS

Weakness in limbs.

HISTORY OF PRESENT ILLNESS

History of Disease

Weakness

- Sudden/insidious onset
- Duration of weakness (i.e. hours to days to weeks/months)
- Mode of onset (ascending or descending) and progression
- Degree of paralysis:
  - Patient able to stand with or without support
  - Able to walk with or without support
  - Noticed any abnormality while walking.
- Type of weakness: Symmetrical or asymmetrical.
  - Upper limb/lower limb
  - Proximal/distal weakness
  - Mainly extensor or flexor involvement (in poliomyelitis extension of lower limbs occur)
  - Unilateral/bilateral weakness.

- Involvement of respiratory muscles: Cyanosis/ decreased chest movements
- Weakness of appendicular muscle
  - Difficulty in reaching for and grasping objects
  - Inability to bear weight on leg.
- Weakness of axial muscles:
  - Inability to sit up
  - Poor head control.

CNS History

- Involuntary movements/altered sensorium
- Wasting of muscles
- Sensory involvement: Numbness, tingling, loss of balance, pain/burning
- Bulbar involvement: Change in voice or difficulty in swallowing, excessive secretions
- Autonomic involvement: Diarrhea, orthostatic dizziness, urinary retention, palpitations, sweating, flushing, disturbed vision
- Facial weakness: Trouble chewing, sucking with straw, blowing
- Extraocular muscle weakness: Diplopia or ptosis
- Respiratory involvement: Dyspnea, orthopnea
- Bladder or bowel involvement (fleeting paralysis of bladder and constipation in polio)
- Raised intracranial tension: Vomiting, headache, convulsions, focal neurological deficits
- Systemic symptoms: fever, weight loss, rash, joint pains.

History of Complications

- Activities of daily living— "DEATH", i.e. dressing, eating, ambulating, toileting, hygiene
- Malena (superficial intestinal erosion in polio)
- Abdominal pain (due to gastric dilatation).

History of Differential Diagnosis

- Guillain-Barré syndrome: Fever and sore throat, 2-3 weeks prior to illness.
- Myositis: Pain in muscles
- Familial periodic paralysis: Loose motions/ vomiting/dehydration.

History of Risk Factors

- Recent illness (diarrhea or respiratory tract infection)
- Recent immunization (oral polio vaccine)
- Recent travel [out of country, to woods (tick bites)]
- Precipitating factors (exertion, carbohydrate loading with periodic paralysis)
- Drug or toxin exposure (canned or 'bad' food, pesticides, 'statins', lead exposure)
- Trauma:Intramuscular injection in gluteal region
- Family history (porphyria)
- Fever with rash (exanthematous illness/viral illness): Herpes/mumps/rubella/influenza/EB virus/HIV/enterovirus.

IMMUNIZATION HISTORY

Take detailed immunization history mentioning pulse polio immunizations also.

GENERAL PHYSICAL EXAMINATION

- Autonomic testing (postural vitals, abnormal sweating, pupillary response, ileus)
- Anthropometry
- Respiratory distress
  - Any irregularity in rate, depth and rhythm of respiration (medullary involvement in polio)
  - Inability to speak without frequent pauses resulting in short, jerky, breathless sentences.
  - Movement of alae nasi and accessory muscle involvement
  - Paradoxical abdominal movement due to diaphragm immobility
  - Relative immobility of intercostals spaces.
- BCG mark

- Neurocutaneous markers: Hypopigmentation, Café-au-lait spot
- Blue line at gums—lead poisoning
- Skin: Rash of Lyme disease (*erythema chronium migrans*), lines on nails with arsenic poisoning (*Mee's lines*), ticks, photosensitivity, *Gottron's papules* (on extensor surfaces) and heliotrope discoloration over eyelids
- Spinal tenderness (with epidural abscess or hematoma, spinal tumor)
- Straight leg rise (radiculopathy)
- Decubitus—especially of involved limb
- Phantom hernia (unilateral bulging on either side of the abdomen due to weakness or paralysis of abdominal wall muscles).
- Rope sign (acute angulation between chin and larynx caused by weakness of hyoid muscles).

SYSTEMIC EXAMINATION

CENTRAL NERVOUS EXAMINATION

- Distribution and degree of weakness.
- Assess power in various group of limb muscles.
- Examine extraocular muscles (ptosis), facial muscles, arms and legs.
- Test neck muscle by doing pull to sit maneuver. There will be head drop if neck muscles are weak.
- *Assess diaphragmatic function:*
  - Depth of respiration
  - Rate of respiration
  - Diaphragmatic paralysis: Respiratory distress on splinting intercostals
  - In intercostal muscle paralysis: Splinting of abdomen causes distress
  - Single breath count.
- Describe the pattern of weakness (e.g. paraparesis, faciobrachial, multifocal) if possible.
- *Assess involvement of bulbar muscles*
  - Nasal twang
  - Inability to swallow: Salivation
  - Ineffective coughing with constant fatigue efforts to clear throat
  - Nasal regurgitation
  - Deviation of palate, uvula or tongue.
- *Sensory loss*
  - To particular modality (vibration/propioception pain/temperature)
  - Look for sensory level
- *Reflexes*
  - Superficial reflexes lost or not
  - DTRs lost (i.e. areflexic) or depressed (In poliomyelitis superficial reflexes are lost before DTRs).

DIAGNOSIS

Right/left; upper limb/lower limb; flaccid, monoplegia/paraplegia affecting proximal/distal (proximal > distal or vice versa) muscles; with/without sensory features/areflexia/autonomic disturbances; most probable etiology being ....

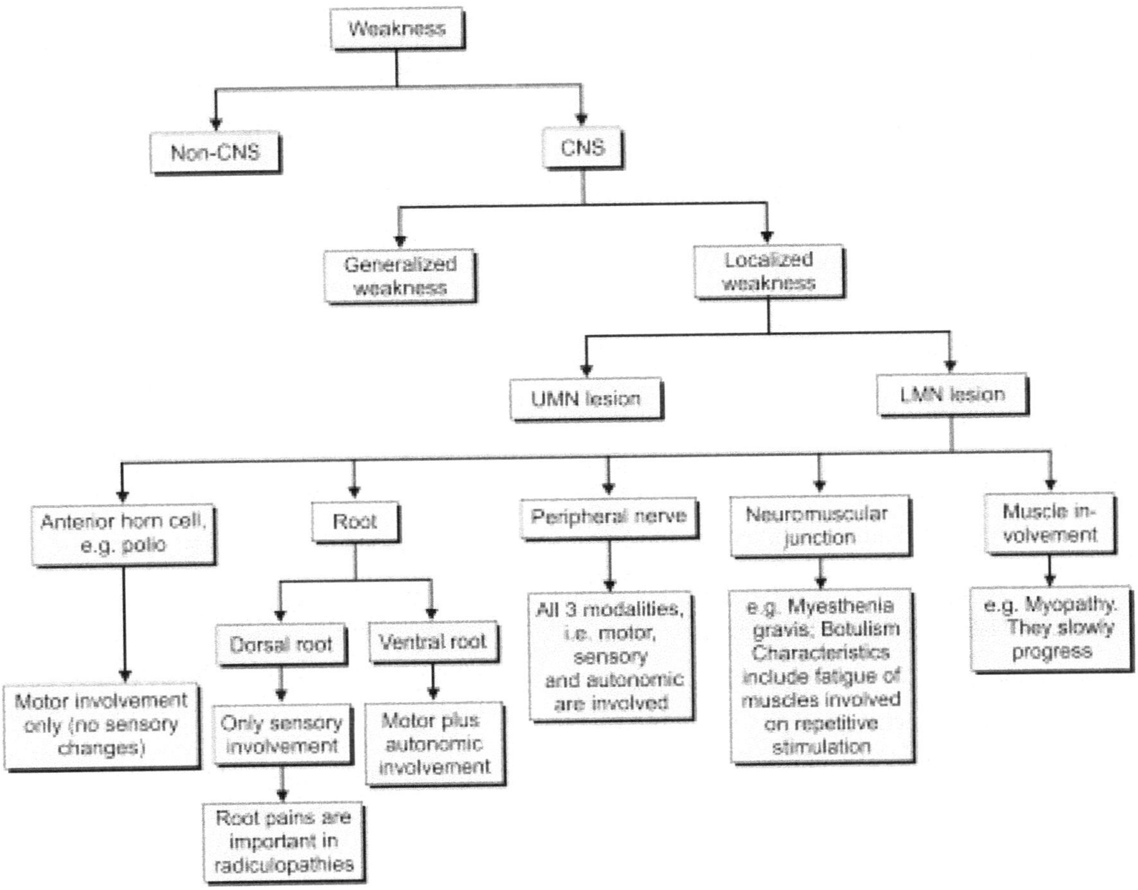

Fig. 18.3: Differential diagnosis of weakness

APPROACH TO AFP

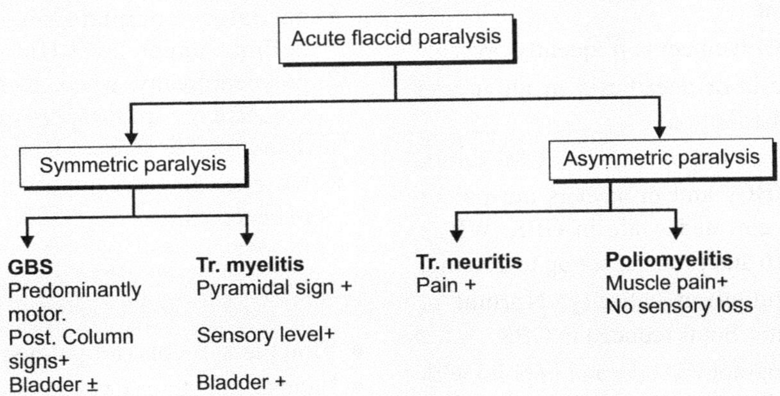

DIFFERENTIAL DIAGNOSIS

POLIOMYELITIS

- Acute onset
- Fever just prior to paralysis—hallmark finding
- Muscle pain
- Asymmetrical paralysis (Proximal muscle involvement/patchy involvement/motor involvement)
- Absent or diminished DTRs
- No sensory loss
- Unimmunized child
- History of intramuscular injection may be there.

GUILLAIN-BARRE SYNDROME

- History of fever 2-3 weeks prior to illness.
- Flaccid, symmetric paralysis with absence or diminished DTRs.
- Commonly, paralysis of GBS is ascending, affecting lower limbs first followed by trunk, then upper limbs.
- Bilateral cranial nerve involvement is common. Facial nerve is most common followed by difficulty in swallowing secondary to 9th and 10th cranial nerve involvement.
- Sensory involvement is frequently present
- Hypoesthesia or anesthesia in glove and stocking distribution.
- CSF findings: In poliomyelitis CSF shows 20-300 WBCs and protein is normal or minimally elevated while in GBS, WBCs usually < 10 and proteins are up to 200 mg.
- Nerve conduction velocity: Normal in poliomyelitis, but is reduced in GBS.
- Electromyography: Abnormal in polio with signs of denervation and giant action potential, while in GBS, it is normal or slightly abnormal.

TRAUMATIC NEURITIS

- Onset of AFP in lower limb occurs 1 hour to 5 days after injection in gluteal region.
- Fever may be present before onset of paralysis as injection is given for preexisting febrile illness.
- Accompanied by pain in gluteal region or affected leg atrophy may appear 40 to 60 days after.
- Knee jerk is present, ankle jerk is absent or diminished. Child walks with a foot drop.

ACUTE TRANSVERSE MYELITIS

- Fever may be present before onset of AFP, but rarely during onset
- Paralysis is symmetrical in lower limbs
- Profound anesthesia to all forms of sensation (sensory involvement)
- Hypotonia and absent DTRs
- Early bladder involvement
- Though behaves like compressive variety, usually there is absence of root pain, spinal tenderness or spinal deformity. Girdle constriction at the level of lesion with zone of hyperesthesia just above may be obtained
- Plantar response is extensor and there is partial or complete sensory loss with definite upper level (In acute infective polyneuropathy, where these two features are: flexor plantar response and no demonstrable sensory loss respectively)
- No cranial nerve involvement/No signs of encephalitis.

INVESTIGATIONS

- Viral titers: Stools (for polio virus)
- Lumbar puncture: Cytoalbuminic dissociation (in GBS)

- ECG: To look for Cardiac involvement
- X-ray spine: If history of trauma
- Blood sugar: To rule out diabetes mellitus
- Serum electrolytes: Hypokalemia for familial periodic paralysis
- Electromyogram
- Nerve conduction velocity.

TREATMENT

Home Management

- Rule out bulbar involvement: Nursing care/Oral hygiene/Ryle's tube feeding
- Bed rest
- Passive movements of the joints
- Hot water fermentation
- If respiratory involvement: Ventilator therapy.
- Frequent change in position. Optimum position for joints
  - Hip—mild flexion
  - Knee—5° flexion
  - Foot—90° dorsiflexion
  - Lateral support to keep limbs opposed.
- Analgesics for muscle pain
- Positive physiotherapy: When muscle pain subsides.
- Bladder care: Warm fermentation, intermittent catheterization.
- Bowel care: Feeding and laxatives.
- For Guillain-Barré syndrome: Intravenous immunoglobulins (400 mg/kg/day for 5 days); Plasmapheresis; steroids.
- Orthotic appliances.

Indications for Hospitalization

- Progressive weakness.
- Respiratory deterioration: Increased respiratory rate and distress, decreased single breath count (< 8), decreased chest expiration (< 2 cm).
- Bulbar involvement: Indicated by feeding problem, nasal regurgitation, pooling of saliva, decreased voice volume.
- Paralysis of upper limbs of < 3 days.

Outcome

- Prognosis is excellent with majority of patients making a good recovery over weeks or months.
- Factors that correlate with poor outcome are:
  - Rapid progression to severe weakness (7 days or less)
  - Need for ventilator support
  - Mean distal compound muscle action potential amplitude less than 20 percent of normal.
  - Preceding *Campylobacter* infection.

DISCUSSION

DEFINITION OF ACUTE FLACCID PARALYSIS

- Paralysis of acute onset (< 4 weeks) duration in a child < 15 yrs of age
- Affected limbs are flaccid with diminished tone
- Cases of acute flaccid paralysis are confirmed as polio, if they:
  - Are associated with isolation of wild poliovirus from the stool of the case OR
  - Have residual neurologic sequelae at 60 days after the onset of paralysis OR
  - Died before follow-up could determine whether residual neurologic sequelae was present at 60 days after onset of paralysis, OR

- Were lost before follow-up could determine whether, compatible residual neurologic sequelae was present at 60 days after onset of paralysis.

MONOVALENT, BIVALENT AND TRIVALENT ORAL POLIO VACCINE

Monovalent oral polio vaccine-1 (mOPV1) is made using only the attenuated strain of type-1 poliovirus and immunizes only against that type (type 1). Except that it does not contain types 2 and 3, mOPV1 is in all other respects similar to trivalent oral polio vaccine (tOPV).

Advantanges of Monovalent Over Trivalent OPV

- Increased immunity to type 1 poliovirus compared to tOPV for the same number of doses. This is because with tOPV there is some interference between the three types of poliovirus.
- Stronger response than tOPV in children being immunized for the first time.
- If children immunized with mOPV1 are subsequently exposed to wild poliovirus type1, they will excrete less virus and for a shorter period of time, limiting the possibility of further transmission.

Bivalent OPV

- Bivalent OPV is effective against types 1 and 3. Type 2 has been eradicated.

WHY MOPV1 IS USED IN SOME AREAS AND NOT OTHERS

Although wild poliovirus type 2 is not circulating anywhere in the world since 1999, type 3 continues to circulate extensively in west and central Africa, and in Pakistan/Afghanistan.

mOPV1 only offers protection against poliovirus type 1, and is therefore only suitable for use in endemic areas where, type 3 poliovirus is no longer circulating, or is at very low levels.

In Egypt and India, population density and birth rates are very high, and the transmission of wild poliovirus type 1 is at its most efficient.

CAUSES FOR POLIO IN FULLY IMMUNIZED CHILD

- Non-maintenance of cold chain
- Diarrhea during vaccination
- Malnutrition and poor sanitation
- HIV
- Enteroviral infection (polio like viruses).

EMG-NCV CHANGES IN POLIO AND GBS

- In Polio—EMG shows giant denervation potential
- In GBS—Nerve conduction is delayed (both sensory and motor).

TOTAL NO OF CONFIRMED POLIO CASES

Year 2009: 1548 total polio cases reported in world in 2009, 703 cases reported in India (Nigeria: 388; Pakistan: 86).

- Uttar Pradesh 571
- Bihar 114
- Delhi 4

Vaccine Derived Polio virus: 16 cases of Vaccine derived polio virus were reported in 2009 in our country due to Polio virus 2, while 2 cases of VDPV were due to Polio virus 1.

Year 2008

559 cases reported in India (75 cases due to Polio virus 1; 484 cases due to Polio virus 3; no case was due to Polio virus 2).

PSEUDOPARALYSIS

Certain conditions present with pseudoparalysis which may be confused with AFP. These conditions are not AFP and should not be reported as AFP.

Hypokalemia: Children are toxic, irritable and present with generalized acute flaccid paralysis of all 4 limbs, neck flop and abdominal distension.

Scurvy: Onset is gradual. History of irritability, digestive disorders and loss of appetite. There is generalized tenderness and child resents handling. Pain leads to pseudoparalysis and legs are kept in frog position.

Acute osteomyelitis, Non specific toxic synovitis, and Congenital syphilitic osteomyelitis are other conditions causing pseudoparalysis.

VIRUS ISOLATION AND SPECIMEN COLLECTION

Stool: Virus can be isolated from feces from 72 hours till 6 weeks after infection, with the highest probability during the first 2 weeks.

Specimen: 8 grams of faeces (approximately thumb sized amount).

Number: Two specimens 24 to 48 hours apart.

When: Within 2 weeks of paralysis onset, no later than 4 weeks.

How: Use clean plastic screw cap container with name, identification number, specimen number and date.

Temperature storage: Less than +8°C.

SURVEILLANCE

Each case of AFP should be investigated within 48 hours of being reported. The steps in the investigation are:

- Collection of demographic and clinical information of the cases
- Filling up of case investigation forms
- Collection of 2 stool samples 24- 48 hours apart from the case
- Sixty day follow-up to see residual paralysis
- Outbreak control should cover entire village in rural areas and the municipal area in urban areas. Children under 5 years of age should receive highest priority to receive one dose of OPV regardless of polio immunization history.

BACKGROUND RATE

- Surveillance is carried out for all cases of AFP, not just for poliomyelitis
- Background rate: 1 case of AFP for every 1,00,000 population children aged <15 years/year
- Background AFP rate is due to other causes of flaccid paralysis (other than polio), e.g. Guillain-Barré syndrome, transverse myelitis, traumatic neuritis.

INDICATORS OF SURVEILLANCE PROGRAM

- Rates of AFP: 1 case of AFP for every 1,00,000 population children aged <15 years/year
- Monthly reporting
- Percentage of AFP cases with 2 stools taken within 2 weeks after onset of paralysis: This percentage should be 80% or greater.

Cerebral Palsy

HISTORY

CHIEF COMPLAINTS

- Delayed milestones
- Convulsions.

HISTORY OF PRESENT ILLNESS

History of Disease

Detailed developmental history: Developmental history should review gross motor, fine motor and verbal milestones from birth until the time of evaluation.

- Course—progressive/static/improving
- Predominant speech delay: Hearing problem, autism, dyslexia
- Predominant motor delay
- Global delay that is nonprogressive (child is achieving milestones but at a later date than expected, child has not lost any achieved milestones)
- Global delay that is progressive
- Development status prior to onset of symptoms
- Any advanced milestones (indicates spastic CP), e.g. early roll over, ability to stand on legs, toe walking
- Current social skills
- Academic performance
- Participation in an early intervention program (if aged < 3 years) or school support (if aged > 3 years) should be reviewed, including resource room assistance
- Physical, occupational, speech and language therapy
- Adaptive physical education
- Standardized cognitive and educational testing can be asked.

CNS History

- Mental retardation, abnormality in behaviour and communication
- Cranial nerves—vision, hearing, speech, drooling of saliva and pooling of secretions
- Motor system—Bulk of muscles/Power (weakness of upper limb/lower limb; proximal or distal involvement)
- Upper limb involvement: Tying shoelaces, buttoning clothes, handwriting, pincer grasp, clumsiness.
- Abnormal posture:
  - Scissoring of legs
  - Arching of body
  - Inequality of movement of limbs
  - Abnormal Fisting
  - Difficulty in handling baby during feeding, bathing and dressing
- Athetosis, i.e. slow, writhing, involuntary movements particularly in the distal extremities
- Chorea (i.e. abrupt, irregular, jerky move ments), choreoathetosis (i.e. combination of athetosis and choreiform movements)
- Dystonia, i.e. slow rhythmic movements with muscle tone abnormalities and abnormal postures
- Response to loud noise
- Follows objects or not
- Speech disturbances
- Sensory system dysfunction
- Bladder/bowel control achievements

- Convulsions
- Vomiting/increasing head circumference/altered sensorium (raised intracranial tension).

History of Complications

CP cases that are generally kept for examinations are admitted due to associated complain like respiratory infections, convulsions, and diarrhea.

- Respiratory difficulty, bedsores, deformities.
- *Nutritional history:*
  - When were oral feeds started
  - Who feeds the child
  - How often
  - How long does it take
  - Associated problems like vomiting, constipation.
- Contractures, behavioral problems, bladder problems.
- Activities of daily living: "DEATH", i.e. Dressing, Eating, Ambulating, Toileting, Hygiene.

History of Early Signs of CP

- Seizures during neonatal period
- Lethargy, absent sucking and rooting reflexes
- Persistent fisting beyond 2 months
- Persistent development reflexes beyond the age at which they should disappear
- Scissoring of legs
- Hand preference before 1 year.

History of Risk Factors

Maternal Risk Factors

- General:
  - Booked case
  - Number of antenatal visits
  - Immunization with tetanus toxoid
  - Iron and folic acid supplementation.
- First trimester:
  - Hyperthermia in first 4-6 weeks (can cause microcephaly, seizures and dysmorphic facies)
  - Rash with fever (rubella)
  - Drug and alcohol intake (fetal alcohol and fetal hydantoin syndrome)
  - Radiation exposure.
- Second trimester:
  - Prenatal exposure to illicit drugs, toxins or infections
  - Acute maternal illness; trauma; radiation exposure
  - Prenatal care and fetal movements
  - Frequent spontaneous abortions.
- Third trimester:
  - Prenatal exposure to illicit drugs, toxins or infections
  - Acute maternal illness; trauma; radiation exposure
  - Prenatal care and fetal movements
  - Antepartum hemorrhage
  - Premature onset of delivery or labor.
- Duration of labor:

Gravida	*1st Stage*	*2nd Stage*
Primi	16 hours	1 hour
Multi	8 hours	30 minutes

- Natal:
  - Place of delivery: Home/Institutional.
  - Person conducting delivery: Trained/ Untrained.
  - Nature of delivery: Normal/ Forceps/ LSCS/ Vacuum.
  - Breech/ abnormal presentation.

Fetal Risk Factors

- Birth weight
- Prematurity
- Birth asphyxia

- American pediatric gross assessment record (APGAR) score
- Meconium stained liquor or instrumentation
- Complications in the neonatal period (intubation, use of surfactant, convulsions, presence of ischemia or hemorrhage on neonatal ultrasound, feeding difficulties, apnea, bradycardia, infection, hyperbilirubinemia).
- Details of placenta.

FAMILY HISTORY

- Age of both parents
- Parental consanguinity
- Duration of married life
- Any similar illness in family
- Any miscarriage, abortion and their reason.

GENERAL PHYSICAL EXAMINATION

- Alertness and interest in surroundings.
- Posture: Decorticate posture, Cortical thumb, ophisthotonus posture.
- Prior to the formal physical examination, observation may reveal abnormal neck or truncal tone; asymmetric posture, strength, or gait; or abnormal coordination.
- Anthropometry.
- Dysmorphic features.
- Involuntary movements.
- Spasticity may be evident in a tendency to keep elbow in a flexed position or hips flexed and adducted with knees flexed and the valgus and ankles in equinus (resulting in toe walking).
- Anterior fontanel/sutural ridging or separation/posterior fontanel/flat occiput.
- Eye changes:
  - Nystagmus.
  - Cataract
  - Strabismus
  - Cortical blindness
  - Optic atrophy
  - Papilledema.
- Vitamin deficiency/dental caries/poor oral hygiene/bedsores/contractures/alopecia/skin and hair changes of protein energy malnutrition.
- Spine.
- Review the patient's equipment or need for equipment such as: Adaptive and communication devices/walkers/seating.
- Neurocutaneous markers:
  - Facial nevus/nodules
  - Café-au-lait spots
  - Tubers/neurofibromas
  - Ash-leaf patch
  - Axillary freckling
  - Shagreen patch
  - Hypo/hyperpigmented spots.
- Primitive reflexes:
  - Asymmetric tonic neck reflex
  - Moro's reflex
  - Rooting and sucking reflex
  - Grasp-Palmar and plantar.
- Autonomic nervous system: Bladder and bowel movements.

SYSTEMIC EXAMINATION

CNS EXAMINATION

Higher mental functions—Alertness/interest in surroundings/inappropriate smiles/does not responds to speech.

Cranial Nerves Examination

- I: Smell sensation.
- II:Head turned to light, optic blink, fundus examination.

- III/IV/VI: Pupils, Extraocular muscle palsies.
- V: Rooting, glabellar tap.
- VII: Facial asymmetry.
- VIII: Acoustic blink, labyrinthine rotation.
- IX, X, XII: Sucking, swallowing, Gag reflex.

Examination of Motor System

Look for Following Signs of Hypotonia

- *Inspection*-Posture: Pithed frog posture—Abduction and external rotation of limbs.
- *Palpation*
  - Muscle feel (shows decreased tone)
  - Decreased resistance to passive movements
  - Increased range of movements along joints
  - Scarf sign
  - Popliteal angle sign
  - Abductor angle
  - On Pull-to-sit: There is Head lag and back is rounded
  - On axillary suspension: There may be telescoping of body
  - On ventral suspension: Head lag is pronounced.

Popliteal Angle (Table 18.8)

With infant in a supine position the thigh is held in the knee chest position by supporting the thigh with examiner's left hand. The leg is then extended by gentle pressure with examiner's right hand index finger placed behind the ankle and popliteal angle is measured.

Scarf Sign (Table 18.8)

Baby is supine and head is maintained in the midline. Arm is held at the wrist and pulled across the chest towards the opposite shoulder.

Abductor Angle

Infant lies supine with legs extended and head in the midline. Both hips are abducted maximally by holding the knee with index finger cutting over the front of thighs. The angle between thighs is the abductor angle.

Table 18.8: Maneuvers to diagnose hypotonia

Tests	*Normal/What to look for*	*Abnormal*
Popliteal angle	90-120°	Greater
Scarf sign	Elbow does not cross midline	Elbow crosses midline
Heel to ear	Does not reach the opposite ear	Reaches the opposite ear
Arm recoil	Brisk	Slow or none

Abnormal Developmental Reflexes

Patients with CP may show the persistence of primitive reflexes (e.g. the Moro or asymmetric tonic neck reflexes) or the underdevelopment or absence of postural or protective reflexes.

A Moro reflex and a tonic labyrinthine reflex should extinguish by the time the infant is aged 4-6 months; palmar grasp by 5-6 months; asymmetric and symmetric tonic neck by 6-7 months; and foot placement before 12 months.

Sensory system examination (for detailed cerebellar examination see chapter on TBM)

Meningeal signs (for detailed meningeal signs see chapter on TBM)

Gait

Developmental examination (will demonstrate spasticity)

- *Pull-to-sit:* Demonstrate tightening of hamstring muscles
- *Prone position:* Head and pelvis touch bed without flexion at the hip joints
- *Ventral suspension:* Head control, Telescoping of body, Scissoring of legs
- *Developmental Reflexes:* In detail.

Assessment of Vision:

- Gross: Micro-ophthalmia, squint, cataract
- Light perception.

Other System: Examined as usual.

DIAGNOSIS

............year old child with delayed development milestones.

Classify:

- Anatomical
- Physiological
- Etiological
- Functional.

With/without mental retardation/convulsions/ blindness/deafness/speech with developmental age of (Gross motor......; Fine motor ......; Language.......; personal social......)

DIFFERENTIAL DIAGNOSIS

NEURODEGENERATIVE DISORDER

- Initial normal development with subsequent slowing of development
- Regression of previously acquired skills
- Unusual body odours
- Family history of similar disorder
- Hypotonia without hyperactive reflexes
- Ataxia
- Movement disorders.

MENTAL RETARDATION

- Children are retarded evenly in all areas as compared to cerebral palsy, who have delayed motor milestones associated with persistence of primitive reflexes
- Motor milestones may be less affected or normal.

MYOPATHIES

- Progressive increase in weakness
- Muscle atrophy or pseudohypertrophy
- Hypotonia
- DTR normal till late stages
- Planters normal.

INVESTIGATIONS

Diagnosis is essentially clinical and laboratory tests are not required to make diagnosis

- Head CT scan identifies congenital malformations, intracranial hemorrhage and periventricular leukomalacia in infants more clearly than ultrasound.

Indications:

  - Focal neurological signs
  - Seizures, Neurocutaneous markers
  - Large head or small head
  - Intrauterine infections.

- MRI brain is the diagnostic neuroimaging study of choice, since it defines cortical and white matter structure and abnormalities more clearly than any other method. It also allows for the determination of appropriate myelination for a given age.
- X-ray skull: No role except when accompanied by microcephaly and craniosynostosis.
- USG skull (if anterior fontanel is open): For detection of intraventricular hemorrhage and periventricular leukomalacia in preterms
- Lumbar puncture: After fundus examination to rule out raised intracranial tension
- Intelligence quotient/Development quotient test
- Vision and hearing assessment: Always screen systematically for visual and auditory problems even if, then may not be clinically apparent
- Chest X-ray: If lower respiratory tract infection or defective drainage of respiratory secretions

due to deformities and bed ridden state of the patient.

TREATMENT

GOALS

- Normal development of child
- Improve skill of child
- Child becomes as much independent as possible.

Line of Management

- Reduction of spasms
- Seizure control
- Appropriate school placement
- Training for any employment
- Young infant simulative program
- Correction of defects
- Explain the prognosis to parents
- Physiotherapy—Both active and passive. To reduce incidence of positional deformities and to recruit whatever muscles are functional so as to decrease the disability to a certain extent.
  - Prevents and retards development of muscle contractures
  - Improves motor functions
  - Improves the strength of muscle
  - Positioning—To reduce primitive reflexes.
- Methods to increase muscle tone:
  - Drugs: Diazepam/nitrazepam, Baclofen, Dantrolene, Levodopa
  - Use of manipulative methods like positioning muscles.
- Treatment of associated disorders:
  - Treatment of epilepsy
  - Treatment of visual problems like squint/myopia
  - Speech therapy for communication problems
  - Psychiatric treatment for behavior disturbances
  - Special education.
- Nursing care and nutritional management
- Orthopedics opinion for the surgical management of hip dislocation, scoliosis and spasticity (tenotomy, a tendon-lengthening procedure)
- Neurosurgery should be consulted for identifying and treating hydrocephalus, a tethered spinal cord or spasticity.

DISCUSSION

DEFINITION

Cerebral palsy is nonprogressive static encephalopathy often associated with convulsions, mental retardation, visual and hearing impairment due to damage to developing brain.

WHAT IS NOT CEREBRAL PALSY?

- Deterioration of acquired motor activity.
- Mild motor dysfunction improving over a period of time.
- Hypertonic child developing hypotonia (while reverse is CP).

MAJOR EVENTS IN HUMAN BRAIN DEVELOPMENT

- Primary neurolation: Weeks 3-4 of gestation
- Prosencephalic development: Months 2-3 of gestation
- Neuronal proliferation: Months 3-4 of gestation
- Neuronal migration: Months 3-5 of gestation
- Organization: Month 5 of gestation to years postnatal
- Myelination: Birth to years postnatal.

CLASSIFICATION OF CEREBRAL PALSY

Topographic (anatomical)	*Physiological*
Monoplegia	Spastic (75%)
Diplegia (LL > UL)	Hypotonic
Triplegia	Dyskinetic (5%)
Quadriplegia	Mixed
Hemiplegia	Ataxia (15%)
Paraplegia	
Double hemiplegia (UL > LL)	
Functional	*Etiological*
Grade 1 No limitation of physical activity	Prenatal
Grade 2 Mild to moderate limitation	Natal
Grade 3 Moderate to severe limitation	Postnatal
Grade 4 No functional ability	

PHYSIOLOGICAL CLASSIFICATION OF CEREBRAL PALSY

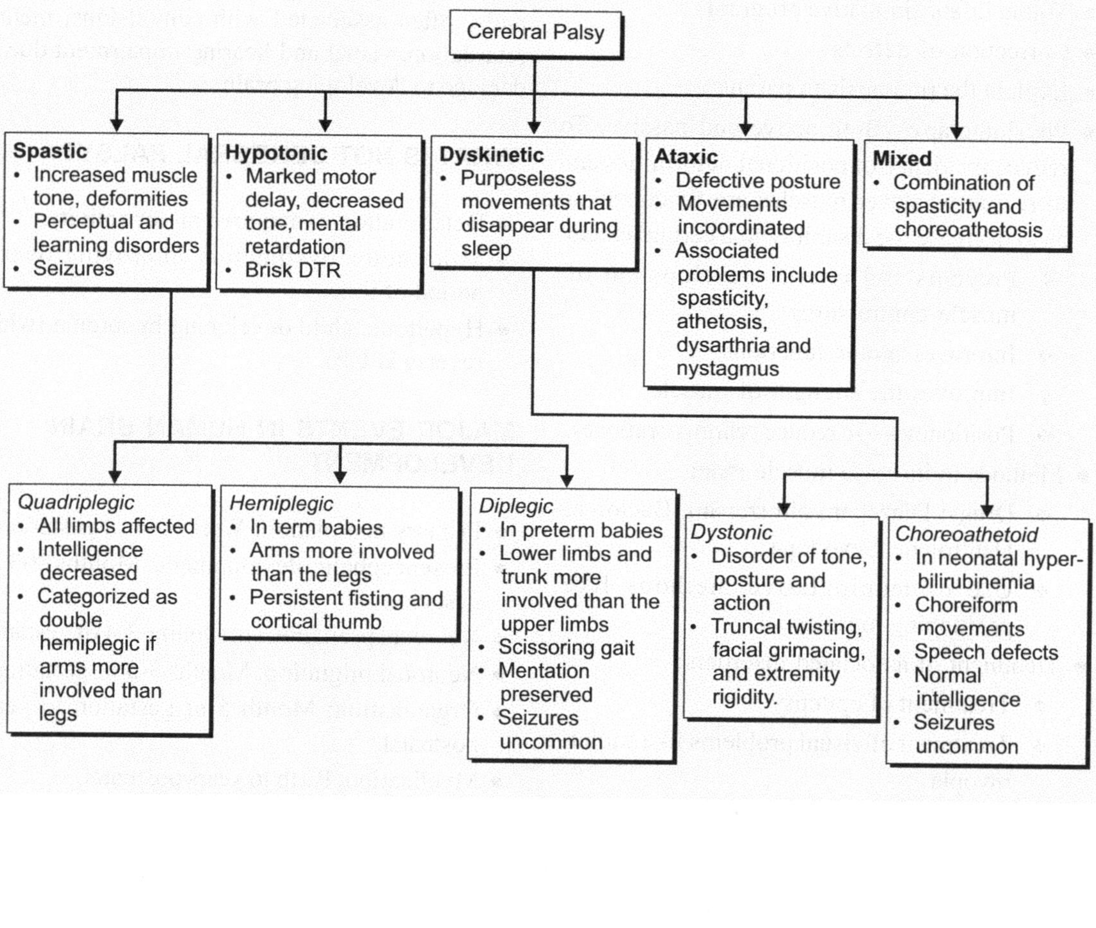

Clinicopathologic Correlation of Cerebral Palsy

CP subtype	*Pathology*	*Etiology*
Spastic diplegia	• Periventricular leukomalacia • Periventricular hemorrhagic venous infarction	• Prematurity
Spastic quadriplegia •	• Multicystic encephalopathy with cortical atrophy Selective neuronal necrosis • Parasaggital cerebral injury • Cerebral malformations	• Perinatal/intrauterine hypoxic ischemia events
Spastic hemiplegia	• Cerebral injury MCA territory (infarction necrosis) • Cerebral malformations	• Genetic • Prenatal events like hypoperfusion haemorrhage
Dyskinetic	• Basal ganglion • Status marmoratus • Bilirubin deposition	• Genetic • Perinatal asphyxia • Neonatal hyperbilirubnemia (kernicterus)
Ataxic, hypotonic	• Cerebellar lesions • Enlarged ventricles	• Prenatal (genetic)

EARLY DIAGNOSIS OF CP

Warning Symptoms

- Lack of alertness
- Increased abnormal movements, seizures
- Feeding problems, drooling
- Poor quality of sleep.

Abnormal Signs

- Reduced head circumference or fall in its growth
- Delayed social smile
- Poor head control present at 3 months of age
- Delayed appearance of postural reflexes and developmental milestones
- Persistent primitive reflexes
- Persistent asymmetric tonic neck response (ATNR)
- Constant fisting after 2 months of age
- Increased tone, scissoring or assumption of equine position of feet
- Visual problems: Roving eyes, no visual following, persistent squint
- Lack of auditory response.

CT SCAN/MRI CHANGES IN CEREBRAL PALSY

- Increase in ventricular size (hydrocephalus due to any congenital malformations) can cause CP
- Periventricular calcifications
- Periventricular leucomalacia
- Periventricular hemorrhages
- Atrophy of gyri and sulci, hygroma
- Congenital malformation/heterotopias
- Infarcts
- Porencephalic cysts
- Craniosynostosis
- Normal CT scan picture.

COMPLICATIONS OF CEREBRAL PALSY

- Gastrointestinal and nutritional
  - ❖ Failure to thrive (FTT) due to feeding and swallowing difficulties secondary to poor oromotor control
  - ❖ Obesity, less frequently than FTT (for wheelchair bound patients)
  - ❖ Constipation
  - ❖ Gastroesophageal reflux.

- Respiratory
  - Aspiration pneumonia because of oromotor dysfunction
  - Bronchial pulmonary dysplasia
  - Bronchiolitis/asthma.
- Skin: Bed sores
- Orthopedic
  - Contractures
  - Hip dislocation
  - Scoliosis.
- Neurological: Seizures
- Cognitive
  - Attention deficit hyperactivity disorder, mental retardation and specific learning disabilities
  - Impact on academic performance
  - Progressive development disorder or autism.
- Hearing loss: In patients with kernicterus
- Vision
  - Visual acuity decreases due to retinopathy of prematurity
  - Visual field abnormalities due to cortical injury
  - Strabismus.
- Sensory integration difficulties.

VISUAL ASSESSMENT

- < 3 years : Miniature toy test
- 3-5 years : Illiterate E test
- > 6 years : Snellen chart
- Cover test : To detect strabismus.

HEARING ASSESSMENT

- 5 months : Behavior observation audiometry
- 6 months : Visual reinforcement audiometry
- 2-5 years : Play audiometry
- >5 years : Audiometry.

MENTAL ASSESSMENT

- Denver development screening test
- Trivardrum Baroda school test
- Boyle's scale
- Weschler intelligence scale.

$$IQ = \frac{\text{Mental age}}{\text{Chronological age}} \times 100$$

$$DQ = \frac{\text{Developmental age}}{\text{Chronological age}} \times 100$$

ATTENTION DEFICIT HYPERACTIVITY DISORDER

- Disobedience
- Destructiveness
- Difficulty in learning languages
- Distractibility (short attention span)
- Defiance.

AUTISM

- Regression in social communication skill
- Normal physical development
- No eye contact
- Abnormal behavior
- Speech: Echolalia and repetitive.

PROGNOSIS

- 90% can reach adolescence
- Life expectancy reduced in severely affected children
- Related to milestones.

Sits Unsupported

- <2 years : 96% walk
- 2-4 years : 50% walk
- > 4 years : 3% walk
- ATNR and dystonia at 4 years: 0% walk.

NEURODEGENERATIVE DISEASES

HISTORY

CHIEF COMPLAINT

Regression of milestones

HISTORY OF PRESENT ILLNESS

History of Disease

Detailed developmental history: Developmental history should review gross motor, fine motor, language and personal, social milestones from birth until the time of evaluation.

- Till what age was the child normal
- Type of onset—acute/insidious/chronic
- Any precipitating factor
- Course—progressive/static/improving
- Predominant speech delay: Hearing problem, autism, dyslexia
- Predominant motor delay
- Global delay that is nonprogressive (child is achieving milestones but at a later date than expected, child has not lost any achieved milestones)
- Global delay that is progressive (child was developing normally, has slowed down in development and ultimately stopped achieving milestones and has lost some of the milestones already achieved)
- Development status prior to onset of symptoms
- Current social skills
- Participation in an early intervention program (if aged < 3 years) or school support (if aged > 3 years) should be reviewed, including resource room assistance
- Physical, occupational, speech and language therapy
- Adaptive physical education
- Standardized cognitive and educational testing can be asked.

CNS History

- Higher mental functions
- Cranial nerves—vision, hearing, speech, drooling of saliva and pooling of secretions
- Motor system—weakness of upper limb/lower limb; proximal or distal involvement
- Upper limb involvement: Tying shoelaces, buttoning clothes, handwriting, pincer grasp, clumsiness
- Cognition, seizures, behavioral disturbances, speech and language (grey matter)
- Tone changes, ataxia, gait difficulties (white matter)
- Athetosis i.e. slow, writhing, involuntary movements, particularly in the distal extremities
- Chorea (i.e. abrupt, irregular, jerky movements); choreoathetosis (i.e. combination of athetosis and choreiform movements)
- Dystonia, i.e. slow rhythmic movements with muscle tone abnormalities and abnormal postures
- Sensory system dysfunction
- Bladder/bowel dysfunction
- Convulsions
- Raised intracranial tension.

History of Complications

- Respiratory difficulty
- Bedsores

- Deformities
- Nutritional history:
  - When were oral feeds started
  - Who feeds the child
  - How often
  - How long does it take
  - Associated problems like vomiting, constipation
- Contractures, behavioral problems, bladder problems
- Activities of daily living: "DEATH", i.e. dressing, eating, ambulating, toileting, hygiene.

History of Risk Factors

Maternal Risk Factors

- Prenatal exposure to illicit drugs, toxins or infections
- Maternal diabetes
- Acute maternal illness, trauma or radiation exposure
- Prenatal care and fetal movements
- Frequent spontaneous abortions.

Fetal Risk Factor

- Preterm child
- Birth asphyxia.

FAMILY HISTORY

- History of consanguineous marriage and affection of other siblings (since most of these disorders are autosomal recessive).
- Make detailed pedigree chart.

GENERAL PHYSICAL EXAMINATION

- Head circumference
- Facies (coarse facies in mucopolysaccharidoses)
- Hair—alopecia, texture, pigmentary changes (wooly hair in Menke's disease)
- Blindness
- Eyes—cataract (Galactosemia, Wilson's), retinitis pigmentosa (Neuronal ceroid lipofuscinosis), cherry red spot (gangliosidosis), optic atrophy (Metachrom- atic leukodystrophy)
- Skeletal examination—joint involvement.

SYSTEMIC EXAMINATION

- Detailed neurological examination
- Abdomen—careful palpation to assess visceromegaly.

INVESTIGATIONS

- Fundus: To look for optic atrophy
- MRI: Good for diseases of basal ganglia, cerebellar atrophies and mitochondrial disorders, demyelination disorders
- Electroretinogram: Abnormal in grey matter disease
- Visual evoked responses: Abnormal in white matter diseases
- Brainstem auditory evoked response: Abnormal in white matter diseases
- After initial evaluation as mentioned above further investigations are advised depending upon suspected clinical diagnosis.

Grey Matter

- Bone marrow for storage cells
- Urine copper and serum ceruloplasmin for Wilson's disease
- Hair microscopy for Menke's disease
- Conjunctival or rectal biopsy for neuronal ceroid lipofuscinosis
- Enzyme analysis for storage diseases
- Urine tests and skeletal survey for mucopolysaccridosis
- Serum and CSF lactate and pyruvate for mitochondrial disorders

- CSF antimeasles antibodies
- HIV.

White Matter

- Aryl sulfatase assay for metachromatic leukodystrophy
- VLCFA for adrenoleukodystrophy
- Acetyl aspartic acid for Canavan's disease
- Galactocerebrosidase estimation for Krabbe's disease
- Nerve conduction studies.

TREATMENT

- Most of them can only be managed symptomatically as course is relentless
- Specific treatment is present only in few conditions, e.g. Wilson's disease, adrenal leukodystrophy, Leigh's disease, Menkes', SSPE and HIV
- Enzyme replacement (Gaucher's) and gene therapy are normal approaches to treatment
- Importance of making a diagnosis is thus mainly for prevention by prenatal diagnosis.

DIFFERENTIAL DIAGNOSIS

NIEMANN-PICKS DISEASE

- Onset below 6 months
- Rapid progression and death by 24 months
- Hepatosplenomegaly
- Cherry red spot and optic atrophy
- Early dementia and spastic paralysis
- Vacoulated lymphocytes
- Foam cells in bone marrow.

GAUCHER'S DISEASE

- Onset below 6 months
- Rapid progression and death by 24 months
- Hepatosplenomegaly/predominant splenomegaly
- Early dementia and spastic paralysis
- Gauchers cells in bone marrow and splenic puncture
- Increased acid phosphatase.

NEURONAL CEROID LIPOFUSCINOSIS

- One of the common grey matter disorder
- Autosomal recessive inheritance
- Variable age at onset: Infantile presents at 0-1.5 years, Late infantile at 1-3 years and Juvenile at 4-9 years
- Loss of skills, dementia
- Progressive visual loss: Retinal atrophy, macular degeneration
- Seizures especially myoclonic, generalized seizures and drop attacks are often hard to control
- Cerebellar ataxia, hypotonia, associated pyramidal and extrapyramidal signs
- No organomegaly
- *Diagnosis:* Demonstration of typical storage material in conjunctival biopsy/rectal biopsy/skin biopsy.
- *Treatment:* None till date, supportive care only, genetic counseling.

TAY-SACHS DISEASE

- Most common of the ganglioside storage disorders
- Normal till 2-6 months
- Then develops apathy towards surroundings
- Loss of acquired motor function with loss of visual ability
- Hyperacusis is very characteristic in early phase
- Generalized, myoclonic seizures
- Associated features: Macrocephaly, cherry red spot

- Vegetative state by 2nd year death by 5 years
- *Diagnosis:* Hexosaminidase assay
- *Treatment:* Supportive.

WILSON'S DISEASE

- Autosomal recessive
- It affects different systems at different ages.
- Hepatic and hematologic manifestation appear early and neurologic manifestations follow later
- Age at onset: During school years but may be variable
- Untreated disease is progressive and there may be a positive family history of a different system involvement.
- *Systemic Manifestations:*
    - Nervous system: Extrapyramidal manifestations—dystonia, choreoathetosis
    - Psychiatric manifestations: Slow dementia, Speech disturbances
    - Eyes: Kayser-Fleischer ring, cataract
    - Hepatic: Acute and recurrent hepatitis, Fulminant hepatic failure
    - Others: Renal tubular acidosis, Rickets, Hemolytic anemia.

Investigations

- Serum ceruloplasmin < 20 mg/dL
- 24 hours urinary copper > 100 µg/24 hours
- D penicillamine challenge: 500 mg of penicillamine is given orally immediately before and 12 hours into urine collection. 24 hours urine copper >1500 µg/24 hours.
- Others: Liver function tests, liver biopsy for copper deposition
- Serum copper is not very useful for diagnosis.

Treatment

- Low copper diet
- Specific treatment—copper chelation
    - *D penicillamine*: 10-30 mg/kg/day orally in 3-4 divided doses 30 minute before meals. It is generally supplemented with pyridoxine and given for life long.
    - *Trientine* may be used in those patients where penicillamine fails or is not tolerated.
    - *Zinc* acts by reducing copper absorption, 75-150 mg elemental zinc per day, in divided doses with meals.

Family Screening

- Families of all index cases should be screened.
- Screening includes clinical evaluation, slit-lamp examination for KF ring, serum ceruloplasmin and 24 hour urinary copper.
- Asymptomatic affected sibs should be put on low copper diet and zinc therapy for life long.

METACHROMATIC LEUKODYSTROPHY (MLD)

Autosomal recessive lysosomal storage disorder due to deficiency of the enzyme arylsulfatase A. MLD is a prototype of white matter degenerative disease.

Late Infantile MLD

- Age of onset of 1-5 years (usually 12-18 months)
- Motor milestones are lost first followed by neurocognitive functions
- Decreased deep tendon reflexes occur late in the disease due to peripheral neuropathy, Ankle jerk may be lost while knee jerk is preserved.
- Optic atrophy
- Patients are bedridden by 3 years of age and death occurs by 5-6 years due to aspiration or bronchopneumonia.

Juvenile MLD

- Age of onset 5-10 years
- Presents with ataxia, spasticity and behavioral problems
- Progression is slower than the infantile variant.

Investigations

- Screening by demonstrating metacromatic granules in urine
- Arylsulfatase A enzyme activity may be decreased in leukocyte or skin fibroblast cultures
- Carriers may be identified and prenatal diagnoses may be made by measuring arylsulfatase A activity
- Brain MRI may be performed to identify white matter lesions and atrophy, which are characteristic of MLD.

Treatment

- Specific—bone marrow transplantation
- Supportive therapy
- Genetic counseling.

DISCUSSION

DEFINITION

A degenerative brain disease is defined as any disorder where there is progressive damage to the brain with or without systemic involvement. Most are genetic (autosomal recessive), while few are acquired, e.g. subacute sclerosing panencephalitis. These diseases are characterized by:

- Progressive loss of previously acquired intellectual, motor or sensory skills
- Delay in attainment of milestones, if damage is slow
- Failure to attain any milestones if insult starts perinatally
- Onset of inherited disease at any age.

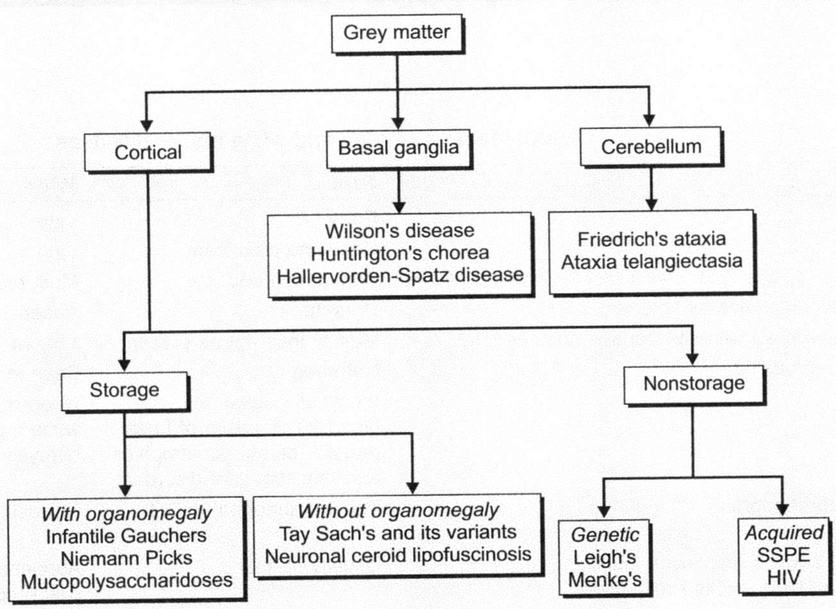

Fig. 18.4 Approach to neurodegenerative disorders

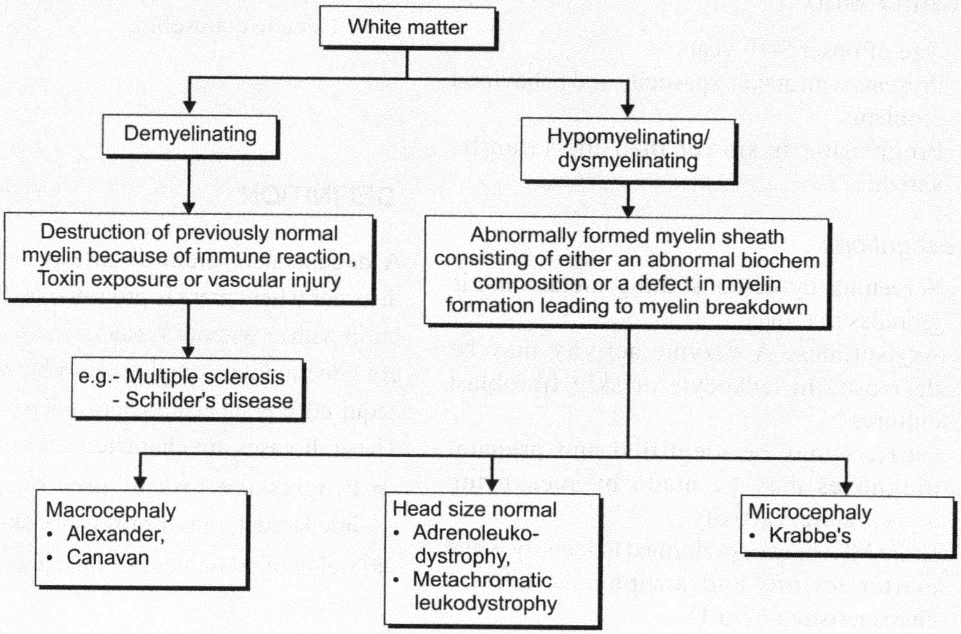

Fig. 18.5: White matter

Table 18.9: Clinical features of grey and white matter diseases

	Grey	*White*
Dementia	Early	Late
Seizures	Early and prominent	Late
Disturbances of tone, gait, ataxia and hyper/hyporeflexia	Uncommon and late	Most prominent feature
Basal ganglia signs and symptoms	Present	Absent
Retinitis pigmentosa with consecutive optic atrophy	May or may not be present	Absent
Peripheral neuropathy	Not seen	Seen in some cases
MRI	Identifies cortical atrophy Good for diseases of basal ganglia, cerebellar atrophies and mitochondrial disorders	Good diagnostic yield for white matter diseases, demyelinations
ERG (Electroretinogram)	May be abnormal (NCL)	Normal
VER (Visual evoked response), BERA (Brainstem auditory evoked response)	Usually normal	Abnormal BERA Dec Amp of V Inc Wave III-IV interpeak latency

FLOPPY INFANT

HISTORY

CHIEF COMPLAINTS

- Paucity of movements—usually lower limbs more than upper limbs (Young infants)
- Delayed milestones (Older children).

HISTORY OF PRESENT ILLNESS

History of Disease (Floppiness)

- Acute onset: Trauma
- Child assuming bizarre posture: Hyper-extensibility
- Posture with which the child lies: Frog like
- History of the child slipping through the fingers.
- Distribution of weakness:
  - Neuropathies have distal weakness except spinal muscular atrophy (SMA)
  - Myopathies have proximal weakness except myotonic muscular dystrophy.

History of Complications

- Poor sucking, recurrent aspiration/infection, neonatal cyanosis suggesting hypoxia
- Activities of Daily Living: "DEATH", i.e. dressing, eating, ambulating, toileting, hygiene
- Cardiac involvement: Palpitation in Duchenne's muscular dystrophy (DMD).

History of Risk Factors

- Trauma
- Vaccination/dog bite (demyelination)
- Immunization status of mother and sibling (neonatal tetanus, polio)
- Progression of weakness
  - Progressive: Spinal muscular atrophy, muscular dystrophy
  - Static: Cerebral palsy, myopathy.
- Postexertion fatigue, diurnal variation in weakness (myasthenia)
- Honey ingestion, constipation, poor feeding, eating outside prepared food (botulism)
- Convulsion (central cause, metabolic myopathy)
- Hoarse cry, dry skin, constipation (hypothyroidism)
- Orthopedic deformities at birth (Spinal muscular atrophy, myotubular myopathy, arthogryposis)
- Sensory symptoms (hereditary motor sensory neuropathy)
- Autonomic symptoms (end stage muscular dystrophy or Riley Day syndrome)
- Loss of acquired milestones (degenerative disorder)
- Recurrent diarrhea (periodic paralysis).

ANTENATAL AND PERINATAL HISTORY

- Onset of quickening (normally 18 weeks in primipara and 16 weeks in multipara), intrauterine fetal movements (less than 10 kicks in 12 hours in late pregnancy is abnormal)
- Gestational and perinatal drug use like sedatives and muscle relaxants
- Intrauterine and perinatal infection
- Detailed history of onset of labor and intrapartum events
- History of prolonged physiological jaundice (Down's syndrome/hypothyroidism)
- Family history of hypotonia, history of weakness in mother.

FAMILY HISTORY

- Important to determine the pattern of inheritance
- Pedigree chart.

GENERAL PHYSICAL EXAMINATION

- Alertness and responsiveness
- Characteristic facies
  - Down facies
  - Coarse features, large tongue (hypothyroidism)
  - Ptosis (myasthenia)
  - Obesity, hypogonadism (Prader-Willi syndrome)
  - Dolicocephalic head, open mouth (CMFTD)
  - Inverted V shaped upper lip, thin cheeks, scalloped temporal fossae (Myotonic muscular dystrophy)
  - Microcephaly/hydrocephalus (TORCH infections).
- Eyes
  - Ophthalmoplegia (myotonic dystrophy, mitochondrial myopathy, Miller Fischer type GBS)
  - Cataract (myotonic dystrophy, TORCH infection)
  - Chorioretinitis (TORCH infections).
- Rash (connective tissue disorder, TORCH infections)
- Orthopedic deformities: Contractures
- Congenital dislocation of hip: Due to laxity
- Pressure sores
- Bell shaped chest (Spinal muscular atrophy, myopathies)
- Neurocutaneous markers
- Undescended testis (Spinal muscular atrophy, myopathies).

SYSTEMIC EXAMINATION

CNS EXAMINATION

- Posture 'Frog like'—hips abducted and externally rotated, knees in contact with bed
- Higher mental functions
- Cranial nerves: Usually spared in spinal muscular atrophy, neuropathies except in Fazio-Londe variant of SMA in which progressive bulbar palsy occurs. Facial asymmetry may be due to weakness and not due to cranial nerve involvement
- Weakness and wasting: Thenar and hypothenar wasting, sternocleidomastoid muscle wasting, neck and facial muscle weakness, muscle hypertrophy and shortening of limbs
- Fasciculation of the tongue and rarely thenar, deltoid, biceps and signs of intercostal muscle paralysis (paradoxical respiration) are pathognomonic of SMA
- Tests specific for confirming hypotonia and hyperextensibility are described in Table 18·10. The whole maneuver is also referred as 180° flip test
- Other Tests
  - Gently shake the hand and feet
  - Passive hip and shoulder abduction
  - Raise and release limbs
  - Made to sit: Rounded back and falls forward.
- Reflexes:
  - Absent in spinal muscular atrophy and other motor neuron diseases
  - Absent distally in neuropathies
  - Diminished but present in myopathies, brisk in atonic cerebral palsy
  - Look for percussion myotonia.
- Sensory findings: Neuropathy

- Autonomic features: May be found in long standing neuropathy, cerebral palsy
- Gait: Usually not elicitable, if required Gower's sign to be looked for
- Examine the sibling if present.

DIAGNOSIS

……… month old floppy male/female child since birth /since…….. months; static/progressive; alert/depressed; with/without normal/delayed development; with/without seizures; with/without other complications.

DIFFERENTIAL DIAGNOSIS

Differential diagnosis will be dependent on presentation and cause of floppy infant.

Causes of Floppy Infant (Table 18.13)

- Central causes (cerebral/ cerebellar/ spinal)
- Alfa motor neuron
- Neurological involvement
- Neuromuscular junction
- Muscular involvement.

Central Nervous System Involvement

Pattern of weakness:

- Axial > Appendicular involvement
- Proximal ≥ Distal involvement
- Deep tendon reflexes: Normal to exaggerated
- Other associated features like seizures are generally present.

Causes:

- Chromosomal disorders
- Inborn error of metabolism
- Cerebral dysgenesis
- Cerebral/ spinal trauma.

Anterior Horn Cell Disease

Pattern of weakness:

- Proximal ≥ distal involvement
- Severe weakness
- Absent deep tendon reflexes
- Fasciculation and fibrillation are generally seen.

Causes:

- Spinal muscular atrophy
- Poliomyelitis

Peripheral Nerve Involvement

Pattern of weakness:

- Moderate to severe weakness
- Distal > Proximal involvement
- Diminished deep tendon reflexes in affected group
- Sensory involvement.

Muscle Involvement (Table 18.14)

Pattern of weakness:

- Mild to moderate weakness
- Arm > Legs involvement
- Distal > Proximal involvement
- Diminished but elicitable deep tendon reflexes.

Causes:

- Congenital myopathies
- Congenital muscular dystrophy
- Congenital myotonic dystrophies.

INVESTIGATIONS

- Hemogram
- Creatine phosphokinase levels

- CSF analysis
- Chest X ray: Prominent hilar markings with scattered infiltrates.

Nerve Conduction Velocity

Nerve conduction velocity (NCV) is a test of the speed of electrical signals through a nerve.

Method

Surface electrodes, similar to those used for ECG, are placed on the skin over nerves at various locations. Each electrode gives a mild electrical impulse to stimulate the nerve.

The nerve's resulting electrical activity is recorded by the other electrodes.

The distance between electrodes and the time it takes for electrical impulse to travel between electrodes is used to determine the speed of the nerve signals.

Electromyography (recording from needles placed into the muscles) is often done at the same time as this test.

Abnormal Results Signifies

- Axonopathy (damage to the long portion of the nerve cell)
- Conduction block (blockage of impulse along the nerve pathway)
- Demyelination (damage and loss of the fatty insulation surrounding the nerve cell).

Electromyography

Electromyography (EMG) is a test that checks the health of the muscles and the nerves that control the muscles.

Method

A thin needle electrode is inserted through the skin into the muscle. The electrode on the needle picks up the electrical activity given off by muscles. This activity is displayed on a special monitor called an oscilloscope, and may be heard through a speaker.

After placement of the electrodes, patient is asked to contract the muscle. The presence, size, and shape of the wave form—The action potential produced on the monitor provides information about muscle's ability to respond, when the nerves are stimulated.

A *nerve conduction velocity* test is usually performed along with an EMG.

Indication

EMG is done for symptoms of weakness, and examination reveals impaired muscle strength. It differentiates primary muscle conditions from muscle weakness caused by neurologic disorders.

Nerve Biopsy

Method

The sural nerve (in the ankle), or the superficial radial nerve (wrist) are the sites most often used for biopsy. A small incision is made under local anesthesia, and a portion of the nerve is removed. The sample is then examined using either a regular (light) microscopic or an electron microscope. Individual nerve fibers may also be examined.

Indication

- Damage to the small nerves
- Demyelination (destruction of parts of the myelin sheath covering the nerve)
- Inflammatory nerve conditions (neuropathies)
- Axon degeneration (destruction of the axon portion of the nerve cell).

Muscle Biopsy

Method

An open biopsy involves making a small cut in the skin and into the muscle. The muscle tissue is then removed.

Indication

- Diseases of the connective tissue and blood vessels (such as polyarteritis nodosa)
- Infections that affect the muscles (such as trichinosis or toxoplasmosis)
- Muscular disorders such as muscular dystrophy or congenital myopathy
- Metabolic defects of the muscle.

DISCUSSION

Floppiness is characterized by
- Abnormal postures
- Diminished resistance of joints to passive movement
- Increased range of movement
- Paucity of spontaneous movements.

WHEN TO SUSPECT A FLOPPY INFANT

- Mother feels the baby is floppy since birth
- Baby is alert but less active
- Delayed development of motor milestones
- Able to walk but falls frequently.

INDICATIONS FOR HOSPITALIZATION

- Progression
- Respiratory and bulbar involvement
- Unsettled diagnosis
- Planning for antenatal diagnosis.

CAUSES OF PSEUDOPARALYSIS

- Congenital syphilis
- Scurvy
- Osteomyelitis
- Fracture
- Dislocation like CDH
- Arthritis.

NEUROMUSCULAR DISEASE IN FLOPPY BABY

Suggested by hypotonia accompanied by weakness. The corroborative features are:
- Paucity of movements
- Week cry
- Poor suck
- Hypoventilation and paradoxical respiration (diaphragmatic weakness) or classically bell shaped chest
- Muscle wasting and winging of scapula.

Table 18.10: Tests specific for hypotonia and hyperextensibility

Test	*Normal/What to look for*	*Abnormal*
Supine	Posture of the baby	Posture: Frog like Less movement
Pull to sit (traction response)	Maintains head in line with trunk	Gross head lag
Sitting	Degree of head holding, degree of trunk control, ability to sit unsupported	Head falls forward, C-shaped spine, cannot sit without support
Vertical suspension and attempted weight bearing	Kicks lower limbs, when foot touches bed tries to bear his own weight	Lower limbs hang limp, cannot bear weight, slides down when held at axilla
Ventral suspension	Holds head at 45° or less Elbows and knees flexed, Back straight or slightly flexed	Hangs limp like an inverted 'U'
Prone position	Lifts the head, roll over, crawl	Lack of head control

Table 18.11: Causes of floppiness in neonates

Well neonate	*Sick neonate*
SMA (type I) Congenital myopathies Congenital muscular dystrophy Down's syndrome Hypothyroidism	Intraventricular hemorrhage Birth asphyxia Sepsis/CNS infection Diazepam/MgSO4 given to mother before delivery

Table 18.12: Causes of floppiness in infancy and childhood

Causes	*Course*
SMA II, III Congenital myopathies Neuropathies Metabolic Hypotonic cerebral palsy	Progressive—**SMA type 1** Congenital muscular dystrophy Indeterminate—**SMA type I, II** Congenital myopathy, Congenital Muscular dystorphy Static—**SMA II, III** Congenital myopathy, Congenital muscular Dystrophy Cerebral palsy Neuropathies

Table 18.13: Clinical features of muscle and nerve disease

	Muscle disease	*Nerve disease*
Wasting	Less	More
Tendon reflexes	Decreased/normal	Areflexia
Fasciculations	Absent	Present
Bulbar involvement	Less	More

SECTION–III

SHORT CASES IN PEDIATRICS

CHAPTER 19

SHORT STATURE

HISTORY

CHIEF COMPLAINTS

Not gaining in height

HISTORY OF PRESENT ILLNESS

History of Disease

- Duration since not gaining height
- Progression—less then 2 inches/year
- Shortest in class, clothes and shoes that used to fit last year are fitting now
- Any aggravating factor
- Previous height measurements.

History of Risk Factors

- Cyanosis/respiratory tract infections (congenital heart disease)
- Cough/breathlessness, edema (congestive heart failure)
- Recurrent cough with expectoration (chronic suppurative lung disease)
- Chronic diarrhea, flatulence, or borborygmi (frequent, discomforting, or even audible peristalsis) suggest malabsorption
- Pain or abdominal discomfort suggests inflammatory bowel disease
- Polyuria, polydipsia, oliguria (renal tubular acidosis)
- Polyuria, polydipsia and weight loss (diabetes mellitus)
- Cough, fever, hemoptysis, poor appetite (tuberculosis)
- Skin changes/hair changes/night blindness/ bleeding gums (vitamin deficiency and malnutrition)
- Chronic steroid use: For asthma, eczema
- Weight gain/constipation/lethargy/mental retardation/feeding difficulties (hypothyroidism)
- Obesity, striae, moon face (Cushing's disease)
- Headache, nausea, vomiting, diplopia (raised Intracranial tension).

DIETARY HISTORY

Detailed dietary history calculating the calorie and protein intake.

ANTENATAL HISTORY

- Birth height, weight
- Gestational age: Preterm, small for gestational age
- Twins/congenital anomalies
- Complications during pregnancy.

FAMILY HISTORY

- Short stature in parents, siblings, relatives
- Make Pedigree chart.

DEVELOPMENTAL HISTORY

Ask for milestones of puberty like onset of menarche, breast development, penile enlargement, pubic hairs.

SOCIOECONOMIC HISTORY

- Emotional deprivation
- Growth often is impaired in migrants and in children emerging from foster care
- The growth pattern with adequate nutrition in a loving environment over time is critical to distinguish pathologic growth failure from normal variant short stature in such patients.

GENERAL PHYSICAL EXAMINATION

Examination relays heavily upon accurate and reliable height assessment

- Vitals: Blood pressure-Cushing's syndrome
- Weigh all patients
- Measure standing height in triplicate using a calibrated wall-mounted stadiometer. In infants, length is determined in triplicate using a tabletop recumbent stadiometer. The mean value of the triplicate data serves as the true measurement.
- For children who cannot stand or recline completely (e.g. those with spina bifida, contractures), arm span is reliable alternative for assessment of long bone growth.
  - Ascertain arm span by facing the child against a flat firm surface (usually the wall), fully extending the arms, and measuring the maximal distance between the tips of the middle fingers.
  - If this positioning is impossible physically, a flexible tape measure may be rolled along the dorsal aspect of the arms and upper back to determine arm span.
  - Arm span/ Height:
    - Increased—vertebral disease (short trunk)
    - Decreased—hypothyroidism, Turner's, achondroplasia.
- With suspicion of short-limb dwarfism, the sitting height can be obtained by measuring the upper body segment, or crown to pelvis, as the child sits upright.
  - Alternatively, the lower segment can be determined by measuring from the superior midline brim of the symphysis pubis to the floor, with the child standing (feet placed together).
  - The upper-to-lower segment ratio (US/ LS) should be close to 1.
  - The ratio is greater than 1 in children with shortened limbs, as it is in individuals with hypochondroplasia or achondroplasia.
- Segmental length
  - Shoulder to elbow length (SE)
  - Elbow to metacarpal length (EMC)
  - Normal SE:EMC=1:1
  - Rhizomelia <0.98, familial
  - Mesomelia (middle segment short); Chondroectodermal dysplasia
  - Acromelia (distal segment short): Ellis van Creveld syndrome.
- Weight/Height:
  - W/H decreased—malabsorption, Malnutrition
  - W/H Increased—growth hormone deficiency, hypothyroidism.
- Measure both biologic parents' height.
- Documenting growth velocity over time, complements the initial height assessment.
  - Calculate growth velocity as the change in standing height over at least 6 months (for children) or in length over at least 4 months (for infants).

- Poor linear growth is defined as linear growth velocity more than 2 SDs below the mean for gender, genetic composition, and chronologic age.

- Body mass index (obesity): Cushing's, growth hormone deficiency
- In infants, measure the head circumference and anterior fontanelle: Large anterior fontanelle is seen in osteogenesis imperfecta, mucopoly saccridosis, rickets, hypothyroidism
- Carefully examine the midface
  - Single, central, maxillary incisor: Defect in midline facial development.
  - Bifid uvula: Submandibular cleft palate
  - Growth hormone deficiency or panhypopituitarism should be considered as a cause of short stature in such patients.
- Dysmorphism/syndromic stigmata
- Dentition: Delayed in growth hormone deficiency, rickets, malnutrition.
- Eyes:
  - Cataract/corneal opacity, intrauterine infection, mucopolysaccridosis
  - Bitot's spot/ corneal or conjuctival xerosis
  - Blue sclera.
- Skin:
  - Dry: Hypothyroid
  - Nevi: Turner's
  - Striae: Cushing's.
- Hair: Flag sign
- Inspect mucous membranes: Ulcerative stomatitis, mineral and vitamin deficiencies
- Visual fields: Pituitary tumors
- Neck: Webbing/thyroid enlargement
- Short 4th metacarpals: Pseudohypoparathyroidism, and Albright's hereditary osteodystrophy.
- Sexual maturity rating.

SYSTEMIC EXAMINATION

As usual

DIFFERENTIAL DIGNOSIS

FAMILIAL SHORT STATURE

Bone age = Chronological age > Height age

- Short stature during the growth period and reduced final height
- Parents or close relatives are short statured
- Bone age is normal
- Normal height velocity, i.e. growth parallel to the growth curve but below it.

CONSTITUTIONAL GROWTH DELAY

Bone age = Height age < Chronological age

- Normal at birth but by the end of infancy, growth falls below the fifth percentile
- Retarded bone age
- Delayed onset of puberty, positive family history of delayed puberty in same sex parent.
- Final height achieved is normal.

ISOLATED GROWTH HORMONE DEFICIENCY

- Birth height and weight are normal.
- Deceleration of growth begins in infancy.
- At birth, males have small testis, under developed scrotum and micropenis.
- Prepubertal growth velocity less than 4 cm per year.
- Bone age below chronological age.
- Height age is less than bone age and chronological age.
- Abnormal 24 hours growth hormone secretory pattern.
- Peak GH levels are less than 10 ng/ml during provocative stimulation test.
- Low IGF-1 and IGFBP-3 levels for age.
- Resumption of growth following growth hormone administration.

INVESTIGATIONS

When to investigate:

- Height between mean and 2SD: Observe
- Height between 2-3 SD:
  - Screening studies
  - Observe growth velocity—if < 25th centile, investigate.
- Height < 3SD below mean or velocity < 25th centile: Screening followed by specific tests.

Screening Studies

- Hemogram: Anemia
- Renal function tests: Chronic renal failure/ Renal tubular acidosis
- Liver function tests: Chronic liver disease
- Blood gas analysis: Renal tubular acidosis
- Calcium/Phosphate/Alkaline phosphatase: Rickets
- Chest X-ray/Mantoux: Tuberculosis
- Urine Routine/Microscopy, Culture/Sensivity
- Stool: ova/cyst, occult blood
- X-ray skull/spine: Mucopolysaccridosis/ Rickets.

Specific Investigations

- *Hypothyroidism:* Thyroid function tests
- *Turner's:* FSH/LH, Ultrasound pelvis
- *Malabsorption:* Anti-endomysial immunoglobulin A (IgA) and immunoglobulin G (IgG), transglutaminase IgG, and antigliadin IgG titers for sprue (gluten enteropathy): For sprue, antiendomysial IgA is more sensitive, and IgG is more specific.
- *Hemolysis:* Hemoglobin electrophoresis
- *Inborn error of metabolism:* Metabolic screen
- *Sweat chloride testing:* Consider in short patients with a history of meconium ileus or pulmonary symptoms to exclude cystic fibrosis.
- *Karyotyping:* Down's syndrome, Turner's syndrome
- *Serum levels of insulin like growth factor-1* (IGF-I), formerly named somatomedin C, and insulin like growth factor binding protein-3 (IGFBP-3)
  - These are useful tests for Growth hormone deficiency, except in patients with brain tumors or during puberty.
  - Consider provocative tests of pituitary function in any euthyroid patient suspected to be growth hormone deficient.
  - Thus, the serum IGFBP-3 concentration has greater specificity than serum IGF-I for the diagnosis of GH deficiency (poor nutrition is associated with low serum IGF-I concentration).
- Cautionary note about measuring serum levels of growth hormone:
  - Beyond the first months of life, endogenous growth hormone is secreted in a pulsatile fashion. These intermittent peaks are greatest after exercise, after meals as blood glucose falls, and during deep sleep.
  - Therefore, measuring a single, random serum growth hormone value is of no use in the evaluation of the short child.
  - Beyond the neonatal period, values obtained during the daytime are unlikely to be detectable.
  - While a random serum growth hormone value greater than 10 mg/dl generally excludes growth hormone deficiency, a random low serum growth hormone concentration does not confirm the diagnosis of growth hormone deficiency.

Imaging Studies

- Assessment of bone age: Films taken before puberty more useful:
  - Newborn: Knee
  - 3-12 months: Shoulder

- 1-12 years: Wrist and hand
- 12-14 years: Elbow/hip.

- Perform renal and cardiac ultrasounds in all patients with Turner's syndrome. The most commonly associated anomalies are horseshoe kidney and bicuspid aortic valve
- MRI of brain for pituitary gland.

Provocative Tests for the Evaluation of Suspected Growth Hormone Deficiency

- Insulin-induced hypoglycemia (associated with fatalities)
- Levodopa
- Propranolol.

TREATMENT

Medical Care

Medical care depends on the etiology of the short stature.

- GH (Growth Hormone) therapy in patients with growth hormone deficiency. GH is given in dose of 0.1 U/kg/day subcutaneous preferably at night.

Indications of Growth Hormone Therapy

- Growth hormone deficiency
- Turner's syndrome
- Chronic renal insufficiency
- Prader-Willi syndrome
- IUGR babies with no catch up growth till 3 years of age.

Surgical Care

- Brain tumors causing hyposomatotropism may require neurosurgical intervention, depending on the tumor type and location.
- Limb-lengthening procedures have been performed but carry enormous morbidity and mortality and are not recommended.

Diet

- Optimize nutrition in patients with gastrointestinal disease.
- Obtain psychologic or psychiatric consultation for patients with eating disorders.
- Forced energy intake in children with normal variant short stature has not been demonstrated to improve short-term growth or final adult height.

Activity

- Do not restrict activity in children with normal variant short stature.

DISCUSSION

DEFINITION OF SHORT STATURE

- Height < 3rd centile or 2 SD of the mean height of that age and sex
- Projected height > 8.5 cm or 2 SD below the mid parental height (target height)
- Growth velocity < 25th centile over 6-12 months of observation
- Fall in height crossing 2 major centiles on growth chart.

Height velocity is based on height measurements made at least 6 months apart since there can be periods of no growth of up to 60 days, in normal children.

BONE AGE, CHRONOLOGICAL AGE AND HEIGHT AGE

- Bone age—this is indicator of skeletal maturation. A child with delayed bone age has a better prognosis than with appropriate or advanced bone age
- Chronological age—actual age of child
- Height age—age which child should have reached his height.

PATHOLOGICAL SHORT STATURE

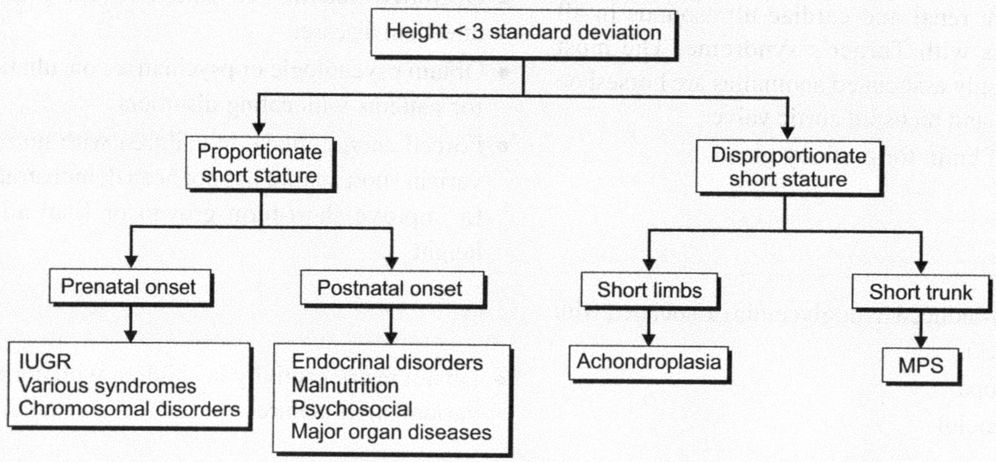

ABNORMAL GROWTH RATES

- Less than 7 cm/year at less than 4 years of age
- Less than 6 cm/year from 4-6 years of age
- Less than 5 cm/year from 6 years till puberty.

HEIGHT/LENGTH

In children < 2 years, supine length should be measured by an infantometer and in children > 2 years age, standing height should be measured by means of a stadiometer.

UPPER SEGMENT/LOWER SEGMENT RATIO

Arm span is usually equal to length or slightly less. In proportionate dwarfs, the US-LS ratio is maintained and arm span is equal to length.

Normal US/LS ratio =

At Birth	1.7: 1
6 months	1.6:1
1 year	1.5:1
2 years	1.4:1
3 years	1.3:1
4 years	1.2:1
5 years	1.1:1
7 years	1:1

Then the lower segment increases slightly as compared to the upper segment (1:1.1).

Interpretation

- If US/LS is increased: Short lower limbs, e.g. skeletal dysplasias, hypothyroidism, achondroplasia.
- If US/LS ratio is decreased: Short trunk, e.g. Scoliosis, or short neck due to Klippel-Feil syndrome or arachnodactyly (e.g. marfan's syndrome, homocystinuria, eunuchs).
- If US/LS ratio normal age: Proportionate dwarf (e.g. pituitary, systemic illness).

CHILD'S ARM SPAN

Distance between tips of middle fingers, when arms are stretched perpendicular to the trunk.

Normal arm span minus height values:

- Birth to 7 years: Height more than arm span by 3cm.
- 8 to 12 years: Height is equal to arm span

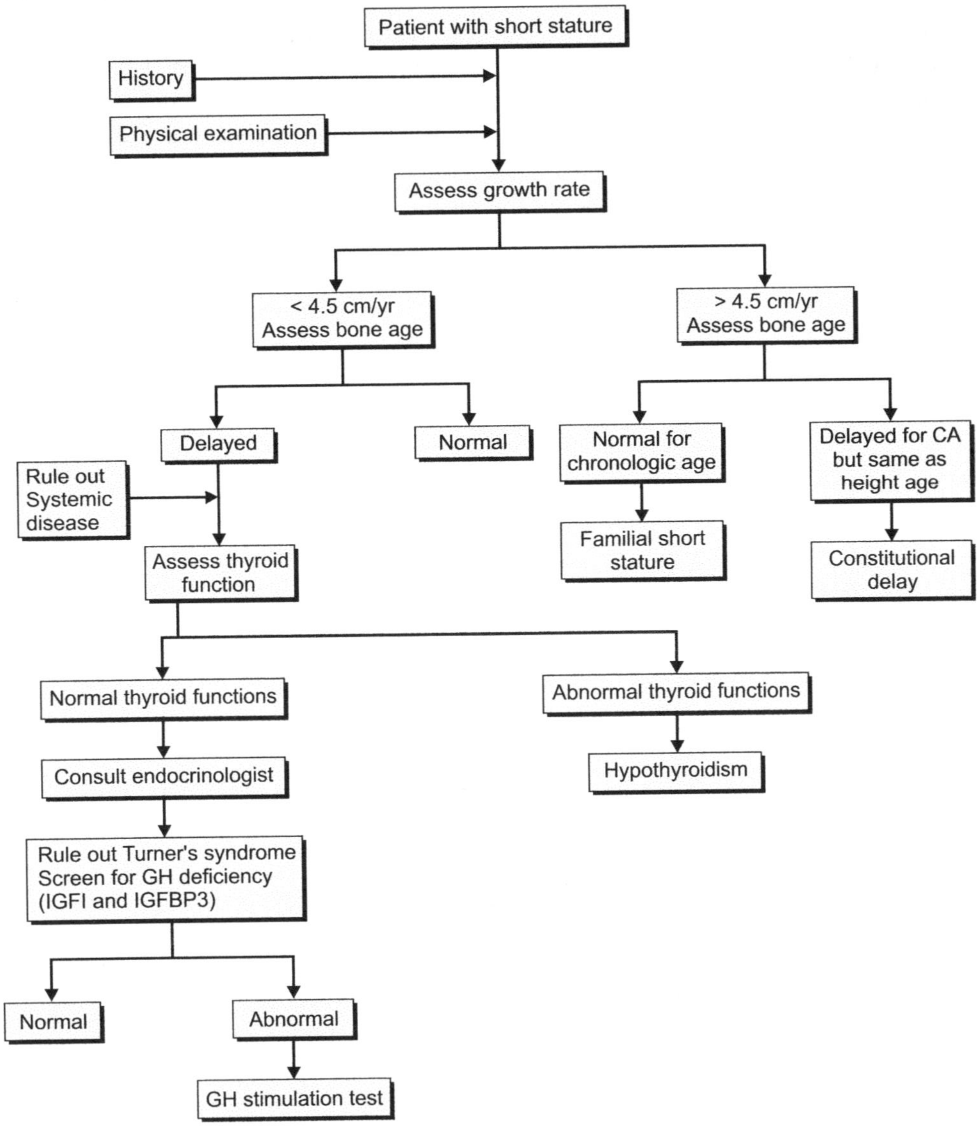

Fig. 19.1: Algorithm for evaluation of short stature

- 14 years: Span is more than height (1cm in girls and 4 cm in boys).

TARGET HEIGHT

- Target height of boy (cm) = Father's height + (mother's height + 13 cm)/2
- Target height of girl (cm) = Father's height + (mother's height – 13 cm)/2.

SEQUENCE OF PUBERTY

In girls:

- Breast development (Thelarche)

- Pubic hair (Puberche)
- Peak growth velocity
- Menarche (two year after start of pubic hair).

In boys:

Testis → Penis → Pubic hair→ Axillary hair appearing.

Peak stage in growth corresponds to 2nd stage in pubic hair in girls and to 3rd stage in boys.

CHAPTER 20

DOWN'S SYNDROME

HISTORY

CHIEF COMPLAINTS

- Symptoms of upper respiratory tract infection
- Delayed milestones.

HISTORY OF PRESENT ILLNESS

History of Disease

- *Delayed milestones:* Developmental history should review gross motor, fine motor, and verbal milestones from birth until the time of evaluation.
  - Predominant speech delay: Hearing problem, autism, dyslexia
  - Predominant motor delay
  - Global delay that is nonprogressive (child is achieving milestones but at a later date than expected, child has not lost any achieved milestones)
  - Current social skills
  - Academic performance
  - Participation in an early intervention program (if aged < 3 yr) or school support (if aged > 3 yr) should be reviewed, including resource room assistance
  - Physical, occupational, speech and language therapy
  - Adaptive physical education
  - Standardized cognitive and educational testing can be asked.

History of Complications

- *Congenital heart disease:*
  - Breathlessness on feeding (suck-rest-suck cycle/sweating)
  - Cyanosis/cyanotic spells
  - Inability to gain weight
  - Repeated respiratory tract infection.
  - Swelling/abdominal pain
  - Seizures.
- *GI complication:*
  - Vomiting (Duodenal atresia)
  - Constipation (Hirschsprung's disease).
- *Leukemia:*
  - Bleeding from any site/rash/bone pains/ weight loss/paleness.
- *Hypothyroidism:*
  - Constipation/lethergy/sleepiness/delayed dentition.

- Impaired hearing/vision
- Inability to gain height (short stature)
- Delay in cognitive abilities, motor development, language development (specifically expressive skills) and social competence
- Difficulty in feeding
  - When were oral feeds started
  - Who feeds the child
  - How often
  - How long does it take
  - Associated problems like vomiting, constipation.

ANTENATAL HISTORY

- Blood tests/ultrasound or invasive tests done during pregnancy.

GENERAL PHYSICAL EXAMINATION

- Vitals
- Anthropometry: Height, length and head circumference
- Behavior: Natural spontaneity, genuine warmth, cheerful, gentleness, patience and tolerance are characteristics
- Signs suggestive of Down's syndrome: described below.

SYSTEMIC EXAMINATION

- As usual
- Do examine **Cardiovascular system** carefully to look out for congenital heart disease.

DIAGNOSIS

Presenting features (usually lower respiratory tract infection) in a child with Down's syndrome with/without congential heart disease with L $\rightarrow$ R or R $\rightarrow$ L shunt; most probably .... with/without delayed milestones; with/without other complications.

INVESTIGATIONS

- Karyotyping to determine the risk of recurrence
- Karyotape of parents if translocation is present
- ECG/Echocardiography (Congenital heart disease)
- T3/T4/TSH (Hypothyroidism)
- Speech evaluation and vision assessment
- X-ray spine with lateral flexion and extension views—done at 3 years of age to rule out atlantoaxial dislocation
- Interphase fluorescence *in situ* hybridization (FISH): FISH may be used for rapid diagnosis. It can be successful in both prenatal diagnosis and diagnosis in the neonatal period.

TREATMENT

No specific therapy exists for the congenital problems of patients with Down's syndrome.

- The treatment is generally directed to the cardiac and respiratory complications or against associated diseases (e.g. leukemia, tumor).
- Dermatologic problems and bacterial infections must be treated with appropriate medicines.
- Specialized institutions may help to teach simple trades to patients with mild retardation.
- Thyroid function test—3 yearly
- Vision/hearing assessment—Yearly
- Speech therapy
- Genetic counselling.

DISCUSSION

Average prevalence (Irrespective of maternal age) = 1: 700-800

Maternal Age (years)	*Risk Incidence*
15- 29	1: 1500
30-34	1: 800

35-39	1: 270
40-44	1: 100
> 45	1: 50

TYPES OF DOWN'S SYNDROME

Trisomy 21(95%): All the body cells of the patient have three chromosomes 21, which happens due to the meiosis nondisjunction.

Mosaic Down's syndrome (1%): Only some cells in body have an extra chromosome 21 (non-disjunction in mitosis).

Translocation Down's syndrome (4%): In this, a part of chromosome 21 is attached to another chromosome. So the patients have two normal chromosomes 21 plus a part of a abnormal chromosome 21. It is seen in more than 10% cases if maternal age is less than 30 years.

INHERITANCE

Most cases of Down's syndrome are not inherited. The trisomy 21 and mosaic type of Down's syndrome happens due to random accidents during meiosis or mitosis (in fetal development).

But in the translocation type, there is a possibility of inheritance. If a parent has a translocated part of chromosome 21 attached in another chromosome, (balanced translocation: a rearrangement of genetic material between chromosome 21 and another chromosome) he may be unaffected, but there is a high risk that his/her children will suffer from Down's syndrome.

Risk of Inheritance in Translocation

Translocation	*Maternal*	*Paternal*
t (14, 21)	12%	<1%
t (21, 21)	100%	100%
t (13, 21)	9%	1%
t (21, 22)	15%	3.5%

Chromosome 13, 14, 15 and 21 are responsible for majority of translocations (fusion of centromeres of above chromosomes results in translocation).

ANEUPLOIDY

- Trisomy: Addition of one chromosome, i.e. 47 chromosomes
- Trisomy of Autosomes:
  - Down's syndrome: Trisomy 21 (47, XY + 21)
  - Edward's syndrome: Trisomy 21 (47, XY + 18)
  - Patau's syndrome: Trisomy 21 (47, XY + 13).
- Addition of one chromosome in sex chromosome:
  - Klinefelter's syndrome: (47, XXY)
  - 47, XYY
  - 47, XXX.
- Monosomy: Loss of one chromosome, i.e. 45 chromosomes.
- Turner's syndrome: (45, X)

CAUSES OF NONDISJUNCTION OF 21 CHROMOSOME

- Increasing maternal age
- More exposure to radiation/viral diseases/ Environmental causes
- Genetic predisposition:
  - The nondisjunction responsible for trisomy 21 arises in the egg in 95% cases and in the sperm in 5% cases.

CHARACTERISTIC FEATURES OF DOWN'S SYNDROME

Craniofacial Characteristics

- Small head (brachycephaly)
- Flat occiput
- Increased interocular distance (hypertelorism)
- Depressed nasal bridge and small nose
- Low set ears/small auricles

- Broad short neck, lose skin folds in posterior neck
- Short hard palate
- Irregular teeth placement
- Protruding tongue
- Open mouth.

Eye Changes

- Mongoloid slant (upward and outward slant)
- Medial epicanthal folds
- Nystagmus
- Strabismus
- Keratoconus
- Refractive errors
- Cataract
- Brushfield's spots: Hypopigmented spots arranged in periphery of iris
- Fundus (in neonate): Spoke wheel pattern.

Central Nervous System Features

- Mental retardation
- Hypotonia
- Seizures
- Alzheimer's disease at early age (< 40 years)
- Cannot write but may be able to read.

Cardiovascular System (40%)

- Endocardial cushion defect (30%)
- VSD, PDA, ASD
- Tetralogy of Fallot.

Gastrointestinal System

- Proturbent abdomen (due to hypotonia)
- Umbilical hernia
- Divarication of recti
- Duodenal atresia.

Hematological Problems

- Increased incidence of leukemia (3 times)
- Decreased T-cell immunity.

Dermatoglyphics

- Single palmar crease (Simian crease)
- Ulnar loop pattern of dermal ridges
- Distal palmar axial triradius
- Plantar crease (*Sandak's crease*) between 1st and 2nd toes.

Skeletal

- Short stature
- Broad, short hands, feet and digits
- Hypoplasia of the mid phalanx of fifth finger: Clinodactyly
- Dysplasia of the pelvis
- Joint laxity
- Wide gap between the first and second toe
- Atlantooccipital instability
- Dysplasia (hypoplasia) of pelvis with shallow acetabular angle (may cause dislocation of hips).

Skin Changes

- Hyperkeratosis
- Cutis marmorata
- Adenomatous malformation of sebaceous glands.

Genitalia

- Hypogenitalism (small penis, scrotum, and testes)
- Hypospadius, cryptorchidism
- Delayed and incomplete puberty.

AGE RELATED FOLLOW-UP

- Newborn: Hypothyroidism
- < 6 months: Cardiac evaluation
- 8 months: Audiologic evaluation
- 4 years: Ophthalmologic evaluation

- > 5 years: Neck radiograph for atlantoaxial dislocation
- T4/TSH: Every 3 yearly
- Evaluate Growth parameters, Vision and Hearing yearly
- Enrolment in various support groups.

NATURAL HISTORY AND COURSE

- Improvement in muscle tone with age
- Intelligence quotient increases with age
- Development enrichment programs improve progress in early years
- Slow growth, late development
- Males infertile; Females rarely fertile.

CAUSES OF MORTALITY AND MORBIDITY IN DOWN'S SYNDROME

- Atlantoaxial dislocation (sudden death)
- Congenital heart disease
- Respiratory tract infections (recurrent)
- Hematological malignancies
- Alzheimer's disease.

PRENATAL DIAGNOSIS

Indications

- Maternal age > 35 years.
- Previous child with Down's syndrome
- Translocation carrier state.

Tests

USG Abdomen and Pelvis

- Short Femur and Humerus
- Thick nuchal fold (approx. 6 mms) at 16 weeks gestation
- Polyhydramnios
- Duodenal atresia
- Congenital heart disease.

Triple Test (16 Weeks)

- Decreased alpha—fetoprotein
- Low unconjugated estriol
- Increased HCG.

Invasive Procedures

- Chorionic villous biopsy (10 weeks)
- Amniocentesis (16 weeks)
- Fetal cord blood sampling for karyotyping.

STEPS TO COUNSEL PARENTS WITH DOWN'S SYNDROME

- Done as soon as possible.
- By someone with sufficient knowledge to inspire credibility.
- With both parents together, if possible.
- With the baby present, if possible and referred to by name.
- In a private, comfortable place, away from disturbances.
- In a straightforward manner, using understandable language, with as much time as needed for questions.
- With a balanced point of view, instead of a listing of problems.
- Parents should be informed regarding natural history of disease, occurrence and recurrence. rate in future pregnancies, prenatal diagnosis and treatment of complications if they arise.
- With follow-up discussion planned and a telephone number to call at any time for information.

- With additional information sources, including contact with other parents, provided and facilitated.
- Followed by uninterrupted time parents and child to remain alone together.

WHAT IS NICE ABOUT THEM DESPITE HANDICAPS

- They are docile, happy, 'good', friendly children.
- They like music and dancing. They need to be stimulated by music and other entertainment.
- They can do repetitive work. Hence, they can be employed in jobs that involve repetitive work like polishing work, making envelope, packing, etc.

CHAPTER 21

RICKETS

HISTORY

CHIEF COMPLAINTS

- Loose motions
- Inability to gain weight
- Deformities
- Convulsions.

HISTORY OF PRESENT ILLNESS

History of Disease

- Irritable child with flabby muscles
- Delayed development with late eruption of teeth
- Recurrent respiratory and gastrointestinal tract infections
- Seizures, tremor, stridor (hypocalcemia)
- Increased sweating over forehead
- White staining of floor by urine (phosphaturia).

History of Complications

- Repeated respiratory infections (due to chest deformity)
- Bony deformities, fractures
- Convulsions: Hypocalcemic convulsions, tetany
- Bone pain, progressive pallor, muscle weakness (renal osteodystrophy).

History of Risk Factors

Nutritional Cause

- Dietary history
- Artificial feeds
- Late weaning
- Prematurity/calcium intake in mother during pregnancy/interval between two successive pregnancies
- Low exposure to sunlight
- Constipation
- Excessive sweating over forehead.

Renal Cause

- Hematuria, dysuria, oliguria
- Polyuria, Polydipsia
- Repeated fractures.

Hepatic Cause

- Jaundice
- Neonatal hepatitis.

Malabsorption Syndromes

- Large quantity, pale, frothy, foul smelling stools
- Inability to gain weight
- Signs of fat soluble vitamin deficiency
- Drug intake—heavy metals, outdated tetracyclines (s/o acquired Fanconi's syndrome), phenytoin, phenobarbitone
- Alopecia—vitamin D dependent rickets Type II
- Fatigue, weight loss, bone pains (tumor).

Family History

- Parental consanguinity
- Family history of similar disorders (all autosomal recessive types of rickets)
- Family history of bone disease, bone defects, short stature
- Deaths in early infancy (infantile hypophosphatasia).

GENERAL PHYSICAL EXAMINATION

- Irritability
- Anthropometry: Growth retardation.

Signs of Rickets

Head

- Craniotabes: Earliest manifestation; there is feeling like compressing a ping pong ball (cracking feeling). It is seen below the age of one year. It is due to small islands of unossified area in the skull.
- Frontal and parietal bossing with large head
- Skull is apparently larger than normal (quadrate skull)
- Widening of sutures
- Delayed closure of anterior fontanelle with late eruption of teeth
- Vitamin deficiency (Vitamin A, D, E, K): Eye changes/petechiae/cheilosis/stomatitis/purpura.

Chest

- Pigeon chest
- Ricketic rosary (swelling or beaded appearance of the costochondral junction)
- Harrison's sulcus (linear transverse depression at insertion of diaphragm)
- Kyphoscoliosis.

Extremities

- Epiphyseal enlargement at wrists and ankles
- Knock knee (genu valgum)
- Genu varum or recurvatum (acrobatic rickets)
- Pelvic deformities (triradiate pelvis—occurs in later childhood and may produce difficulties during childbirth)
- Double malleolus.

Spine: Kyphoscoliosis

Bony deformities: Bow-legs/knock-knee/rib cage anomalies

Signs of Tetany

Chvostek's Sign

Elicitation: Tapping on the face at a point just anterior to the ear and just below the zygomatic bone.

Positive response: Twitching of the ipsilateral facial muscles, suggestive of neuromuscular excitability caused by hypocalcemia.

Trousseau's Sign

Elicitation: Inflating a sphygmomanometer cuff above systolic blood pressure for 3 minutes. Positive response: Muscular contraction including flexion of the wrist and metacarpophalangeal joints, hyperextension of the fingers, and flexion of the thumb on the palm, suggestive of neuromuscular excitability caused by hypocalcemia.

Erb's Sign

Increased electrical excitability of the peripheral nerves to the galvanic current.

DIAGNOSIS

.... year old child with signs of rickets–most probably due to.......... (etiology); with/without protein energy malnutrition; with/without deformities.

INVESTIGATIONS

To Prove Rickets

- Biochemistry:
  - S. Calcium—usually normal (may be decreased in some cases)
  - S. Phosphorus—decreased or normal (because Parathormone decreases phosphorus reabsorption in kidney)
  - S. Alkaline phosphatase increased
  - 25 hydroxy cholecalciferol levels (sensitive and reliable) are decreased.
- X-ray features of classical rickets are: (Usually seen in the bones of the wrist)

– Increased distance between the epiphysis and the metaphysis (loss of zone of provisional calcification)

– Metaphysis
  - "Fraying" (margin of metaphysis become blurred)
  - "Splaying" (metaphysis becomes widened)
  - "Cupping" of the metaphysis.

– Osteoporotic changes (decrease in density of bone)

– Deformities—"bending" of the bones or 'fracture' (pathological fracture) (Fig. 21.1).

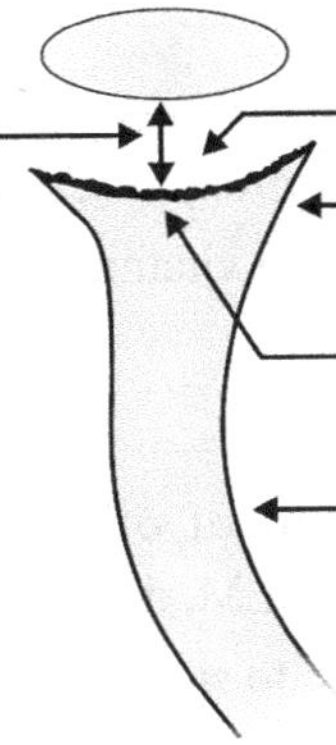

Fig. 21.1: Bone deformities

Etiological Investigations

- Hemogram with ESR
- Kidney function test with serum electrolytes
- SGOT/SGPT, serum proteins, serum bilirubin.

Refractory Rickets

Levels of Calcium, Parathormone and Vitamin D are important in distinguishing Vitamin D dependent rickets from Hypophosphatemic rickets. While hypocalcemia and raised parathormone point towards Vitamin D dependent Rickets; normal calcium and parathormone levels are suggestive of hypophosphatemic rickets. Low blood pH suggests renal tubular acidosis.

TREATMENT

Vitamin D (Stross Regime)

- Vitamin D 6 Lac units (15,000 µg), given orally
- Repeat X-ray wrist after 3-4 weeks
- White line appears at zone of preparatory calcification-continue 400 units Vitamin D_3 everyday for 3 months.
- Healing not seen
  - Repeat Vitamin D 6 Lac IU
  - Continue Vitamin D 400 IU daily.

Calcium Supplementation

- 100 mg/kg/day of calcium
- Diet rich in vitamin D and calcium.

Supportive Treatment

- Treatment of other etiology (if present)-Anemia, PEM, diarrhea, infections
- Exposure to sunlight
- If baby is breastfeeding—mother should also receive vitamin D and calcium supplementation.

DISCUSSION

DEFINITIONS

Rickets: Demineralization of growing bone.

Osteomalacia: Demineralization of adult bone (after growth ceases).

Osteolysis: Breaks in fully mineralized bone.

Osteoporosis: Proportionate loss of bone volume and mineral, which in children is due to excessive use of corticosteroid.

VITAMIN D METABOLISM

- Sunlight converts 7 dehydrocholesterol (precursor of vitamin D_3 present in skin) to cholecalciferol.
- Vitamin D (cholecalciferol) is converted in liver to 25 hydroxy cholecalciferol. It is the main circulating vitamin D metabolite and its plasma concentration is best indicator of vitamin D status in the body.
- 25 (OH) D_3 is further hydroxylated in kidney, forming 1, 25$(OH)_2D_3$ (calcitriol) which is most potent vitamin D metabolite. It increases calcium and phosphate absorption from intestine.

RICKETS

- Rickets results from either calcium or phosphorus deficiency, since both are necessary for bone mineralization.
- Important cause of calcium deficiency is insufficient vitamin D. Parathormone levels are almost raised in such cases.
- Vitamin D deficiency results from poor dietary intake, insufficient sunlight exposure and malabsorption like in chronic liver disease.
- Even anticonvulsants can lead to Vitamin D deficiency states and thus rickets, by inducing hepatic cytochrome P-450 oxidase that leads to conversion of 25$(OH)D_3$ into its inactive metabolites.
- Rickets can also occur secondary to dietary deficiency of Calcium, such patients have normal 25 $(OH)D_3$ but elevated 1,25$(OH)_2D_3$. Calcium supplements alone can treat rickets in such cases.
- Rickets is called 'Refractory' if no radiological healing is observed after second 6 lakh IU course of vitamin D. It does not refer to one particular disorder.

CAUSES OF REFRACTORY RICKETS

Calcium deficiency (Raised Parathormone Levels)

- Vitamin D dependent rickets type I and II
- Chronic renal failure
- Distal renal tubular acidosis

Phosphate Deficiency (Normal Parathormone Levels)

- Familial hypophosphatemic rickets
- Proximal renal tubular acidosis
- Fanconi syndrome.

VITAMIN D DEPENDENT RICKETS TYPE I AND II

These are rare autosomal recessive conditions.

VDDR type I, characterized by deficiency of 25 hydroxyvitamin D_1 alpha hydroxylase, results in hypocalcemia, hypophosphatemia and very low $1,25(OH)_2D_3$ levels.

VDDR type II, has similar features but due to end organ resistance, has high $1,25(OH)_2D_3$ levels.

Treatment with high doses of alpha-calcidiol or calcitriol, and calcium and phosphate supplements may be useful in some.

FAMILIAL HYPOPHOSPHATEMIC RICKETS

- The tubular defect results in impaired proximal tubular reabsorption of phosphate.
- This defect is inherited as X linked dominant, with mutation in PHEX gene (phosphate regulating gene).
- Severe rickets, growth retardation and dental abnormalities are typically present.
- Hypophosphatemia with low levels of $1,25(OH)_2D_3$ and normal 25 $(OH)D_3$ are characteristic. Serum calcium levels are normal.
- Urinary phosphate excretion is increased.
- Treatment is with phosphate supplementation and vitamin D analog.
- Hypercalciuria and nephrocalcinosis are frequent complications.

CLINICAL MANIFESTATIONS OF HYPOCALCEMIA

Increased Neuromuscular Irritability

- Chvostek sign
- Trousseau sign
- Erb's sign
- Paresthesias in circumoral and acral areas (fingers, toes)
- Muscle stiffness, myalgias, d spasms; in severe cases, laryngeal spasms may occur, which may lead to respiratory arrest.

Neuropsychiatric Symptoms

- Seizures (all types, but most commonly grand mal)
- Mental retardation
- Emotional problems (anxiety, depression, irritability, psychosis)
- Extrapyramidal symptoms
- Calcifications of basal ganglia (in long-standing disease)
- Papilloedema (raised intracranial tension).

Cardiovascular Symptoms

- Prolongation of QT interval
- Congestive heart failure
- Hypotension
- Arrhythmias.

Autonomic Symptoms

- Biliary colic
- Bronchospasm
- Diaphoresis.

Other Symptoms

- Cataract
- Dry and coarse skin, dermatitis, hyperpigmentation, and eczema
- Steatorrhoea (due to loss of calcium-stimulated secretion of biliary and pancreatic enzymes), which leads to vitamin D deficiency
- Gastric achlorhydria.

CHANGES IN SEQUENCE OCCURRING IN RICKETS

Biochemical Changes Occur 1st, Followed by Radiological Changes

- Raised alkaline phosphatase
- Decrease phosphate
- Hypocalcemia
- Radiological change (1st occurs in ulna).

With Treatment

- Radiological changes revert to normal 1st followed by biochemical changes followed by clinical changes (deformities may persist)
- Last to improve is S. alkaline phosphatase—if, it comes back within normal range then rickets is treated.

INTERPRETATION OF SERUM CALCIUM LEVELS

- Total calcium in serum (8.8 to 10.4 mg/dl) includes: free ions, ions bound to albumin, and to a small extent, diffusible complexes.
- The concentration of free calcium ions, averaging 4.8 mg/dl, influences many cellular functions and is subjected to tight hormonal control, especially through parathormone.
- In a patient with hypocalcemia, raised serum albumin leads to reduction in ionized serum calcium, or to the diagnosis of "factitious" hypocalcemia, meaning decreased total, but not ionised, calcium.
- It is thus more useful to measure serum *free calcium ion levels*.
- If ionised calcium cannot be measured, an approximation can be used to estimate the protein-bound and ionized fractions.
- The correction is to add 1 mg/dl to the serum calcium level for every 1 g/dl by which the serum albumin is below 4 g/dl.

IMPORTANCE OF VITAMIN D_3 LEVELS IN RICKETS

- Low 25 hydroxy and 1,25 dihydroxy vitamin D_3—Nutritional rickets
- Low 25 hydroxy vitamin D_3—Hepatic rickets
- Low 1 hydroxy vitamin D_3—Renal rickets.

Table 21.1: Differential diagnosis

	Ca	*P*	*Alk. PO_4*	*PTH*	*GSá*	*On Exogenous adm, PTH*
Hypoparathyroidism	↓	↑	N or ↓ (PTH acts on osteoclasts which causes release of Alk. phosphatase)	↓	Normal urinary cAMP and PO4	↑
Pseudohypoparathyroidism IA	↓	↑	↑	↑	Mutation (mat. Transmission)	No increase
IB	↓	↑	↑	↑	N	No increase
II	↓	↑	↑	↑	Defect distal to cAMP because it is normally activated but cell is unable to respond to signal ↓ (mutation)	Urinary cAMP ↑, no increase in PO_4
Pseudohypoparathyroidism	N	N	↑	↑		
Rickets	↓	N or ↓	↑	(slightly)		

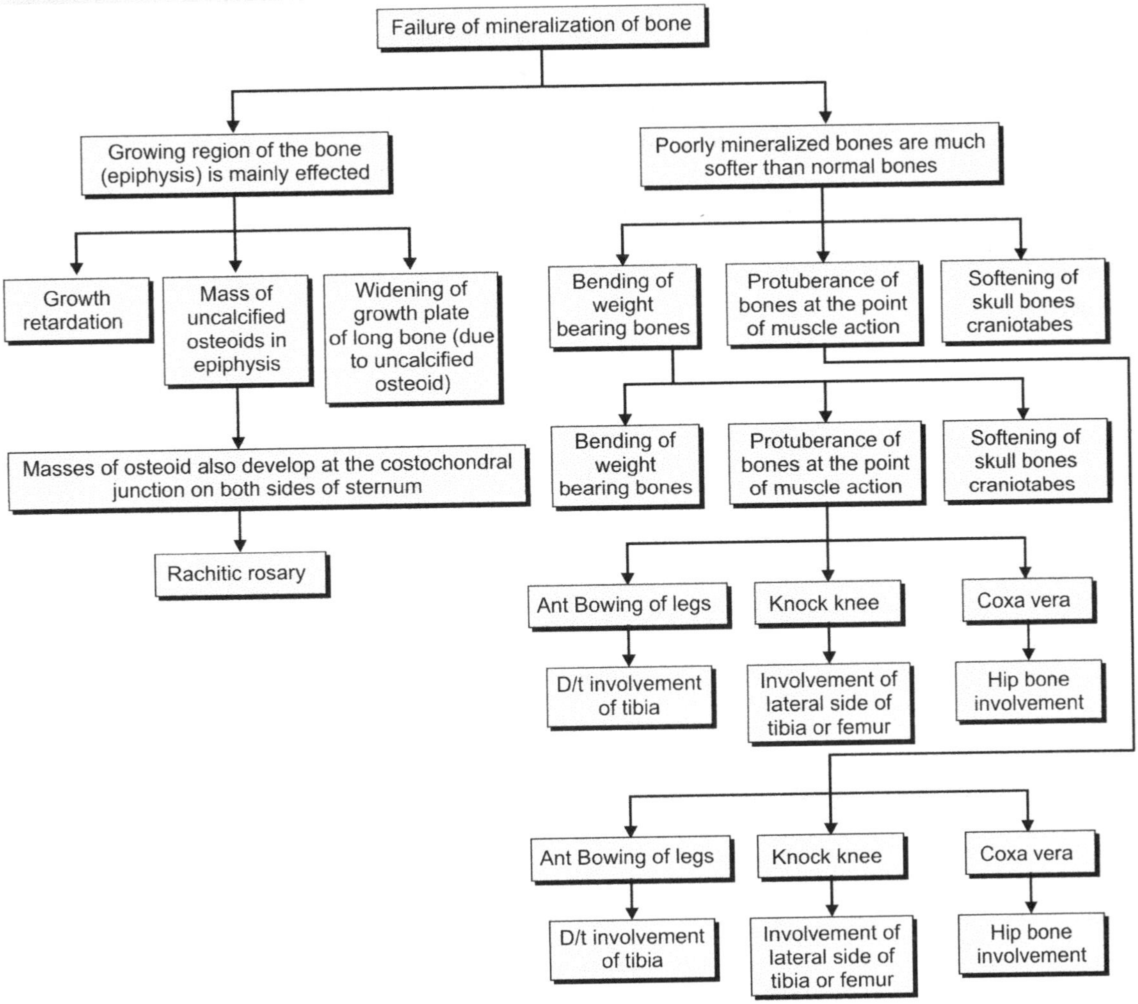

Fig. 21.2: Pathogenesis of rickets

ATROPHIC RICKETS—OCCURS IN PEM

Cupping, splaying, fraying which are classically seen on X-ray are less visible, but they come up with treatment of PEM.

CAUSES OF MENTAL RETARDATION IN A PATIENT WITH RICKETS

- Lowe's syndrome
- Cystinosis
- Galactosemia
- Tyrosinemia
- Wilson's disease
- Fructose intolerance.

COMMONEST CAUSE OF VITAMIN D DEFICIENCY IN INDIA

- Malabsorption.

CLOSURE OF FONTANELLES

- Anterior fontanelle closes by 9-18 months
- Posterior fontanelle closes by 3-6 months.

DELAYED CLOSURE OF ANTERIOR FONTANELLE

- Rickets
- Cretinism
- Syphilis
- Hydrocephalus
- Protein-energy malnutrition.

CHAPTER 22

NORMAL NEONATE

HISTORY

INTRODUCTION

Baby of ......(mothers name), a ....hours/days old, male/female child born to a G......... P....A...... mother, resident of .... brought with chief complaints of jaundice/inability to feed/ excessive crying etc.

HISTORY OF PRESENT ILLNESS

Take detailed history of following complaints in a sick neonate:

- Fever
- Difficulty in respiration
- General activity: Lethargic or excessively irritable
- Excessive crying
- Refusal of feeds
- Rash
- Progressive pallor, jaundice, cyanosis
- Bleeding manifestations
- Details of passage of urine and stool
- Vomiting
- Abdominal distension.

BIRTH HISTORY

Antenatal History

- Age of mother at conception
- Registered at which month of pregnancy
- No. of antenatal visits, one visit in each trimester (booked/unbooked)
- Maternal immunization: Number of doses of tetanus toxoid taken, duration between two doses, second dose taken at least two weeks before delivery or not.
- Maternal diseases

  First trimester: Hyperemesis, radiation exposure, fever with rash or neck swellings, bleeding per vaginum

  Second trimester: Quickening, vaginal bleeding

  Third trimester: Vaginal bleeding, edema, blurring of vision, headache, seizures, pallor, anemia, genital infections, jaundice.
- Caloric and protein intake during pregnancy
- Weight gain during pregnancy (malnutrition as cause of IUGR)
- Vitamins/mineral supplements taken during pregnancy

- Maternal medications (Sulphonamides and other oxidant drugs can precipate hemolysis in G6PD deficient neonates)
- Investigations done during pregnancy (Hemoglobin, TORCH, urine, blood group, ultrasound)
- Screening: HIV, Thalassemia.

Labor History

- Place of delivery, delivery conducted by doctor/nurse/dai
- Spontaneous/Induced labor after rupture of membranes
- No. of times per vaginal examination done, PV done by gloved hands or ungloved hands
- Whether oxytocin used to augment labor (oxytocin is known to increase jaundice)
- Liquor meconium stained or not
- Presentation—vertex/breech
- If LSCS—indication and anesthesia
- History of fetal distress
- Whether cried immediately after birth or not
- Developed cyanosis, required resuscitation, and required admission to intensive care unit.
- Birth weight
- Passed urine
- Passed meconium.

Immediate Postnatal History

- Feeding/urination/stools
- No. of day's child kept in NICU or given to mother for feeding
- Child developed fever/seizures or any other complications
- Whether kept under warmer, phototherapy machine
- Treatment received in NICU: intravenous fluids, antibiotics, oxygen
- Investigations done during admission in NICU
- If breastfeed
  - Frequency
  - Duration of each feed
  - Adequacy of breastfeeding (child gains weight; sleeps adequately between feeds, there is a minimum interval of 2-3 hours between feeds, passes urine at least 6 to 8 times per day, Let-down reflex occurs from the opposite breast on feeding).
- If top-fed:
  - Milk used
  - Dilution
  - Mode of feeding (bottle-fed or katori spoon fed)
  - Vitamin supplements given or not.
- Immunization.

PAST OBSTETRIC HISTORY

- GPAL
- Full-term/preterm
- Complications in previous delivery
- Family planning measures used.

FAMILY HISTORY

- Anemia, jaundice and epilepsy in siblings
- Cardiopulmonary disorders
- Thalassemia trait
- Sickle cell disease.

GENERAL PHYSICAL EXAMINATION

- Posture: Frog like, semiflexed extremeties, pelvis flat or high up
- Vitals: Temperature/heart-rate/respiration/CFT.
- Anthropometry: Length (US/LS)/head and chest circumference/weight.
- Skin: Color, jaundice, cyanosis, mongolion spots.

- Cry: Depressed, high pitched, weak cry.
- Skull:
  - Anterior fontanelle: Open, closed, size, bulging.
  - Posterior fontanelle.
  - Caput, cephalhematoma.
  - Sutures.
- Signs of sepsis: Petechiae, sclerema, edema, circumoral grey discoloration, pallor, capillary refilling time.
- Eyes: Subconjuctivial hemorrhage, epicanthic folds, cataract
- Mouth: Cleft lip, cleft palate, oral thrush, epstein pearls.
- Facial dysmorphism and congenital malformation: Ear, nose, neck.
- Umbilical cord:
  - No. of arteries/veins.
  - Dried cord/shriveled/fallen off.
  - Discharge/meconium stained/redness around the base of cord.
- Genitalia: Undescended testis/incomplete cover of labia majora by minora.
- Anus: Imperforate anus.
- Spine and back: any sinus tract.
- Extremeties: Congenital dislocation of hip, talipes equinovarus.

SYSTEMIC EXAMINATION

RESPIRATORY SYSTEM

- Chest movement
- Tachypnea
- Grunting
- Stridor
- Breath sounds with any additional sounds
- Pleural rub.

CARDIOVASCULAR SYSTEM

- Pulse—rate, rhythm, volume, peripheral pulses
- Murmur
- Signs of congestive cardiac failure.

ABDOMEN

- Distension
- Hepatosplenomegaly
- Any mass in abdomen
- Umbilicus
- Genitalia
- Bowel sounds.

CNS

- Cry
- Tone
- Activity
- Reflexes
- Assessment of gestational age by New Ballard scoring.

NEONATAL REFLEXES (TABLE 22.1)

Rooting or Search Reflex

- When baby's cheek comes in contact with mother's breast, baby seeks the nipple.
- When upper lip, lower lip or cheeks are stimulated the baby will turn to that side to find the source of milk.
- It is present in normal full term babies and disappears by three months.
- *Importance:* This reflex action helps the baby for finding the breast as there is no neck control at birth. So baby cannot voluntarily turn to source of milk. This reflex disappears, when baby develops neck control and can voluntarily turn and find the breast.

Table 22.1: Various developmental reflexes

Level of control	Reflexes	Appears at	Disappears at
Spinal cord	Flexor withdrawal Extensor withdrawal Crossed extensor Gallant	Birth	2 weeks
Brainstem	Asymmetric tonic neck Symmetric tonic neck Tonic labrynthine Positive supporting Negative supporting	2 weeks	6 months
Midbrain	Neck correcting body Optical correcting body	4 months	2 years
Cortical or cerebellar	Various balancing reflexes	2 years	
Stretch receptors of neck	Moro	Birth	6 months
Semicircular canal	Parachute, Landau		

Sucking and Swallowing Reflex

- Sucking reflex can be elicited by introducing finger into the baby's mouth. Baby starts sucking vigorously.
- It appears at 28 weeks of gestation. Sucking gets well synchronized with swallowing at 34 weeks.
- *Importance:* Its absence suggests developmental defect.

Moro's Reflex

- With baby in supine position and back of head supported on palm of hand, flex the neck by 15 degrees. Release the head to initiate the reflex. Head should be in midline and hands should be open.

Components of Reflex

Phase 1: Abduction of arms at shoulder and extension of arms at elbows with hands open.

Phase 2: Adduction of arms and flexion of forearms. In preterm babies phase two is absent because of weakness of antigravity muscles.

- Moro's reflex is a vestibular reflex.
- It appears at 28 weeks of gestation. Reflex is complete after 32 weeks of gestation. It disappears by 3 months.
- Persistence is seen in cerebral palsy while asymmetrical reflex is seen in Erb's palsy, Spastic hemiplegia, Fracture of humerus or clavicle, closed hand.

Grasp Reflex

- Touch the ulnar side of palm of baby by your index finger to initiate grasp reflex. As you lift your index finger, flexor muscles of forearm of baby become tight, and baby supports his whole weight. Phase 2 is present only in term babies.
- It appears at 34 weeks of gestation and disappears by three months.
- Persistence is seen in spastic cerebral palsy and reflex is asymmetrical in hemiplegia and cerebral damage.

ATNR (Asymmetrical Tonic Neck Reflex)

- Passive rotation of head in supine position leads to extension of upper limbs on same side and flexion of contralateral knee.
- It appears at birth and disappears by three months.
- Persistence is seen in spastic cerebral palsy.
- *Importance:* Prevents baby from rolling. So it must disappear, when baby learns to turn prone voluntarily.

STNR (Symmetrical Tonic Neck Reflex)

- Passive extension of head in prone position leads to extension of both upper limbs and flexion of lower limbs.
- It appears at three months and disappears by six months.
- Persistence is seen in cerebral palsy.
- *Importance:* When baby learns to turn to prone position, choking over bed may asphyxiate him. So if baby lifts the chin by extension of neck, automatically both upper limbs are extended and choking is avoided however; this reflex must disappear if, baby has to crawl, as that will require voluntary flexion and extension of upper and lower limbs. So it disappears by six months.

Landau Reflex (Position Reflex)

- Passive extension of neck in ventral suspension leads to extension of spine, lower and upper limbs. Passive flexion of neck leads to flexion of spine, lower limbs and upper limbs.
- It appears at 6 months and disappears at 9 months.
- *Importance*: Absent in cerebral palsy.

Parachute Reflex (Position Reflex)

- In ventral suspension with head low position, baby is brought down towards ground from height, as if baby is falling. This leads to extension of both upper limbs in attempt to avoid injury to face.
- It appears at 9 months and Never disappears. Persists all through life.
- *Importance:* Absent in cerebral palsy.

Neck Righting Reflex

- If neck is turned sideways, body as a whole follows.
- It appears at birth, strong at three months and disappears by six months.
- *Importance:* Before the development of neck control, (age < 3 months) passive movement of neck sideways can cause twisting of neck which is prevented by this reflex.

  At three months neck control is achieved but there is no control on trunk. When neck is turned voluntarily, again twisting could occur. This is avoided by neck righting reflex.

  At six months, control over trunk muscles develops as baby starts turning prone. Thus, body can voluntarily follow neck movement in sideways, so the reflex disappears.

Body Righting Reflex

- Change of posture of body in vertical direction leads to neck movement following in the same direction. Thus, head moves along the trunk in vertical direction.
- Appears at 6 months (as neck righting reflex wanes), gradually becomes stronger. Strong at nine months and disappears by 12 months.
- *Importance:* When body moves, the neck flexion or extension will automatically follow the body. Thus "spatial" head position is well maintained. When child starts standing alone, and walking with little support, (good control over trunk and lower limbs), the need for this reflex is over and it disappears by the age of 12 months.

DIAGNOSIS

..........hours/days old full term AGA/SGA or Preterm AGA/SGA, male/female born to a G..... mother with gestational age of ....weeks with no antenatal/intra/post natal complication with/without icterus, birth asphyxia, etc.

DISCUSSION

NORMAL FULL-TERM

- 50 cm long, head circumference 35 cm; chest circumference 3 cm less than head circumference; Upper segment/Lower segment ratio 1.7:1.
- Flexion attitude, sleeps 20 hours
- Heart rate 120-140/min; RR 35-40/min
- Voids urine within 24 hours, meconium black and passed within 72 hours
- Losses up to 10% weight in first week and regains by 10th day, then gains 30 gram/day up to 3 months.

PREMATURITY

Child is premature (i.e. < 37 weeks) when:

- Sole creases absent or present in anterior 1/3rd
- Testes at external ring, small scrotum with few rugacities/labia majora widely separated exposing labia minor and clitoris
- Breast nodule < 5 mm diameter
- Ear cartilage deficient and poor elastic recoil
- Hair wooly.

CEPHALHEMATOMA

- Subperiosteal collection of blood
- Does not cross suture line, unlike caput succedaneum
- Reaches maximum size by 3rd day
- Usually parietal bone is most commonly affected
- When bilateral, it may be associated with skull fracture
- Disappears by 4 to 6 weeks.

CAPUT SUCCEDANEUM

- Diffuse soft boggy swelling of scalp
- Seen at birth
- Crosses suture line
- Disappears by 1-2 days.

OPHTHALMIA NEONATORUM

- Conjunctivitis with discharge during 1st to 2nd weeks of life
- Appears sticky within 2-5 days after birth
- Corneal damage if untreated
- *Etiology:* Neisseria gonorrhea, Chlamydia trachomatis
- *Prophylaxis:* Clean eyes immediately, 1% silver nitrate solution, 1% tetracycline ointment.

BIRTH WEIGHT

- AGA: Birth weight between 10th to 90th percentiles for the gestation
- SGA (IUGR): Birth weight less than 10th percentile for their gestational age
- LGA: Birth weight more than 90th percentile for their gestational age
- LBW: Birth weight less than 2500 grams irrespective of gestational age.

INTRAUTERINE GROWTH RETARDATION

Asymmetrical (Malnourished)	*Symmetrical (Hypoplastic)*
Insult in later part of gestation	Insult in early part of gestation
Head Circumference and brain weight-normal	Head circumference and brain weight—less than normal
Ponderal index < 2	Ponderal index > 2
No increase in congenital anomalies	Increased congenital anomalies

PONDERAL INDEX

$$\frac{\text{Weight (gm)}}{\text{length (cm)}^3} \times 100$$

JAUNDICE IN NEONATES

Physiological Jaundice

- Appears after 30 hrs of life (30-72 hrs)
- In term neonates-Peaks in 3-4 days (12 mg %), returns to normal in 7 to 10 days
- In preterm neonates- Peaks in 5-7 days (15 mg %), returns to normal in 10 to 14 days
- Usually no treatment required.

Pathological Jaundice

- Appearing in less than 24 hrs of life
- Rate of rise > 0.5 mg/dl/hr of serum bilirubin
- Total bilirubin > 15 mg%
- Direct bilirubin > 2.0 mg% or more than 15% of total bilirubin
- Jaundice persisting for 2 weeks in term and 3 weeks in preterm infants
- Any elevation requiring phototherapy.

Breast Milk Jaundice

- Due to inhibitory substances (preganendiol and free fatty acid) in the breast milk that interferes with conjugation
- Onset on day 4 of life, peaks by day 14 of life, can persist upto 4 to 6 weeks of life.

Breastfeeding Jaundice

Early onset, due to inadequate feeding leads to increased enterohepatic circulation and thus increased bilirubin levels.

Causes of Jaundice in First 24 Hours

F Fetomaternal blood group incompatibility (Rh, ABO)
I Intrauterine infection
R RBC enzyme defect
S Spherocytosis
T α-thalassemia
Crigler-Najjar syndrome
Lucey-Driscoll syndrome.

WORK UP OF JAUNDICED BABY

- Maternal and perinatal history: Intrauterine infection, Infant of diabetic mother, Oxytocin infusion during delivery
- Physical examination: Prematurity, IUGR, Cephalhematoma, Hepatosplenomegaly, Sepsis
- Family H/o liver disease s/o galactosemia, α-1-Antitrypsin deficiency, Criggler-Najjar syndrome
- Lab studies:
  - Serum bilirubin—total, direct and indirect
  - Blood grouping and Rh typing
  - Hematocrit, reticulocyte count
  - Direct Coomb's test on baby
  - Sepsis screen
  - Liver function and thyroid function test
  - TORCH assay.

CLINICAL CRITERIA TO ASSESS JAUNDICE

- Head and neck 5 mg/dl
- Trunk 10 mg/dl
- Thighs 15 mg/dl
- Arms and lower legs 20 mg/dl
- Palms end soles > 25 mg/dl.

APPROACH TO JAUNDICED BABY

- Determine birth weight, gestation, postnatal age in hours
- Check baby's and mother's blood group, see if ABO incompatibility (Mother O; baby A/B/AB) or Rh incompatibility (Mother Rh negative and baby Rh positive)
- Assess clinical condition (well or ill)
  - Decide jaundice is physiological or pathological: If physiological and baby well, only observation is required.
  - If deeply jaundice, look for kernicterus (lethargy, poor feeding, absent Moro's reflex, hypertonia, convulsions).

WHEN TO SUSPECT CHOLESTASIS

- Jaundice: During neonatal period and infancy
- Urine: High coloured
- Diaper stained with urine
- Stool: Clay colored
- Jaundice persisting for >14 days.

PROLONGED JAUNDICE

- >10 mg/dl after 2 wks of age.

Causes

- Breast milk jaundice
- Hypothyroidism
- Cephalhematoma
- Ongoing hemolysis
  - Enzymatic defects—G6PD and pyruvate kinase deficiency
  - Membrane defects—hereditary spherocytosis.
- Gilbert's syndrome
- Down's syndrome
- Hirschsprung's disease.

MECHANISM OF PHOTOTHERAPY

In decreasing order of importance

Structural Isomerization

Bilirubin is converted to lumirubin, which is excreted in bile and urine. This is irreversible reaction and hence produces rapid decline in bilirubin.

Photoisomerization

Less toxic photoisomers are formed which are excreted in bile but they can revert back to unconjugated bilirubin and can get reabsorbed from gut if baby is not having stools.

Native bilirubin in 4Z15Z; first bilirubin that is formed is 4Z15E which is more polar therefore more water soluble and excreted in bile.

Photo-oxidation

Converts bilirubin into small polar products that are excreted in urine.

PRECAUTIONS WITH BABY ON PHOTOTHERAPY

- Shield the eyes and genitalia
- Source of light must be 45 cm above baby. In intensive phototherapy, source of light may be brought at 20 cm with changing the position of baby more often.
- Increase fluid intake by 20-40 ml/kg/hour.
- Blue lamp with wavelength of 425-475 nm are used and irradiance of 6-12 $\mu W/cm^2/nm$
- Give feeding every 2 hours and frequently change posture
- No role of prophylactic phototherapy since bilirubin must be present in skin for phototherapy to be effective.

CHOICE OF BLOOD FOR EXCHANGE TRANSFUSION

ABO Incompatibility

- Give O blood group, Rh compatible with baby
- Ideal is Group O blood cells suspended in AB plasma.

Rh Incompatibility

- O Rh negative cells cross matched with mother's blood.
- Ideal is group O blood cells suspended in AB plasma.

INDICATIONS FOR TRANSFER TO NICU

- Birth weight < 1800 gram
- Gestation < 34 weeks
- Unable to feed
- Sick neonate.

Table 22.2: Growth and calories requirements

	Daily wt.gain (g)	Length (cm/ month)	Head Circum (cm/month)	Calories/ kg/day
0-3 months	30	3.0	2	115
3-6 months	20	2.0	1	110
6-9 months	15	1.5	0.5	100
9-12 months	12	1.2	0.5	100
1-3 years	8	1	0.25	100
4-6 years	6	3 cm/yr	1 cm/yr	90-100

Table 22.3: Age estimation by X-ray

Age of the infant	Area of which X-ray should be taken
0-3 months	X-ray knee joint, foot
3-9 months	Shoulder
1-13 years	Hand and wrist
12-14 years	Elbow, hip joint
18 years	Elbow and knee joint

CRITERIA OF DISCHARGE FROM NICU

- Accepting feeds well
- Adequately gaining weight
- No danger signs.

DANGER SIGNS IN NEWBORNS

- Lethargy/refusal to feed
- Hypothermia
- Tachypnea
- Grunting/apnea
- Seizures/vacant stare
- Persistent vomiting
- Abdominal distention
- Bleeding from umbilical stump
- Icterus over palms and soles.

HYPOTHERMIA

- Normal temperature 36.5-37°C
- Cold stress (mild hypothermia) 36-36.5°C
- Moderate hypothermia 32-36° C
- Severe hypothemia < 32°C.

Table 22.4: Distinguishing preterm baby from a term baby

Preterm baby	Term baby
From LMP/growth charts	Same as but findings will be different
Deep crease on ant 1/3rd of foot	Deep crease present on 2/3rd of foot or more
Pinna of ear devoid of cartilage so remains folded	Pinna of ear recoils back
No rugae on scrotum	Deep rugae on scrotum are present
Labia are well separated not covering minora and prominent clitoris	Covers the minora

Table 22.5: Problems of preterm and IUGR babies

Preterm	IUGR
Respiratory distress syndrome	Birth asphyxia
Hypothermia	Meconium aspiration syndrome
Birth asphyxia	Hypothermia
Apneic cells	Hypoglycemia
Metabolic problems	Infections
Infections	Polycythemia

Treatment

Cold Stress

- Warm clothes and cover adequately
- Warm room and bed (28-32°C)
- Bedding in with mother
- Skin to skin contact
- Frequent breastfeeding
- No extra heat source required.

Moderate Hypothermia

- Provide extra heat with warm towels, 200 W bulb, heater, radiant warmer
- Monitor temperature every 15 minutes.

Table 22.6: Feeding schedule

	Wt. < 1200 gms Gestation < 30 weeks	Wt:1200-1800gms Gestation: 30-34 weeks	Wt >1800 gms Gestation> 34 weeks
At birth	Start on IVF	Tube feeds	Breastfeeds
3-7 days	Move to gavage feeds	Katori spoon feeds	If not satisfactory katori spoon feeds
1-2 weeks	Katori spoon feeds	Breastfeeds	

Severe Hypothermia

- Warm rapidly under radiant warmer till temperature reaches 34°C
- Once temperature reaches 34°C slow down warming
- Give 100% oxygen by hood
- Investigate for sugar, sepsis screen, blood culture and hemogram
- Start Intravenous fluids
- Administer appropriate antibiotics
- Give injection vitamin K
- Measure temperature every 30 minutes.

HYPOTHERMIA PREVENTION: TEN STEPS OF WARM CHAIN

- Warm delivery room
- Immediate drying
- Warm resuscitation
- Skin to skin contact
- Breast feeding
- Postpone bathing
- Appropriate clothing and bedding
- Mother and baby together
- Warm transportation
- Training/awareness of health persons.

CAUSATIVE ORGANISM IN NEONATAL SEPSIS

Early onset (0-7 days)	*Late onset (> 7 days)*
E. coli	*Klebsiella*
Klebsiella	*Staph. aureus*
Group B *Streptococcus*	*Pseudomonas*

CHARACTERISTICS THAT DISTINGUISH JITTERINESS FROM SEIZURE

- Jitteriness is stimulus sensitive
- In jitteriness movements cease with restrain
- Associated abnormal eye movement are not present in jitteriness
- Quality of movement is tremor like in jitteriness while it is clonic jerking in seizures.

SUMMARY OF SAFE TRANSPORT OF NEONATES

Prepare Well Before Transport

- Assess
- Communicate
- Correct hypothermia
- Stabilize
- Write a note
- Encourage mother to accompany
- Arrange a provider to accompany.

Ensure Warm Transport

- Skin to skin care (kangaroo mother care) or
- Cover the baby or
- Improvised containers or
- Transport incubator.

Provide Other Care during Transportation

- Ensure warm feet
- Ensure an open airway
- Check breathing
- Provide feeds.

CHAPTER 23

HIGH-RISK NEONATE

HIGH-RISK BABIES

- Very low birth weight
- Neurological disorders
    - Perinatal asphyxia
    - Intraventricular hemorrhage
    - Meningitis
    - Persistent seizure
    - Neurological abnormality on discharge.
- Ventilated neonates
- Neonatal sepsis
- Hyperbilirubinemia requiring exchange transfusion.

CORRECTED GESTATIONAL AGE

- Growth is monitored by using corrected gestational age.
  Corrected age = Chronological age – No. of weeks born prematurely.

LENGTH

- Preterm infants show catch up growth in 1st 3 years
- Asymmetric IUGR shows complete catch-up growth mostly in 6-12 months of age
- Symmetric IUGR shows catch-up growth up to 3 years of life or they never achieve full catch-up growth.

IMMUNIZATION

- All vaccines can be given as per schedule according to chronological age, irrespective of birth weight or period of gestation
- Very LBW and preterm babies can be given immunization after initial stabilization
- Previously, Hepatitis B vaccine was not recommended below 2 kg because of poor immunogenicity.

LOW BIRTH WEIGHT: FLUIDS AND FEEDING

Weight < 1200 grams; Gestation <30 weeks

- Start initial Intravenous fluids
- Introduce nasogastric feeding once stable
- Shift to katori spoon feeds over next few days later on breastfeeds.

Weight 1200 -1800 grams; Gestation 30-34 weeks

- Start initial nasogastric feeds
- Introduce Katori spoon feeds after 3-7 days
- Shift to breast feeds as soon as baby is able to suck.

Weight >1800 grams; Gestation > 34 weeks

- Start breastfeeding
- Katori spoon feeding, if sucking not satisfactory on breast
- Shift to breastfeeds as soon as possible.

Feeding Schedule

- Begin milk at 60 to 80 ml/kg/day
- Increase by 15 ml/kg/day
- Maximum of 180 to 200 ml/kg/day
- Give feeds 2 hourly.

Fluid Schedule

- Give 60 to 80 ml/kg/day on first day
- Increase by 15 ml/kg/day till day 7
- Add 20-30 ml/kg/day for infants under radiant warmer and phototherapy
- Maximum of 150 ml/kg/day.

NUTRITIONAL SUPPLEMENTATION IN PRETERMS

- The peak of fetal accumulation of mineral and vitamins occurs after 34 weeks of gestation
- So calcium, phosphorus, iron, multivitamins needs to be supplemented
- Calcium (100 mg/kg/day) and phosphorus (40-50 mg/kg/day) is supplemented when full feed is achieved at 150 ml/kg/day. It is supplemented in 1.5 : 1 to 2:1.

RDA OF CALCIUM AND PHOSPHORUS IN PRETERM INFANTS

Calcium 100-200 mg/kg/day

Phosphorus 50-150 mg/kg/day

- ❖ Human milk provides 25 mg/dl of calcium, 14 mg/dl of phosphorus and vitamin D 12-50 U/L
- ❖ Supplements to be continued to 40 weeks of corrected gestation.
- ❖ Supplements to be given until weight reaches 3-3.5kg.
- ❖ European society for pediatric gastroenterology and nutrition recommends vitamin and mineral content to be added at 2 weeks of age.

Multivitamin Supplementation

- Supplements should provide the vitamins in the following amounts each day:

Vitamin A	1000-1500 IU
Vitamin D	400 IU
Vitamin E	25 IU
Vitamin C	40-50 mg
Vitamin B_1	1000 µg
Vitamin B_{12}	3-5 µg
Niacin	5-10 mg
Folic acid	50 µg
Zinc	1-2 mg/kg/day.

- Supplements are added when full feed is achieved at 150 ml/kg/day and to be continued upto 40 weeks of gestational age
- Visyneral Z drops—0.6 ml once a day.
- Vitamin E has controversial role in prevention of Retinopathy of prematurity, bronchopulmonary dysplasia and Intra ventricular hemorrhage.

CAUSES OF INADEQUATE WEIGHT GAIN IN PRETERM BABIES

- Chronic cold stress
- Decreased caloric intake
- Poor sucking
- Abnormal oral motor development
- Severe bronchopulmonary dysplasia requiring high caloric intake
- Faulty feeding (due to dilution, bottle feeding)
- Anemia of prematurity

- Infection
  - Urinary tract Infection
  - Fungal infection
  - Sepsis.
- Late hyponatremia
- Late metabolic acidosis
- Patent ductus arteriosus.

PROBLEMS IN VERY LOW BIRTH WEIGHT BABIES

- Developmental disability
  - Major handicaps (cerebral palsy and mental retardation)
  - Sensory impairments (hearing loss, visual impairment)
  - Minimal cerebral dysfunction (language disorder, learning disability, hyperactivity, attention deficit, behavioral disorders).
- Retinopathy of prematurity
- Chronic lung disease
- Poor growth
- Increased rates of postneonatal illnesses and rehospitalization
- Osteopenia of prematurity.

ASSESSMENT OF VERY LOW BIRTH WEIGHT BABIES ON FOLLOW-UP

- Growth – weight, length and head circumference
- Neurodevelopmental assessment
- Immunization
- Ophthalmologic screening for Retinopathy of prematurity
- Hearing screening
- Nutritional supplementation
- Ultrasound cranium for Intraventricular hemorrhage.

HEARING SCREENING OF LOW BIRTH WEIGHT BABIES

- Prematurity – Risk factor for sensorineural and conductive hearing loss
- All VLBW infants require screen both in neonatal period and again at 1 year of age
- *Risk factors*
  - Family history of sensorineural or conductive hearing loss
  - Bacterial meningitis, TORCH infection
  - Hyperbilirubinemia requiring exchange blood transfusion, persistent pulmonary hypertension, treatment with mechanical ventilation
  - Recurrent or persistent otitis media with effusion for at least 3 months.
- *Screening test:* Auditory brainstem responses
- *Treatment* by hearing aids or cochlear implants.

ANEMIA OF PREMATURITY

Occurs at 2-4 weeks of the postnatal age.

Causes

- Inadequate erythropoietin by preterm liver
- Frequent blood sampling in neonatal period for stabilization of vital signs
- AAP recommends iron supplementation at 4 weeks of age at the dose of 2 mg/kg/day and continue up to 1 year.

RETINOPATHY OF PREMATURITY (ROP)

- Multifactorial, vasoproliferative retinal disorder.

Whom and When to Screen

- All infants BW < 1.5 kg or Gestational age < 32 weeks
- > 32 weeks with severe respiratory distress syndrome, hypotension requiring pressor

support or surgery in first several weeks of life

- ❖ Infants born before 32 weeks of age should be screened at 32 weeks of age, i.e:

Gestation	*Screening done at*
<26 weeks	6 weeks
27-28 weeks	5 weeks
29-30 weeks	4 weeks
>30 weeks	3 weeks

Stages for Severity

- ❖ Stage 1: A *demarcation line* as a thin white line between normal retina and undeveloped avascular retina
- ❖ Stage 2: *Ridge* of fibrovascular tissue
- ❖ Stage 3: *Ridge with extraretinal fibrovascular proliferation*, abnormal blood vessels and fibrous tissue develop on the edge of the ridge
- ❖ Stage 4: *Partial retinal detachment* outside the macula (4A) and involving macular (4B)
- ❖ Stage 5: *Complete retinal detachment.*

Plus Disease

- ❖ Presence of *vascular dilatation and tortuosity* of the posterior retinal vessels in at least *two quadrants.*

Treatment

- ❖ Laser therapy
- ❖ Cryotherapy.

PERINATAL ASPHYXIA

Neurodevelopmental Assessment

- Most common cerebral palsy (CP) in preterm infants—spastic diaplegia
- Risk factors are:
  - ❖ Intracranial hemorrhage
  - ❖ Periventricular white matter injury
  - ❖ Neonatal complications like bronco-pulmonary dysplasia, brain injury.
- Most cases of cerebral palsy are not related to perinatal asphyxia
- Only 3-13% of infants with cerebral palsy have evidence of intrapartum asphyxia
- Presence of seizure increases risk of cerebral palsy by 50-70 folds.

Stopping Anticonvulsants

- Detection of low voltage activity, electrocerebral inactivity or burst suppression pattern on EEG shows poor outcome
- When infant's condition has been stable for 3-4 days, all anticonvulsants are weaned except phenobarbitone
- If seizures have resolved, neurological findings and EEG normal then anticonvulsants should be stopped at 14 days of life
- If this is not the case, anticonvulsants are continued for 1-3 months, then if neurological findings are normal with no recurrent seizure and nonepileptiform EEG, phenobarbital is tapered over 4 weeks
- If result of neurological examination is not normal and EEG was done, which shows no electrographic seizure activity then phenobarbital is tapered over 4 weeks, even if, infant has abnormal neurological signs.

Imaging

- CT scan is most useful: 4-6 weeks after asphyxia
  - ❖ Acute: Diffuse cerebral hypodensity with loss of gray white differentiation
  - ❖ Chronic: Changes in basal ganglion and thalamus.
- Cranial ultrasound
  - ❖ Acute: Periventricular leukomalacia
  - ❖ On follow-up: Evolution of echolucencies, cyst, ventricular dilatation secondary to tissue loss.

- MRI: Very sensitive for demonstration of all HIE regions subsequent to neonatal period.

Follow-up

- Preterm infants manifest CP later as corrected gestational age completes around 3 months
- Neurological assessment if normal at 4 months, it indicates almost normal latter developmental outcome
- Neuromotor assessment is done by: Neurological examination including milestones.

CRANIAL ULTRASOUND

Routine cranial ultrasound studies should be performed in:

- All infants < 32 weeks
- Infants born > 32 weeks with
  - Perinatal asphyxia
  - Abnormal neurological signs
  - Hypotonia, seizures
  - Full fontanelle
  - Apnea.

CHAPTER 24

KALA-AZAR

HISTORY

CHIEF COMPLAINTS

- Fever and weakness
- Heaviness in the left upper abdomen.

HISTORY OF PRESENT ILLNESS

History of Disease

Fever

- Onset: Sudden, insidious
- Associated with chills and rigour
- Associted with sweating
- Associated with malaise or apathy
- Accompanied by loss of appetite
- Documented or not
- Intermittent, remittent, continuous.

Abdominal Pain

- Duration of pain
- Localised to left side of abdomen
- Nature of pain: Dragging (due to splenomegaly)
- Radiation or migration of pain
- Progression
- Aggravating and relieving factors
- Pain on severity scale: Considering 0 for no pain and 10 for maximum pain.

Associated Complaints

- Vomiting, change in bowel habits, painful micturition (TRO other abdominal conditions)
- Jaundice
- Multiple swellings over body (lymphadenopathy)
- Paleness of body (anemia)
- Skin- Dry, thin and scaly and loss of hairs
- Black pigmentation on hands, feet, abdomen and face
- Weight loss
- Difficulty in food intake due to oral lesions.

History of Complications

- Diarrhea or dysentery; rarely jaundice in late stage (GIT system)
- Dry cough, chest pain or bronchopneumonia due to superadded infection (Respiratory system)
- Hemoptysis (To look for pulmonary tuberculosis)
- Palpitation (CVS involvement)

- Bleeding gum or epistaxis (hemorrhagic manifestations)
- Cancrum oris and diffuse black pigmentation of the whole body
- Lymph node swelling (very rare in India).

History of Differential Diagnosis

- Jaundice, hematemesis or malena (cirrhosis of liver and portal hypertension)
- Repeated blood transfusions, progressive paleness (thalassemia)
- Tuberculosis (kala-azar may be complicated by tuberculosis)
- Any swelling in neck, axilla or groin (lymphoma)
- Exposure to toxins like Copper, Arsenic, Vinyl chloride (portal hypertension).

PAST HISTORY

- Past history of typhoid fever, tuberculosis, Jaundice (It gives clue to present diagnosis).
- Whether patient was on any drugs or not.
- History of Umbilical sepsis, Umbilical catheterization, Blood transfusion, Dehydration, Neonatal sepsis (Extrahepatic portal hypertension).

GENERAL PHYSICAL EXAMINATION

- Vitals
- Anthropometry
- Appearance: Look for emaciation and alopecia
- Tongue: Coated or moist
- Look for mucosal lesions in mouth and nose which appear as nodules or ulcers and can lead to perforation of nasal septum (rare in India)
- Dry rough pigmented skin
- Pallor (cirrhosis/thalassemia)
- Clubbing/cyanosis/edema feet
- Lymphadenopathy (lymphoma/leukemia/ infectious mononucleosis)
- Jaundice (cirrhosis/thalassemia)
- Hemorrhagic manifestation: Examination of gum and nose is necessary (for gum bleeding and epistaxis)
- Protuberant abdomen, thin legs with edema feet
- Leg ulcers (congenital hemolytic anemia)
- Sternal tenderness (acute leukemia)
- Signs of liver cell failure:
  - Fetor hepaticus
  - Parotid enlargement
  - Spider nevi.
- Signs of portal hypertension:
  - Ascites
  - Splenomegaly
  - Dilated veins over abdomen
  - Caput medusae
  - Esophageal varices.
- Signs of vitamin A deficiency
  - Conjunctival/corneal xerosis
  - Bitot's spots.
- Signs of vitamin B deficiency
  - Angular stomatitis
  - Cheilosis.
- Signs of vitamin D deficiency—rickets
- Signs of vitamin E deficiency—petechiae, purpura.

SYSTEMIC EXAMINATION

ABDOMINAL EXAMINATION

Done with emphasis on description of following points (For detailed examination see chapter on gastrointestinal system).

Description of Splenomegaly

- Enlarged ….. cm below the left costal margin along its long axis and has crossed the umbilicus towards the right iliac fossa
- Nontender (tenderness is seen in splenic infarction, especially in a very big spleen)
- Notch in the anterior border
- Consistency: Firm
- Moves freely with respiration
- Surface: Smooth
- Margin: Sharp
- Fingers cannot be insinuated between the spleen and the left costal arch
- Neither bimanually palpable nor ballottable
- No colonic resonance over the mass
- No splenic rub (present in case of splenic infarction)
- Auscultate for any bruit.

Description of Hepatomegaly

- Enlarged …. cm below the right costal margin at right mid clavicular line
- Upper border of liver dullness is at right 5th ICS at right mid clavicular line
- Moving with respiration
- Firm in feel
- Nontender
- Smooth surface
- Margin is sharp and regular
- Left lobe is not palpable
- No pulsation/rub/bruit.

RESPIRATORY SYSTEM

- Crepitations due to secondary infection.

CARDIOVASCULAR SYSTEM

- Tachycardia, murmur due to anemia.

GI TRACT

- Hepatosplenomegaly, jaundice (at last stage).

SKIN

- Increased black pigmentation (so the name kala-azar) or rarely cancrum oris (ulcerative lesion around mouth).

RETICULOENDOTHELIAL SYSTEM

- Sternal tenderness (due to severe anemia) and palpable lymph nodes (very rare in India, found in African form).

DIAGNOSIS

Splenomegaly with mild (to moderate) hepatomegaly and fever, probably due to kala-azar.

DIFFERENTIAL DIAGNOSIS

KALA-AZAR

- ❖ Patient comes from endemic zone
- ❖ Appetite is preserved inspite of fever and loss of weight
- ❖ Splenomegaly: Massive, firm, nontender
- ❖ Hepatomegaly: Moderate enlargement, firm, nontender
- ❖ Alopecia, pigmentation.

MALARIA

- ❖ History of exposure in Malaria endemic zone
- ❖ High rise of temperature associated with chills and rigor. Fever generally comes on alternate days periodically
- ❖ Splenomegaly-moderate to massive, firm and nontender

- Malaise, headache, myalgia, nausea, vomiting
- Characteristic parasites in RBCs identified in thick and thin blood smears.

TUBERCULOSIS

- Gradual onset with vague ill health, high fever with sweats and loss of weight
- Cough, breathlessness and anorexia
- Tachycardia, paucity of signs in chest
- Mild to moderate hepatosplenomegaly.

TROPICAL SPLENOMEGALY SYNDROME

- Patient comes from hyperendemic area
- More common in females
- Splenomegaly: Massive enlargement
- Hepatomegaly: Mild to moderate enlargement
- Signs of portal hypertension may be present without evidence of cirrhosis of liver.

EXTRA-HEPATIC PORTAL HYPERTENSION

- Recurrent attacks of hemetemesis
- Anemia
- Splenomegaly
- Absence of signs of liver cell failure
- Ascites may develop later.

INTRA-HEPATIC PORTAL HYPERTENSION

- Signs of liver failure
- Ascites
- Firm liver
- Signs of portal hypertension.

BUDD-CHIARI SYNDROME

- Sudden development of ascites
- Sudden enlargement of liver and spleen
- Liver is soft and tender.

INVESTIGATIONS

Kala-Azar

See Figure 24.1.

- Direct evidence of leishmaniasis: The gold standard is detection of parasite from peripheral

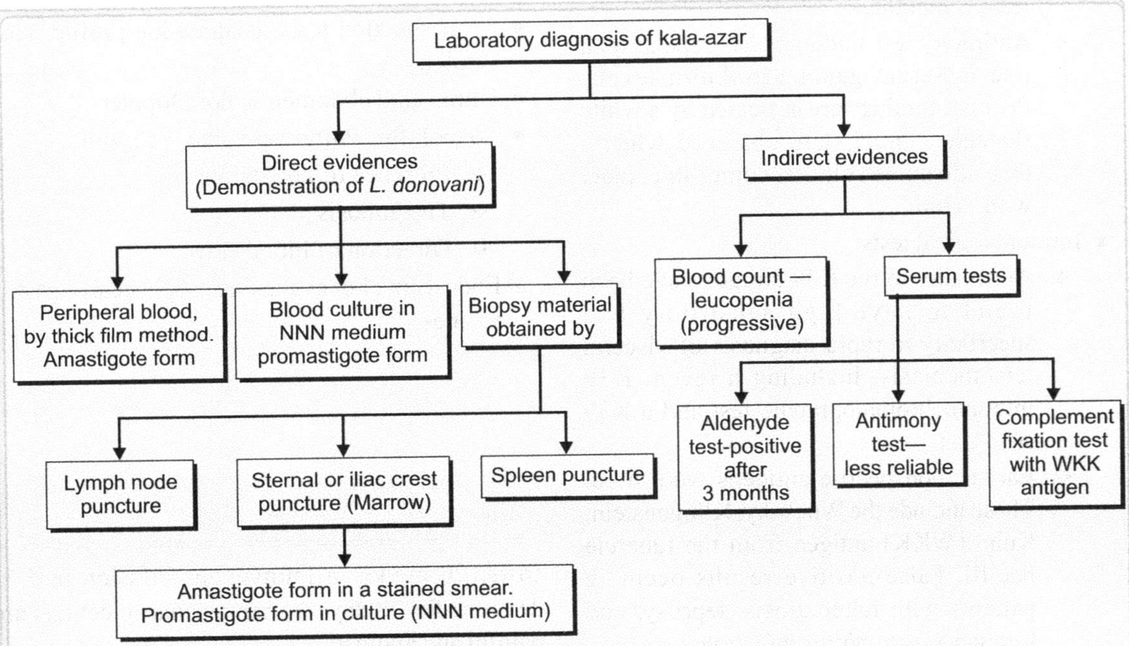

Fig. 24.1: Laboratory diagnosis of kala-azar

blood, bone marrow, or splenic aspirates. The smears are stained in Leishman, Giemsa, or Wright stains and examined under oil immersion microscope.

- ❖ Peripheral blood smear: Amastigotes are revealed inside the circulating monocytes and neutrophils.
- ❖ Culture: Obtaining a culture is time consuming, and findings take approximately a month. Cultures are made using a Novy-McNeal-Nicolle medium.

- Indirect evidence of infection
  - ❖ Detection of hypergammaglobinemia
  - ❖ The aldehyde test and the antimony test were the initial tests used to diagnose kala-azar.
  - ❖ Aldehyde test results reveal increased gamma globulin levels. Take approximately 1 mL of blood in a small glass tube and add 1-2 drops of 40% formalin. The formation of milky white like opacity and jellification indicates a positive result. Aldehyde test findings are not positive unless the disease has been present for at least 3 months.
  - ❖ Antimony test findings also depend on a rise in serum gamma globulin levels. Positive findings are indicated by a white flocculent precipitate observed when a urea stibamine solution comes in contact with serum.
- Immunological tests:
  - ❖ Antibodies to the K39 antigen have been found to have high sensitivity and specificity in rapid diagnosis of visceral leishmaniasis, including a recent K39 immunochromatographic test and a K39 strip test.
  - ❖ Earlier, nonspecific antigens were used. These include the Witebsky, Klingenstein, Kuhn (WKK) antigen from the tubercle bacilli. False-positive results occur in patients with tuberculosis, leprosy, and tropical *Eosinophilia infection.*
- Skin test:
  - ❖ Leishmanin skin test (Montenegro test) is a delayed hypersensitivity reaction. It is performed by intradermally injecting 0.1 mL of killed promastigote antigen. The test results are available after 72 hours. The leishmanin skin test results are negative during active visceral leishmaniasis and usually become positive only after successful therapy. The test results are also positive in patients with dermal leishmaniasis. This test is useful only for epidemiological purposes, indicating prior exposure to infection.
- Supportive tests: Hematological parameters include the following:
  - ❖ Normochromic normocytic anemia
  - ❖ Leukopenia, neutropenia
  - ❖ Thrombocytopenia
  - ❖ Elevated gamma globulin levels
  - ❖ Reversal of the albuminglobulin ratio.

Tests to Rule out Portal Hypertension

- Liver function tests, coagulation profile, viral serology.
- Ultrasound abdomen/ color Doppler
- To look for: Portal vein size > 15 mm
  - ❖ Presence of collaterals
  - ❖ Thrombosis
  - ❖ Direction of blood flow.
- Endoscopy: For evaluating esophageal or gastric varices.

TREATMENT

Sodium Antimony Gluconate: Drug of Choice

Dose: 20 mg/kg in intravenous infusion in 5 % dextrose for 28 days. Intramuscular injections are painful and avoided.

An initial clinical response to therapy usually occurs in the 1st week of therapy, but complete clinical healing (regression of splenomegaly and normalization of cytopenias for VL) is usually not evident for weeks to a few months after completion of therapy. Now, lower initial cure rates have been noted recently in regions where clinical resistance to antimony therapy is common, such as India. It also shows very low cure rate in children < 5 yr of age.

Side effects: Vomiting, arthralgia, myalgia, elevated serum transaminase, abdominal discomfort and mild hematologic changes (slightly decreased leukocyte count, hemoglobin level, and platelet count).

For Resistant Cases

Amphotericin B

- Amphotericin B desoxycholate and the amphotericin lipid formulations are very useful in the treatment of VL or ML, and have replaced antimony as 1st line therapy.
- Amphotericin B desoxycholate at doses of 0.5-1.0 mg/kg every day or every other day for 14-20 doses achieved a cure rate for VL of close to 100%, but the renal toxicity commonly associated with amphotericin B was common.
- The lipid formulations of amphotericin B is better for treatment of leishmaniasis because the drugs are concentrated in the reticuloendothelial system and are less nephrotoxic.
- Liposomal amphotericin B (3 mg/kg on days 1-5, and again on day 10) has been shown to be highly effective, with a 90-100% cure rate for VL in immunocompetent children, some of whom were refractory to antimony therapy.

Miltefosine

Miltefosine, has been recently developed as the 1st oral treatment for VL and has a cure rate of 95% in Indian patients with VL when administered orally at 2.5 mg/kg/day for 28 days. Gastrointestinal adverse effects are frequent.

Recombinant Human Interferon

Used in seriously ill patients or in treatment failures). Recombinant human interferon has been successfully used as an adjunct to antimony therapy in the treatment of refractory cases of leishmaniasis. It is not effective alone and has the frequent side effects of fever and flu-like symptoms.

Adjunctive splenectomy in some drug resistant kala-azar.

DISCUSSION

ACUTE KALA-AZAR

- Early kala-azar of 2-6 weeks duration
- Aldehyde test is negative in acute kala-azar
- Others: Leukopenia, positive complement fixation test
- Demonstration of parasite in blood smear, blood culture and bone marrow aspiration (at this stage spleen is not sufficiently enlarged to be punctured).

CAUSES OF ANEMIA IN KALA-AZAR

- Autoimmune hemolysis
- Hypersplenism
- Ineffective erythropoiesis
- GIT blood loss.

POST KALA-AZAR DERMAL LEISHMANIASIS

- Causative organism: *L. donovani*
- This generally follows treatment of visceral leishmaniasis in 10% cases.

- Hypopigmented macules and papules appear over face, extensor surfaces
- These patients act as reservoir of infection.

SIDE EFFECTS OF ANTIMONY PREPARATIONS

- Nausea, vomiting and diarrhea
- Anaphylaxis (after 6th or 7th injections)
- Hepatitis
- Tachycardia
- Cyanosis, rapid and irregular pulse, dyspnea and shock-known as 'Nitritoid crises'.

ASSESSMENT OF PROGRESS IN KALA-AZAR

- Alleviation of symptoms
- Measurement of splenic size
- Hemoglobin estimation
- Serum albumin level.

UNUSUAL CLINICAL PRESENTATION OF KALA-AZAR

- Pancytopenia without splenomegaly
- Generalized lymphadenopathy without hepatosplenomegaly
- Massive hepatic necrosis
- Retinal hemorrhages.

RESISTANT VISCERAL LEISHMANIASIS

Resistance can be caused by:

- Delayed diagnosis (prolonged illness)
- Interrupted and low dose treatment
- Immunological failure
- Emergence of resistant strains of parasites
- Leishmaniasis associated with AIDS.

PROGNOSIS IN KALA-AZAR

- Prognosis depends on nutritional and overall immune status of the host and on the precise species of infection.
- With early treatment, the cure rate is higher than 90%.
- If untreated, death occurs in 3-20 months.

CHAPTER 25

THALASSEMIA

HISTORY

CHIEF COMPLAINTS

- Abdominal pain
- Yellowish discoloration of eyes
- Progressive paleness.

HISTORY OF PRESENT ILLNESS

History of Disease

Abdominal Pain

- Type of pain
- Localised to left side of abdomen
- Nature of pain: Dragging (due to splenomegaly)
- Associated with mass in abdomen.

Progressive Paleness

- Child becomes increasingly pale with age
- Weakness, fatigue
- Giddiness
- Anorexia
- Palpitation, breathlessness
- No response to iron therapy.

Jaundice

- Mild jaundice which increases from time to time
- Yellowish tinge of sclera
- Acholuric urine, i.e. freshly passed urine is of normal color as no bilirubin is present in urine but turns dark yellow soon due to conversion of urobilinogen to urobilin by oxidation.
- High colored stool due to excess amount of stercobilinogen and stercobilin.

History of Complications

- Respiratory distress—exertional or not and whether associated with purulent expectoration
- Palpitation—exertional
- History of leg ulcers or bipedal swelling (edema)
- Growth impairment
- Delay in appearance of secondary sexual characteristics (delayed puberty)
- Cold intolerance (hypothyroidism).

History of Differential Diagnosis

- Fever (chronic malaria and kala-azar)
- Colicky abdominal pain (pigment stones)
- Resident of Bihar or Uttar Pradesh (kala-azar)
- Gum bleeding, epistaxis, hematemesis, malena and hemoptysis (malignancy).

Treatment History

- Blood transfusion
  - Frequency of blood transfusion
  - Amount of blood given per transfusion, i.e. number of bags each time
  - Any adverse reaction to blood transfusion
  - Calculate requirement of blood/kg/year
  - Has annual requirement of blood increased as compared to last year
  - Calculate rate of fall of hemoglobin.
- Blood transfusion alleviates his sufferings.
- Drug intake for the present disease (e.g. desferrioxamine, deferiprone or deferasirox)
- Surgery (pigment stone removal or splenectomy)
- Does child follows dietary iron reduction like avoiding iron rich food
- Consumption of tea with every meal
- Investigated for HBsAg, Hepatitis C and HIV
- Immunized with Hepatitis B or not
- Frequency of getting serum ferritin and what was his last serum ferritin.

FAMILY HISTORY

- Health of parents and other siblings
- Thalassemia or hemophilia in family
- Cause of death in family if any
- Tuberculosis in family.

GENERAL PHYSICAL EXAMINATION

Look for following physical signs relevant to abdomen:

- Icterus
- Pallor
- Thalassemic facies
  - Frontal bossing (prominent forehead due to marrow hyperplasia)
  - Depressed nasal bridge (due to hyperplasia of lesser wing of sphenoid)
  - Hypertelorism (wide separated eyes)
  - Apparent mongoloid slant of eyes
  - Malar prominence (due to marrow hyperplasia)-*Chipmunk facies*
  - Dental malocclusion with prominent incisors.
- Bleeding manifestations
- Lymphadenopathy
- Signs of liver cell failure
- Edema
- Enlarged jugular venous pressure
- Clubbing
- Sternal tenderness
- Nutritional status.

SYSTEMIC EXAMINATION

ABDOMINAL EXAMINATION

Abdomen is divided into 9 quadrants by 2 vertical and 2 horizontal lines.

Vertical lines: Two vertical lines are drawn passing through the tips of both the ninth costal cartilages above and the femoral arteries below.

Horizontal lines: First horizontal line passes through lowest points of both the costal margins while the second horizontal line passes through both the iliac tubercles.

9 quadrants of abdomen from above downwards are:

i. Right hypochondrium, epigastric and left hypochondrium;
ii. Right lumbar, umbilical and left lumbar; and
iii. Right iliac, suprapubic and left iliac.

Inspection

Skin and Subcutaneous Tissue

- Any visible swelling or erythema: Gross enlargement of the liver may be seen as a bulge in the right upper quadrant;

- Gross enlargement of the spleen may be seen as a bulge in the left upper quadrant
- If superficial veins are engorged—their location

Umbilicus-Everted (ascites): Displaced upwards or downwards by ascites or swelling.

Contour of abdomen: Movements—visible peristaltic or any pulsatile movement.

Palpation

- If superficial veins are engorged: Their direction of blood flow.

  Empty the vein of blood by placing two fingers side by side over the vein. Move one finger away while keeping the other fixed.

  Now, release the finger one by one to see the direction through which the blood fills the vein. If direction of flow of blood is towards the umbilicus, it suggests inferior vena cava obstruction while the direction of blood flow away from the umbilicus suggests portal hypertension.
- Superficial and deep palpation to look for any tenderness: Tenderness is pain elicited by the palpating hand, when pressure is applied to the abdomen wall. It is a sign that the peritoneum under the abdominal wall or the underlying organ is inflamed.
- Rebound tenderness is pain elicited when pressure applied to the abdomen wall by the palpating hand is suddenly released. It is a sign that the underlying peritoneum is inflamed.

Description of Splenomegaly

- Enlarged ….. cm below the left costal margin along its long axis and has crossed the umbilicus towards the right iliac fossa
- Nontender (tenderness is seen in splenic infarction, especially in a very big spleen)
- Notch in the anterior border
- Consistency: Firm
- Moves freely with respiration
- Surface: Smooth
- Margin: Sharp
- Fingers cannot be insinuated between the spleen and the left costal arch
- Neither bimanually palpable nor ballotable
- No colonic resonance over the mass
- No splenic rub (present in case of splenic infarction)
- Auscultate for any bruit.

Description of Hepatomegaly

- Enlarged …. cm below the right costal margin at right mid clavicular line
- Upper border of liver dullness is at right 5th ICS at right mid clavicular line
- Moving with respiration
- Firm in feel
- Nontender
- Smooth surface
- Margin is sharp and regular
- Left lobe is not palpable
- No pulsation/rub/bruit.

Percussion

- During abdomen percussion, always proceed from a tympanitic or resonant site towards a dull site. The middle finger should be positioned so that it receives the strike parallel to the anticipated border and not perpendicular to it.
- To delineate the liver borders, start percussing along the midclavicular line at the 4th intercostal space. The percussion note will change from resonant to dull at the 5th intercostal space, where the upper border of the liver normally lies. This dullness will continue till the lower border of liver which is just below the costal margin in a normal subject.

Puddle Sign

If the fluid in the peritoneal cavity is minimal, make patient prone so that he bears weight over his knees and elbows and the abdomen is off the couch. When the patient assumes this posture, the fluid gravitates down around the centre and percussion over the umbilicus will give a dull note.

Fluid Thrill

Fluid thrill is demonstrable only if a large volume of ascitic fluid is present.

1. Lay the subject supine and place one hand flat against his flank on one side.
2. Ask an assistant to place the ulnar aspect of his hand firmly in the midline of the abdomen.
3. Now, tap the opposite flank of the abdomen with your other hand. If ascitic fluid is present, the impulse generated by the tap will be transmitted to your hand on the flank. The hand on the abdomen is to prevent transmission of the impulse through the subcutaneous fat of the abdominal wall.

Shifting Dullness

1. Expose the abdomen and ask the child to lie supine. Keep the plexor finger perpendicular to the midline at a point between the xiphisternum and umbilicus. Percussing here, normally elicits a resonant note.
2. Percuss downwards from this point towards the umbilicus up to suprapubic region. The note should remain resonant. A dullness suggests an underlying full urinary bladder. Ask the child to void so that the bladder becomes empty.
3. After the percussion note at the umbilicus is resonant, keep the plexor finger at the umbilicus in the direction of the midline.
4. Start percussing from the umbilicus and go laterally towards the right or the left flank.
5. If the note remains resonant throughout up to the flanks, this indicates absence of significant fluid in the peritoneal cavity. A dull note in the dependent flanks suggests presence of fluid because of gravitation.
6. If the flanks are dull, turn the patient towards the opposite side without removing your plexor finger. Wait for some time to let the fluid shift to the other flank because of gravity. Percuss again over the same area. A resonant note now confirms that the fluid has shifted to the dependent area.

Auscultation

Auscultation is generally done over the abdomen to hear the bowel sounds. They are exaggerated in intestinal obstruction. The abdomen will be silent in patients of ileus or peritonitis.

A renal bruit may be heard in patients with renal artery stenosis like hypertension or arteritis.

CARDIOVASCULAR SYSTEM

- Effect of anemia on CVS with special reference to hemic murmur
- Look for features of heart failure.

RESPIRATORY SYSTEM

- Occasional rhonchi and crepitations due to respiratory tract infection.

NERVOUS SYSTEM

- Paraplegia (rarely) due to extramedullary hematopoiesis in the paravertebral region in thorax.

RETICULOENDOTHELIAL SYSTEM

- Anemia
- Tonsils may be enlarged
- No lymphadenopathy
- No bleeding manifestations in skin
- Hepatosplenomegaly

- Rarely, sternal tenderness may be present (due to severe anemia).

DIAGNOSIS

Moderate anemia with splenohepatomegaly probably from thalassemia major.

DIFFERENTIAL DIAGNOSIS

THALASSAEMIA

- Patient is usually child or young adult with positive family history
- History of recurrent blood transfusions
- Thalassemic facies (Frontal bossing, Depressed nasal bridge, Hypertelorism, mongoloid slant of eyes, Malar prominence)
- Stunted growth, massive splenomegaly with moderate hepatomegaly
- Severe anaemia, mild jaundice, leg ulcers over malleoli of foot.

MALARIA

- Patient from endemic zone
- High rise of temperature associated with chills and rigour.
- Fever generally comes on alternate days periodically
- Splenomegaly—moderate to massive, firm and nontender.

KALA-AZAR

- Patient comes from endemic zone
- Appetite is preserved inspite of fever and loss of weight
- Splenomegaly—massive, firm, nontender
- Hepatomegaly—moderate enlargement, firm, nontender
- Alopecia, pigmentation.

LYMPHOMA

- Progressive painless lymphadenopathy
- Fever, loss of weight, weakness, anaemia
- Splenomegaly—moderate enlargement, nontender
- Hepatomegaly—moderate enlargement.

TROPICAL SPLENOMEGALY SYNDROME

- Patient comes from hyperendemic area
- More common in females
- Splenomegaly—massive enlargement
- Hepatomegaly—mild to moderate enlargement
- Signs of portal hypertension may be present without evidence of cirrhosis of liver.

TUBERCULOSIS

- Gradual onset with vague ill health, high fever with sweats and loss of weight
- Cough, breathlessness and anorexia
- Tachycardia, paucity of signs in chest
- Mild to moderate hepatosplenomegaly.

INVESTIGATIONS

- Peripheral blood smear
  - Anisocytosis (variation in size), poikilocytosis (variation in shape), microcytic hypochromic anemia, target cells, tear-drop cells, cigar-shaped cells, basophilic stippling.
  - Reticulocytosis.
- Hemogram with indices
  - Hemoglobin—Low
  - Total leucocyte count—Mildly increased
  - Platelet count—Normal
  - MCV and MCH—Decreased
  - MCHC—Normal.
- Hemoglobin electrophoresis is diagnostic: shows presence of HbF (>2% of total

hemoglobin) and variable amount of HbA_2 and HbA (HbA_2 is increased more in thalassemia minor than in major and more than 3.5% is suggestive of thalassemic carrier).

- DNA mutation and Gene mapping: This is done to confirm the diagnosis and determine presence of coinheritant alpha globin gene defects.

Supportive Investigations

- Alkaline denaturation test—HbF is resistant to alkaline denaturation (i.e. the test is positive)
- Osmotic fragility decreased: Increased resistance of red cells to osmotic lysis (osmotic fragility is increased in hereditary spherocytosis).
- Iron studies:
  - Serum iron increased
  - Serum ferritin increased
  - Transferrin saturation—increased.
- Liver function tests:
  - Increased indirect bilirubin.
  - Increased AST (SGOT)—due to hemolysis.
  - Increased ALT (SGPT).
- Bone marrow: Hypercellular with erythroid hyperplasia with increased erythroblasts and sideroblasts.
- Cr_{51} labelled red cell survival studies: Lifespan of RBC's decreased (6.5-19 days), normal life span is 25-35 days.
- Radiology
  - X-ray of skull—*Hair on end appearance* (separation of two tables of skull with perpendicular trabeculae in between)
  - X-ray of small bones of hands—*Mosaic -patterns* (widening of medullary space with thinning of cortex and criss-cross trabeculae in between).

Antenatal Diagnosis

DNA analysis of chorionic villus in early pregnancy (10 weeks) and also by amniocentesis (16 weeks) should be done. This is appropriate, if both the parents are known to be carriers, i.e. β- thalassemia minor. Genetic counseling is a must.

Carrier Detection

- Microcytic hypochromic anemia
- Increased HbA_2
- *NESTROF test (Naked Eye Single Tube Red Cell Osmotic Fragility Test):*

Principle

This test is based on the principle that microcytic red blood cells are resistant to lysis, when exposed to hypotonic solutions.

Method

4 drops of blood taken in EDTA vial is added to 5 ml of 0.36% buffered saline in test tube. Tube is shaken and left at room temperature for 30 min. Tube is shaken again and immediately held in front of piece of paper with text.

Interpretation

If the words on the paper are clearly visible through the tube, the test is negative; whereas if the words are not clearly visible the test is positive (thalassemia trait) due to turbidity of the solution. The test is positive in both beta and in thalassemic carriers, and iron deficiency anemia. False positive results are obtained in patients with iron deficiency and therefore positive NESTROF needs further investigation to define diagnosis.

TREATMENT

Transfusion Therapy

a. Hypertransfusion—Hb level is kept > 10 gm/dl
b. Supertransfusion—Hb level is kept > 12 gm/dl.

Chelation Therapy

Desferrioxamine

- Dose: 25-50 mg/kg/day, subcutaneous continuous infusion via portable pump over 10-12 hours (overnight).
- Side effects: Pruitus, local swelling, sore arm.

Deferiprone

- Oral iron chelating agent
- Dose: 75- 100 mg/kg/day in 2-3 divided doses
- Side effects: Arthropathy, Agranulocytosis.

Splenectomy

Patients with thalassemia intermedia invariably develop splenomegaly due to extramedullary hematopoesis and reticuloendothelial hyperplasia. Inadequately transfused thalassemia major patients may also present with splenomegaly. Sometimes it may evolve into hypersplenism. It results in increased blood requirement, increased iron load, leucopenia and thrombocytopenia.

Indications

- Annual requirement of blood transfusion increased 1.5 times or more of previous year value.
- When transfusion requirement >250 ml/kg/year
- Presence of leucopenia or thrombocytopenia, i.e. hypersplenism.
- Symptoms of splenic enlargement and danger of rupture.

Surgical Approaches

- Total splenectomy
- Partial splenectomy.

Splenectomy should preferably be postponed till 5th year of age. Patient should be immunized against Pneumococcal, Meningococcal A and C and Hemophilus infuenzae (Hib) at least 4 weeks prior to operation.

Postsplenectomy

- Prolonged Penicillin prophylaxis Injection. Benzathaine Penicillin 6-12 lakhs every 3 weeks till 5 years of age or 2 years postoperative whichever is later.
- Patient should be given Aspirin 50-100 mg/day if platelet count exceeds 8,00,000/mm^3.
- Postsplenectomy infections should be dealt with broad spectrum antibiotics.
- Genetic manipulation is done by Azacytidine, Myelaran, Hydroxyurea which increases the production of HbF (increased HbF in thalassemia is associated with less severe clinical course).
- Allogenic bone marrow transplantation as and when necessary.
- Folic acid and Antibiotic supplementation as and when necessary.

DISCUSSION

DEFINITION

Heterogeneous group of genetic disorders in which the production of normal Hb is partly or completely suppressed because of defective synthesis of one or more of globin chains.

Two Types

a. α (reduction or absence of α-chain synthesis), and
b. β (reduction or absence of β-chain synthesis)—commonest.

α-Thalassemia (Chromosome 16)- 4 α Globin Genes

1. Silent carrier : Deletion of one α gene
2. α-thalassemia trait: Deletion of 2 α genes
3. Hb constant spring: Abnormal α chain variant
4. HbH disease: Deletion of 3 α genes
5. Hydrops fetalis: Deletion of all 4 α genes.

β-Thalassemia (Gene on Chromosome 11) - 2 β Globin Chains

1. β^0 Thalassemia: no detectable β chain synthesis.
2. β + Thalassemia: Reduced β chain synthesis.
3. δβ Thalassemia: Both the α and β chains are deleted.
4. E β-Thalassemia: Hb E(lysine → glutamic acid at 26) and β chain genes deletion.
5. Hb lepore: fusion of globin leads to unequal crossover of α and β genes.

Clinical Classification

1. Silent carrier (α/ β) – Hematologically normal.
2. Thalassemia trait (α/ β) – Mild anemia, microcytic hypochromic cells.
3. HbH disease (α) – Moderate to severe hemolytic anemia, Icterus, Splenomegaly.
4. Hydrops fetalis (α) – Severe anemia, Death in-utero.
5. Thalassemia major (β) – Transfusion dependent.

CLINICAL PRESENTATION OF THALASSEMIA

- Normal at birth and manifest during second 6 months of life
- Usually presents with persistent and progressive pallor
- Poor appetite, weakness, letharginess
- Failure to thrive
- Splenohepatomegaly
- Jaundice
- Facio skeletal changes
- Osteoporosis and pathological fractures
- Skin changes
- Leg ulcer
- Growth retardation
- Delayed puberty
- Endocrine abnormalities
- Infections
- Thromboembolic complications
- Spinal cord compression.

RED CELL DISTRIBUTION WIDTH

- RDW is coefficient of variation of red cell volume distribution
- It is objective documentation of subjective anisocytosis
- Normal range 11.5-14.5%.

	MCV decreased	*MCV normal*	*MCV high*
RDW Normal	Thalassemic Trait	Normal	Aplastic Anemia
RDW High	Iron Deficiency anemia	Chronic Liver Disease, Myelofibrosis	Megaloblastic anemia

INCREASED HBF IN THALASSEMIA MAJOR

Due to reduction of β-chain production, excess of α-chain synthesis occurs which forms inclusions within the RBC precursors in bone marrow. This leads to abnormality in membrane permeability and marked shortening of the life span of circulating RBC. There is also a compensatory increase in a chains which combine with excess of a chain to form a stable tetramer of HbF (α_2 α_2). Patients with thalassemia major who have relatively high rate of α-chain synthesis (i.e. more HbF), have less severe clinical course.

CRISES IN HEMOLYTIC ANEMIAS

- *Hemolytic crises:* Sudden hepatosplenomegaly with rapidly developing anemia.
- *Aplastic crises:* Occurs in the presence of infection and/or folic acid deficiency and may be seen even in thalassemia major.
- *Vasoocclusive or infarction crises:* Painful crises and appear with explosive suddenness. They attack various parts of the body like abdomen, chest, joints, etc.
- *Sequestration crises:* Causes RBC sequestration

In hemolytic crises, reticulocyte count increases, but in other crises reticulocyte count does not increase from the basal level.

RATE OF FALL OF HEMOGLOBIN IN THALASSEMIA

- Rate of fall of hemoglobin should not exceed 1 g/dl/week for splenectomised patients and 1.5 g/dl/week for non-splectomised patients.
- If hemoglobin falls at a greater rate, rule out:
  - Hypersplenism
  - Alloimmunization to RBC
  - RBC transfused shorter life span
  - Bleeding from gut
  - Increased RBC destruction
  - Folate deficiency.

PAIN ABDOMEN IN THALASSEMIA MAJOR

- Dragging pain due to splenomegaly
- Vasoocclusive crises
- Biliary colic (due to pigment stones from hemolysis)
- Splenic infarction.

EVALUATION PRIOR TO BLOOD TRANSFUSION

- ABO and Rh blood cell typing
- Screening of patients for Hepatitis B, Hepatitis C and HIV
- Initiation of Hepatitis B vaccination
- Family studies by HPLC for genetic counseling
- Mutation identification.

WHEN TO START TRANSFUSION

- As soon as diagnosis established (except in children >18 months of age)
- If age >18 months, a period of observation is required to rule out thalassemia intermedia
- If Hb drops <7gm% regular transfusion regimen.

IDEAL BLOOD FOR TRANSFUSION

- Group and type specific packed red cells (Hematocrit 65 to 75%)
- Triple saline washed red cells or filtered RBCs
- Compatible by indirect antiglobulin test (coombs cross matched)
- Not more than 4 to 5 days old.

BLOOD PRODUCTS FOR SPECIAL SITUATIONS

- Irradiated Red Cells: For transplant aspirants.
- Washed red cells:
  - IgA deficient patients and
  - Patients having severe allergic reactions.
- Frozen red cells/ deglyceralized red cells: patients with rare RBC antigen.
- Neocyte transfusion, i.e. transfusion of young low-density RBC; the neocytes increase the interval between the two transfusions and reduce iron overload. Now outdated, no longer recommended.

PREVENTION OF INFECTION IN THALASSEMICS

- Strict donor selection
- Hepatitis B vaccination
- Screening for HBsAg, HCV and HIV
- Malaria prevention
- Use leucodepletion for blood transfusion to prevent CMV infection
- Stop desferrioxamine and initiate cotrimoxozole or aminoglycosides in case *Yersinia* infection is suspected.

ADVERSE REACTIONS OF BLOOD TRANSFUSION

See Table 25.1.

Table 25.1: Adverse Reactions of Blood Transfusion

Reaction	Cause	Treatment
Nonhemolytic Febrile transfusion reaction	Leukocytes	Anti-pyretic
Allergic reaction	Plasma protein	Washed red cells
Acute hemolytic reaction	Faulty typing and Crossmatching	1. Stop blood transfusion. 2. Intravenous fluids with diuretic. 3. Maintain vitals
Autoimmune Hemolytic Reaction	Alloimmunisation	1. Steroid. 2. Immunosuppresives 3. Intravenous Immunoglobulin
Delayed hemolytic transfusion reaction	Alloantibody	-do-
Transfusion related acute lung injury	Anti-neutophil or Anti-HLA antibodies	1. Oxygen 2. Steroid. 3. Diuretic
Transfusion Transmitted infection	HIV, Hepatitis B, Hepatitis C, CMV, malaria	Treat as per cause

SOURCE OF IRON OVERLOAD IN THALASSEMIA

- Transfused red cells (thalassemia major)
- Increased absorption from gut (thalassemia intermedia).

IRON OVERLOAD REDUCTION STRATEGY

- Chelation therapy
- Splenectomy for hypersplenism to reduce frequency of transfusion
- Inhibiting GIT absorption by:
  - Keeping pretransfusion hemoglobin by >9
  - Avoiding Iron rich food
  - Consumption of tea with every meal.

MONITORING IRON OVERLOAD

- Serum ferritin:
  - Target recommendation <1000 μg/L
  - Trend of level more important than single value.
- Liver iron (best method).
  - Techniques: Liver biopsy/ MRI/SQUID
- T2 Cardiac MRI: Only method of assessing severity of cardiac iron overloading.

CHELATION THERAPY IN THALASSEMIA

When to start?

- Serum ferritin >1000 μg/L
- After 15-20 transfusions
- Liver iron concentration >3.2 mg/gram of dry weight of liver.

DESFERRIOXAMINE

- Standard Recommendation: Slow subcutaneous over 8-12 hours using infusion pump.
- Strength: 10%
- Site:
  - Anterior abdominal wall
  - Lateral side of thigh
  - Deltoid.

Continuous Intravenous administration of Desferrioxamine is recommended in special situations like significant cardiac disease.

SIDE EFFECTS OF DESFERRIOXAMINE

- Local skin reaction
- Severe sensivity reaction
- Infection: *Yersenia,* mucormycosis and *Klebsiella*

- Ototoxicity
- Ocular toxicity
- Growth retardation and skeletal changes.

DEFERIPRONE

- It chelates iron from parenchymal tissue, reticuloendothelial cell, transferrin
- Dose = 75 mg/kg/day in 2-4 divided doses orally
- Side effects:
  - Neutropenia
  - Agranulocytosis
  - Arthropathy
  - Gastrointestinal symptoms
  - Zinc deficiency.

COMBINATION THERAPY (DESFERRIOXAMINE + DEFERIPRONE)

- *Shuttle effect:* Low molecular weight deferiprone enters cell and transfers intracellular iron to desferrioxamine in plasma.
- Beneficial for patients with cardiomyopathy on desferrioxamine.
- No additional side effect.
- Regimens:
  - Deferiprone daily + Desferrioxamine – 2 days/week
  - Deferiprone daily + Desferrioxamine – 2 to 6 days/week
  - Deferiprone – 4 days/week + Desferrioxamine 2 days/week.

DEFERASIROX (ICL 670)

- New class of oral iron selective synthetic chelator
- Twice as effective as subcutaneous desferrioxamine
- Chelates iron from parenchymal tissue, reticuloendothelial cell, myocardial cell.
- Dose = 20-30 mg/kg once daily
- Administer on empty stomach at least 30 minutes before food
- To be dispersed in a glass of water or orange juice
- Not to be taken with milk or carbonated water
- Side effects: GI disturbances, skin rash, mild nonprogressive increase in serum creatinine.

DIET IN THALASSEMIA

- High calorie and high protein diet
- Avoid Iron rich foods e.g meat, liver, kidney, egg yolk, green vegetables, jaggery etc.
- Do not cook in iron utensils
- Do take bread, cereals, moong dal, soya beans to reduce Iron absorption
- Avoid vitamin C rich foods with meals
- Take strong tea/coffee with meals
- Take milk/milk products frequently.

ROLE OF VITAMIN C IN THALASSEMIA

Vitamin C is Usually used with Desferrioxamine

- Increases the availability of the chelatable iron to desferrioxamine.
- Generally started after, desferrioxamine therapy in progress for one month.
- Should be administered 30-60 minutes after starting infusion.
- Dose: 50 mg (not to exceed 2-3 mg/kg/day)
- Not to be given in patients with cardiomyopathy.

OBJECTIVE OF DIAGNOSING THALASSEMIA CARRIER

- To inform couple about risk of having thalassemic child.
- To prevent unnecessary long time treatment with iron therapy to improve hemoglobin.

MENTZER INDEX

This is used to differentiate Thalassemia from Iron deficiency anemia. In Thalassemia RBC count is preserved but MCV is low. The formula is to divide MCV by RBC count. If the value is more than 14 it is iron deficiency anemia.

LABORATORY FEATURES OF HEMOLYSIS

- High serum bilirubin (unconjugated > conjugated)
- High urinary urobilinogen
- Low plasma haptoglobin
- Increased methemalbumin in blood (Schumm test)
- High urinary hemosiderin
- Fragmented red cells in peripheral blood
- Reticulocytosis
- Hyperplastic bone marrow.

CAUSES OF MICROCYTIC–HYPOCHROMIC ANEMIA

- Iron deficiency anemia
- Thalassemia
- Sideroblastic anemia (often responses to pyridoxine)
- Lead poisoning.

FETAL HEMOGLOBIN LEVELS

During Gestation

8th week	HbF is predominant hemoglobin
24th week	HbF constitutes 80% of hemoglobin
At birth	HbF constitutes 70% of hemoglobin

HbA Levels

16-20 week	HbA can be detected prenatally
24th week	HbA 5-10% of hemoglobin
At term	HbA is 30% of hemoglobin

This means switch mechanism (from fetal to adult hemoglobin) begins at 16-20 weeks and is completed by 38th week of gestation.

COMPLICATIONS OF SPLENECTOMY

Sepsis

Risk Factors of Sepsis in Splenectomised Patient

- Age < 2 years
- First 4 years of splenectomy
- Iron overload
- Desferrioxamine therapy
- Associated G6PD deficiency.

Organisms responsible for sepsis: Streptococcus pneumoniae – 75%

Others – Haemophilus infuenzae, N. meningitis, etc.

Presentations: Sudden onset of fever with chills, vomiting, headache, progression to hypotensive shock and DIC.

Preventive Measures of Sepsis

- Immunoprophylaxis: Vaccination (at least 4 weeks before):
  - 23 valent pneumococcal vaccine
  - *Haemophilus influenzae,* meningococcal and typhoid vaccine.
- Chemoprophylaxis:
  - Benzathaine penicillin 6-12 lakhs every 3 weeks till 5 years of age or 2 years post-operative, whichever is later.
- Education: To parents and to physician.

Other complications of Splenectomy

- Bleeding
- Atelectasis
- Subphrenic abscess
- Postoperative thrombocytosis.

EVALUATION PRIOR TO BONE MARROW TRANSPLANTATION

- Serologic testing for HIV, Hepatitis A, Hepatitis B, Hepatitis C
- Liver function test
- Immunize against Hepatitis B and Hepatitis A
- CMV serology
- HLA typing of all siblings
- Extended red cell antigen typing that includes at least C, c, E, e and Kell.

NEWER MODALITIES IN MANAGEMENT OF THALASSEMIA

Bone Marrow Transplantation

- Donor – HLA – A, B, DR identical (Blood group – not essential).
- Donors marrow is harvested and transfused through peripheral vein in recipient.

Peripheral Bloodstem Cell Transplants

- Same as bone marrow transplantation except method of collection of stem cells.
- Granulocyte colony stimulating factor is administered 4-5 days prior which leads to high circulating stem cells which are collected by cell separator.
- No anesthesia and less painful procedure.
- Rapid engraftment but more chances of Graft versus host disease.

Cord Bloodstem Cell Transplants

- Good results with even 1-2 HLA antigen mismatch
- Number of stem cells are very less
- Engraftment takes longer time and some have found higher early morbidity
- Advantage: Incidence and severity of Graft versus host disease is less.

PROGNOSTIC FACTORS FOR BONE MARROW TRANSPLANTATION

Children who have following parameters have better outcome:

- Absence of hepatomegaly
- Absence of hepatic fibrosis
- Serum ferritin around 1000-2000 ng/ml.

ALTERNATIVE APPROACH TO BONE MARROW TRANSPLANTATION IN THALASSEMIA

Modulation of Fetal Hemoglobin

- Cytotoxic agents: Hydroxyurea/5-azacytidine/ Cytosine arabinoside
- Butyric acid derivatives
- Others: Erythropoetin.

MONITORING IN THALASSEMIA

Transfusion Day

- Date
- Amount of blood to be transfused
- Pretransfusion hemoglobin
- Liver/spleen enlargement
- Desferrioxamine/deferiprone dose
- Date of next transfusion.

Quaterly

- Weight
- Height
- Serum ferritin
- Calcium/phosphate/alkaline phosphatase
- Serum creatinine
- Liver function tests.

Yearly

- HBsAg
- Anti-HCV
- HIV serology

- Bone density
- Audiogram (if on desferrioxamine)
- Eye examination (if on desferrioxamine)
- Cardiac evaluation (ECHO).

COMPLICATIONS OF THALASSEMIA MAJOR

Endocrine Complications

- Growth impairment
- Delayed puberty
- Hypothyroidism
- Hypoparathyroidism
- Osteoporosis
- Diabetes mellitus.

Cardiac Complications

Iron induced myocardial damage results in cardiac failure, arrhythmias and sudden death in thalassemics. Average age of presenting cardiac symptoms in nonchelated thalassemic is 6-18 years.

Ankle Ulcers

It often starts with bruise just above the ankle. It can be prevented by:

- Avoiding injury over ankles
- Wearing toweling socks (turned down top) socks.
- Using wrist bands on ankles
- Raising foot end by 10 cm while sleeping
- Raising lower limbs above heart level at least 2 hours in a day while sitting.

EVALUATION IN THALASSEMIC CHILDREN

- 5 years onwards annually:
  - Glucose tolerance test
  - Thyroid function test
  - Serum calcium and phosphorus.
- 10 years onwards:
  - Height/ weight velocity
  - Cardiac work up
  - Bone studies.

MONITORING FOR BONE DISEASE

- Calcium, phosphate, alkaline phosphatase is poor indicator
- DEXA scan for bone density is ideal
- Urine calcium/creatinine ratio (> 0.2) and urine phosphate/creatinine ratio (> 0.6) are cheap and reliable screening test.

TREATMENT OF OSTEOPENIA IN THALASSEMIC CHILDREN

- Hormone replacement therapy: Females-estrogen; Males-hCG
- Calcitonin-inhibitor of osteoclasts
- Hydroxyurea, bisphosphonates and intravenous pamidronate
- Diet rich in calcium and vitamin D
- Moderate exercise.

PRENATAL DIAGNOSIS

- DNA based mutation studies
- Globin chain synthesis studies.

DNA Based Mutation Studies

For this fetal tissue is taken by chorionic villous biopsy (best method) or amniotic fluid or cord blood. Chorionic villous biopsy is performed at 11-14 wks of gestation and 10-20 gm of sample is taken under ultrasound guidance. Maternal tissue is cleaned and DNA is extracted. Sample is then tested for parental mutations. If not informative, do globin chain synthesis studies or HPLC using cord blood.

Gene Therapy

Lenti viral vector derived from human immuno-deficiency virus where a large fragment of human beta gene and its locus control region, has been introduced is in experimental stage.

PREVENTION OF THALASSEMIA IN INDIA

The birth of a thalassemic child places strain not only on affected child and family but on society at large. Therefore there is emphasis for shift from treatment to prevention of birth of such children in future. This can be achieved by:

- Population education: About the prevalence and the difficulties in management of this condition.
- Mass screening of high-risk communities for thalassemia minor: Screening young people amongst all high-risk communities before marriage is the right way to go. If screening is performed in childhood, it is often forgotten around the time they get married.
- Genetic counseling of those who test positive for thalassemia minor.
- Prenatal diagnosis: All at-risk couples need to be counseled about the prenatal diagnosis to confirm the thalassemic status of the fetus. If the fetus is not affected, the pregnancy should be continued. If the fetus is affected, the choice of terminating the pregnancy is offered.

Each and every person MUST get his/her thalassemic status tested to save his/her family and our society from the trauma of thalassemia.

CHAPTER 26

LYMPHOMA

HISTORY

CHIEF COMPLAINTS

- Fever
- Multiple swellings over the body.

HISTORY OF PRESENT COMPLAINT

History of Disease

Lymph Node Enlargement

- Position or anatomical region affected (situation and extent)
- Number and size
- Discrete or matted (margin)
- Tenderness
- Consistency—Soft, rubbery, firm or hard
- Mobility—Fixity to skin and surrounding structures (muscles, vessels, nerves or with any viscus)
- Rise of local temperature
- Skin changes (sinus or peau d'orange or any sign of inflammation).

Fever

- Onset: Sudden, Insidious
- Associated with chills and rigour
- Associcted with sweating
- Documented or not
- Intermittent, remittent, continuous.

Abdominal Pain

- Duration of pain
- Localised to left side of abdomen
- Nature of pain—Dragging (due to splenomegaly)
- Radiation or migration of pain
- Progression
- Aggravating and relieving factors
- Pain on severity scale—Considering 0 for no pain and 10 for maximum pain.

History of Complications

- Bleeding manifestations
- Breathlessness, cough
- Pruritis
- Facial swelling, dysphagia (signs of mediastinal compression).

GENERAL PHYSICAL EXAMINATION

- Anemia
- Any hemorrhagic manifestation (hemorrhage into skin, epistaxis, gum bleeding, hemarthrosis, hematuria)
- Details of lymph nodes examination as mentioned below
- Examination of the mouth (oral cavity) and skin thoroughly
- Sternal tenderness (absent in lymphoma)
- Ophthalmoscopic examination for any retinal hemorrhage, exudate, papilledema, Roth spots.

EXAMINATION OF SWELLING

Inspection

- Situation or anatomical region affected
- Shape
- Size and number
- Surface
- Color
- Edge
- Number
- Pulsation
- Impulse on coughing
- Skin over the swelling—any signs of inflammation.

Palpation

- Number
- Position
- Temperature
- Shape, size, surface
- Discrete or matted
- Fluctuation
- Consistency—Soft (abscess), rubbery (Hodgkins), firm or hard
- Mobility—Fixity to skin and surrounding structures.

Auscultation

- To exclude bruit.

Lymph Node Examination

Nodes are palpated symmetrically on both sides of the body from above downwards.

Lymph Nodes in Neck

Palpated from 'behind' with patient in sitting or standing with the head bending forward.

Upper circular group is palpated by both hands in following order:

- Submental
- Submandibular
- Preauricular
- Postauricular and
- Occipital.

Lower horizontal or Supraclavicular group of lymph nodes—They are divided into medial, intermediate and lateral groups.

Vertical chain in the middle of the neck—The glands in the (i) anterior triangle, and (ii) posterior triangle are palpated (the triangles are divided by the Sternomastoid muscle).

Axillary Lymph Nodes

The examiner sits in front of the patient (only subscapular group is palpated from behind).

- *Central group*—The patient's arm is abducted and the hand of the examiner is placed in the axilla with palm directed towards the chest. Now the arm is adducted and allowed to rest on the examiner's forearm. The other hand of the examiner is placed on the patient's opposite shoulder. The central group is palpated by sliding the fingers.

- *Apical group*—The same method is applied but fingers are pushed as high as possible.
- *Pectoral group*—These glands are situated under the anterior axillary fold. The nodes are palpated with the help of the thumb and fingers.
- *Brachial group*—Here the left hand is used for the left side and the right hand for the right side. This group is palpated against the upper part of the humerus with the examiner's palm directed laterally.
- *Subscapular group*—This group lies on the posterior axillary fold. It is a palpated from behind when the hand insinuates within the latissimus dorsi, keeping the patient's arm horizontally forward.

Epitrochlear Lymph Nodes

Keep elbow of patient slightly flexed, forearm supinated and wrist of patient fixed by the examiners opposite hand. The glands are palpated in the anterior-medial region of the lower part of arm (in between the groove of biceps and brachialis muscle) adjacent to the elbow.

Inguinal Lymph Nodes

Examined in supine position after extending the thighs.

Popliteal Group of Lymph Nodes

Examined in supine position with flexed legs. The popliteal fossa is felt with the fingertips of either hand, the fingers of both hands being buried into the popliteal fossa.

Mediastinal Group of Lymph Nodes

Their presence can be detected indirectly by percussion of the sternum.

Abdominal Lymph Nodes (Pre and Para-aortic, Retroperitoneal)

- This group will present as lump in the abdomen.

SYSTEMIC EXAMINATION

RESPIRATORY SYSTEM

- Pleural effusion (often bilateral), collapse of the lung due to mediastinal lymphadenopathy.

CARDIOVASCULAR SYSTEM

- Superior mediastinal syndrome, pericardial effusion.

NERVOUS SYSTEM

- Cranial nerves involvement, paraplegia.

GI TRACT

- Hepatosplenomegaly, jaundice, ascites, intestinal obstruction.

MUSCULOSKELETON SYSTEM

- Diffuse bone pain, swelling of bones.

SKIN

- Skin lesions, generalized pruritus, herpes zoster.

GENITOURINARY SYSTEM

- Hematuria, renal lump, hydronephrosis; Occlusion of renal vein may produce nephrotic syndrome.

DIAGNOSIS

Generalized lymphadenopathy most probably lymphoma, probably Hodgkin's disease:

DIFFERENTIAL DIAGNOSIS

LYMPHOMA

- Commonly cervical group is involved first then gradual painless lymphadenopathy
- Discrete, rubbery or firm, nontender lymphadenopathy
- Fever, night sweats, loss of weight.
- Hepatosplenomegaly.

ACUTE LYMPHATIC LEUKEMIA (ALL)

- Fever may be very high
- Discrete, nontender adenopathy.
- Moderate splenomegaly with hepatomegaly
- Short course of disease
- *Anemia*: Pallor, fatigue, tachycardia, dyspnea and occasional cardiovascular decompensation.
- *Leukopenia*: Low to marked temperature elevation with infections.
- *Thrombocytopenia*: Petechiae, mucosal bleeding and epistaxis.
- Presence of sternal tenderness, bone pains.

MILIARY TUBERCULOSIS

- High rise of temperature with drenching sweats, loss of weight, progressive anemia, cough.
- Matted, painless lymphadenopathy but may be painful, firm, without any rise of local temperature: rarely there may be sinus in the skin with formation of cold abscess underneath.
- Paucity of signs in the chest. Often few crepitations are heard late in the disease.
- Mild hepatomegaly with mild, tender splenomegaly.
- Choroidal tubercles seen in the retina by ophthalmoscopy.

INFECTIOUS MONONUCLEOSIS

- Cervical adenitis (posterior cervical group), may be generalized. Glands are slightly tender
- Fever, malaise, headache, sore throat
- Acute onset with a maculopapular rash (like drug rash)
- Splenomegaly.

CHRONIC LYMPHADENITIS

- Common in cervical and inguinal lymph nodes
- Primary focus is usually present
- Moderately enlarged, firm, mildly tender (rarely matted)
- There may be rise of temperature.

HIV

- History of receiving blood transfusion or presence of HIV in parents
- Thirty percent present with persistent generalized lymphadenopathy (PGL) or AIDS—related complex (ARC). Patient with ARC may have chronic diarrhea, weight loss and oral candidiasis.
- Rapid downhill course
- Biopsy of lymph nodes shows reactive hyperplasia.

INVESTIGATIONS

- Blood examination:
  - Anemia (normocytic normochromic)
  - Leukemoid reaction and eosinophilia in Hodgkin's disease
  - Lymphocytopenia
  - High ESR.
- Lymph node biopsy:
  - FNAC (fine needle aspiration cytology)—Often not informative

- Excision biopsy—**'Most important'** investigation. It gives the accurate diagnosis and helps in evaluation of prognosis.
- Chest X-ray: Mediastinal widening (Hodgkins disease), pleural effusion or involvement of lung.
- Ultrasonography: Abdomen to look for liver, spleen, free fluid, lump.
- CT Scan: Identifies both nodal and extranodal sites of involvement and can provide approach to monitoring response to therapy
- MRI: Particularly useful in identifying bone and CNS involvement, can reveal meningeal involvement when gadolinium is used.
- Gallium scans: Used for resolving difficulties in determining response to therapy, more accurate in evaluating supradiaphragmatic rather than infradiaphragmatic sites because of colon uptake of the gallium.
- Positron emission tomography (PET) scanning: Has same sensitivity and specificity as gallium scanning.
- Pleural aspiration, ascetic tap or lumbar puncture.
- Bone marrow examination: Helps in the diagnosis and staging of the disease (bone marrow involvement indicates stage IV disease).
- Biochemical: LDH, Liver function tests.
- Skeletal survey by X-ray: Usually osteosclerotic lesion is seen in HD—ivory vertebra', and osteolytic lesion in NHL variety.

TREATMENT

HODGKIN'S DISEASE

Regimes of Chemotherapy

- ABVD (Adriamycin, Bleomycin, Vinblastine and Decarbazine)
- MOPP (Nitrogen mustard, Vincristine, Prednisolone and Procarbazine)
- MVPP (Only Vinblastine replaces the vincristine of MOPP regimen).

Indication of Radiotherapy

- Stage I and II A with 3 or less areas of involvement
- Lesions causing serious pressure symptoms, e.g. superior vena cava syndrome.

Indication of Chemotherapy

- All patients with B-symptoms
- Stage II with > 3 areas of involvement, stage III and stage IV diseases.

NON-HODGKIN'S LYMPHOMA

Regimes of Chemotherapy

- CHOP (Cyclophosphamide, Hydroxyadriamycin, Vincristine and Prednisolone).
- BACOP (Bleomycin, Adriamycin, Cyclophosphamide, Vincristine and Prednisolone). These drugs are given on a 28-day cycle (one pulse) for a minimum of '6 pulses' and up to 9, if necessary.

Indications of Radiotherapy

- Superior vena cava syndrome (obstruction of blood flow through superior vena cava)
- Spinal cord compression due to paraspinal disease.

Cranial irradiation or prophylactic intrathecal chemotherapy is given in stage III or IV disease

- Bone marrow transplantation is a new modality of treatment in lymphoma.
- Monoclonal antibodies (Rituximab) are the latest addition against B-cell lymphoma.

- Patients with lymphoblastic lymphoma who remain relapse free for 30 months after diagnosis are considered as cured.

DISCUSSION

DEFINITIONS

Lymphoma: These are group of malignant disease of lymphoreticular origin.

Lymphadenopathy: Inflammatory or non-inflammatory enlargement of lymph nodes.

Generalized lymphadenopathy: Involvement of three or more noncontiguous lymph node areas.

Persistent generalized lymphadenopathy: Presence of enlarged lymph nodes (>1 cm) in two or more extrainguinal sites for more than 3 months.

Significant lymphadenopathy can be defined as:

- Axillary lymph node—1 cm in size
- Cervical lymph nodes—1 cm in size
- Inguinal lymph nodes—1.5 cm in size
- Palpable lymph nodes at multiple sites
- Lymph nodes which are red/tender/matted/ulcerated
- Enlarged lymph nodes associated with a focus of infection
- Enlarged lymph nodes associated with systemic signs and symptoms.

B-SYMPTOMS OF LYMPHOMA

- Fever above 38°C
- Night sweats and/or
- Unexplained loss of 10% or more of body weight in the previous 6 months.

B-symptoms Indicate bad Prognosis

Fever in Lymphoma

- Low grade fever unaccompanied by chills and rigor.
- Occasionally it is a swinging fever (with ups and downs)
- Classical 'Pel-Ebstein' fever (in HD) is not seen now. It is a cyclical fever where several days or weeks of fever alternate with afebrile period.

CAUSES OF PARAPLEGIA IN LYMPHOMA

Thoracic vertebrae is most commonly involved:

- Vertebral body involvement with collapse
- Invasion of the epidural space from retroperitoneal lymph nodes with cord compression
- Compression of the vascular supply of the spinal cord.

DESCRIPTION OF LYMPH NODE ENLARGEMENT IN LYMPHOMA

Hodgkin's Disease

- Cervical nodes are initially affected. Other nodes are involved in course of time.
- These are enlarged, nontender with rubbery feel, smooth surface, not fixed to skin or deeper structures, discrete, no sinus or no rise of temperature in the overlying skin, there is no softening or any suppuration.

Non-Hodgkin's Lymphoma

- Enlargement of lymph nodes may affect any area initially.
- There is more chance of involvement of epitrochlear nodes and Waldeyer's ring.
- These are enlarged, nontender (rarely tender) with firm or variegated feel, smooth or nodular surface, may fix to deeper structures, discrete,

without any sinus in the overlying skin, often the local skin temperature is raised and there is neither softening nor any suppuration.

REED-STERNBERG CELL

Features of R-S Cell (Looks Like Owl's Eye)

- Large cell with abundance of acidophilic cytoplasm
- Mirror image nuclei with vesicular pattern
- Chromatin is loosely woven
- Multiple nucleoli with perinuclear halo.

R-S Cells or Cells Simulating R-S Cells

- Hodgkin's disease
- Infectious mononucleosis
- Burkitt's lymphoma
- Mycosis fungoides.

SMALL ROUND CELL TUMOR

- Non-Hodgkin's lymphoma
- Rhabdomyosarcoma
- Neuroblastoma
- Medulloblastoma
- Reticuloblastoma
- Ewing' sarcoma.

TUMOR LYSIS

- Caused by rapid release of cellular contents from cell death.
- Usually occurs after chemotherapy, but can occur with steroid treatment alone.
- Uric acid release causes renal damage/failure
- Hyperphosphatemia causes hypocalcemia, then seizures.
- Hyperkalemia leads to arrhythmias, death.
- Treatment:Hydration, allopurinol, urine alkalization, treatment of hypocalcemia.

CYTOGENETICS

- Normal karyotype 46XY or 46XX
- Abnormal karyotype often found in malignant cells
- Prognostically important in leukemia – t (9; 22); t (4;11); t(12; 21); t(8; 14) in Burkitts lymphoma; t (11; 22) seen in Ewing's sarcoma
- 1p depletion in neuroblastoma associated with poor prognosis.

Table 26.1: Clinical differentiation between HD and NHL

	Hodgkin's disease	*Non-Hodgkin's lymphoma*
• Frequency	Less common (30%)	More common (70%)
• Age	Two peaks:Youngsters and elderly	Any age; more frequent with increasing age
• Constitutional symptoms (B-symptoms)	Early and prominent (only in 20% cases)	Late and non-prominent
• Anemia	Late	Early
• Lymph node involvement		
❖ Presentation	90% nodal and 10% extranodal	60% nodal and 40% extranodal
❖ Size	Smaller	Larger
❖ Rate of growth	Slow	Fast
❖ Consistency	Rubbery elastic	Variegated or firm
❖ Matting	Rare	Often early
❖ Local temperature	Normal	May be raised
❖ Tenderness	Absent	May be present
❖ Epitrochlear nodes involvement	Less common	Common
❖ Waldeyer's ring involvement	Less common	Common
❖ Mediastinal lymph node involvement	More common	Less common
• Splenomegaly	More common	Less common
• Gastrointestinal involvement	Uncommon	Common
• CNS involvement	Uncommon	Common

CHAPTER 27

LEUKEMIA

HISTORY

CHIEF COMPLAINTS

- Fever
- Recurrent infections
- Bleeding manifestations.

HISTORY OF PRESENT COMPLAINT

History of Disease

The history should be elicited keeping in mind following clinical points:

- Fever
- Pallor
- Bleeding manifestations
- Lump in the abdomen
- Swelling in the neck
- Convulsions.

Fever

- Onset: Sudden, Insidious
- Associated with chills and rigor
- Associated with sweating
- Documented or not
- Intermittent, remittent, continuous.

Progressive Paleness

- Patient becomes increasingly pale with time
- Weakness, fatigue
- Giddiness
- Anorexia
- Palpitation, breathlessness
- No response to iron therapy.

Abdominal Lump

- Duration of lump
- Localization
- Associated with pain or not
- Radiation or migration of pain
- Progression.

History of Complications

- Bleeding manifestations—Petechiae (< 2 mm), purpura (2-10 mm), ecchymosis (>10 mm) (thrombocytopenia), gum bleeding, epistaxis, hematemesis, malena and hemoptysis.
- Pallor (anemia), fever (infection)
- Signs of congestive cardiac failure:
  - Edema feet
  - Pain abdomen

- Difficulty in respiration
- Feeding difficulties
- Failure to thrive.

- Pruritis
- Facial swelling, dysphagia (signs of mediastinal compression).

GENERAL PHYSICAL EXAMINATION

- Vitals
- Anthropometry
- Pallor
- Clubbing/cyanosis/edema feet
- Lymphadenopathy (lymphoma/leukemia/ infectious mononucleosis)
- Jaundice
- Sternal tenderness (acute leukemia)
- Any hemorrhagic manifestation (hemorrhage into skin, epistaxis, gum bleeding, hemarthrosis, hematuria)
- Details of lymph nodes examination (if present) as mentioned in chapter on lymphoma
- Examination of the mouth (oral cavity) and skin thoroughly
- Ophthalmic examination for any retinal hemorrhage, exudate, papilledema.

SYSTEMIC EXAMINATION

ABDOMEN EXAMINATION

Inspection

- Contour of abdomen
- Skin and subcutaneous tissue
- Any visible lump in abdomen
- Umbilicus: Everted (ascites)
  - Displaced upwards or downwards by ascites or lump.
- Bone marrow aspiration/biopsy mark.

Palpation

- Superficial and deep palpation to look for any tenderness
- Fluid thrill
- Shifting dullness
- Description of abdominal lump
- Palpation of abdominal organs: Spleen and liver.

Description of Splenomegaly

- Enlarged ….. cm below the left costal margin along its long axis and has crossed the umbilicus towards the right iliac fossa
- Non-tender (tenderness is seen in splenic infarction, especially in a very big spleen)
- Presence of notch in the anterior border
- Consistency: Firm, soft
- Moves freely with respiration
- Surface: Smooth, nodular
- Margin: Sharp, rounded
- Fingers cannot be insinuated between the spleen and the left costal arch
- Neither bimanually palpable nor ballotable
- No colonic resonance over the mass
- No splenic rub (present in case of splenic infarction)
- Auscultate for any bruit.

Description of Hepatomegaly

- Enlarged …. cm below the right costal margin at right midclavicular line
- Upper border of liver dullness is at right 5th ICS at right midclavicular line
- Moving with respiration
- Nontender
- Surface: Smooth, granular, nodular
- Consistency: Soft, firm, hard
- Margins: Sharp, rounded
- Left lobe is not palpable
- No pulsation/rub/bruit

- Ascites (presence or absence of free fluid in abdomen should be noted).

CARDIOVASCULAR SYSTEM

- Effect of anemia on CVS with special reference to hemic murmur
- Look for features of heart failure.

RESPIRATORY SYSTEM

- Occasional rhonchi and crepitations due to respiratory tract infection.

NERVOUS SYSTEM

- Paraplegia (rarely) due to extramedullary hematopoiesis in the paravertebral region in thorax
- Fundus examination is must.

DIAGNOSIS

Mild/moderate/severe hepatomegaly; with/without splenomegaly (mild/moderate/severe); with/without signs of bleeding manifestations; with/without pallor;

Most probable etiology being acute lymphoblastic leukemia.

DIFFERENTIAL DIAGNOSIS

- Leukemoid reaction:
  - Bacterial infection, acute hemolysis, tuberculosis, sarcoidosis, histoplamosis or metastatic tumors
  - Increased WBC (up to 50 × 10^9/l) and peripheral immature granulocyte precursors are seen.
- Lymphocytosis:
  - Pertussis and other viral infections
  - Infants and small children often have physiological lymphocytosis.
- Infectious mononucleosis
- Aplastic anemia:
  - Pancytopenia and hypoplastic bone marrow.
- Idiopathic thrombocytopenic purpura (ITP):
  - Patients with ITP do not have anemia (with exception of children with severe bleeding) and have normal morphology of white blood cell differentiation.
- Bone marrow infiltration by a solid tumor (metastatic disorder):
  - Neuroblastoma (increased level of urine catecholamines)
  - Non-Hodgkin lymphoma (NHL with more than 25% of blasts in the bone marrow are defined as leukemia)
  - Rhabdomyosarcoma and retinoblastoma may have a similar infiltration of the bone marrow as leukemia, but they generally have clusters of malignant cells.
- Rheumatoid fever and rheumatoid arthritis can often be confused with leukemia (because bone pain is present in 25% of leukemia cases), but alteration of peripheral blood cell count and bone marrow abnormalities are not seen.

INVESTIGATIONS

Red Cells

- The level of hemoglobin is often moderate to low
- Low number of reticulocytes.

White Blood Cell Count

- Number of white blood cells can be normal, low or high
- In children with leucopenia, few or no atypical lymphoblasts are detected

- In children with a high WBC leukemic blast cells are often present
- In children with a high WBC (more than 100×10^9 white blood cells/L) the lymphoblasts are predominant (together with marked visceromegaly).

Platelets

- The platelet count is usually low: in 50% of children less than 50×10^9/L
- Spontaneous hemorrhage appears in children with less than 20-30 $\times 10^9$ platelets/L.

Serum Chemistry

- Hyperuricemia: Uric acid level is often high initially.
- Hyperkalemia (due to massive cell lysis)
- Hypokalemia (potassium level may be low in malnourished or due to renal tubular loss)
- Hypocalcemia (due to renal insufficiency or due to calcium binding to phosphate released by leukemic cells)
- Hypercalcemia (due to marked leukemic bone infiltration)
- Abnormal liver function tests like increased level of transaminases with/without hyperbilirubinemia (due to liver infiltration by leukemic cells or as a side effect of treatment)
- Serum immunoglobulin levels: In 20% of children with ALL low serum IgG and IgM levels.

Bone Marrow Analysis

- Bone marrow analysis serves to characterize the blast cells and to determine hyper or hypocellularity
- It can be used for morphological, immunological, biochemical, and cytogenetic analyses.
- To rule out aplastic anemia and myelodysplastic syndrome.

Cytochemical Reactions

See Table 27.1.

Table 27.1: Cytochemical Reactions

	Lymphoblasts	*Myeloblasts*
Peroxidase	–	+
Sudan black	–	+
Periodic acid-Schiff	++	±
Esterase	–	± (positive in Acute monocytic leukemia)
Terminal deoxynucleotidyl transferase	+ (negative in L3)	–

Cytogenetic Characterization

- In 85% of children with leukemia, an abnormal karyotype in the malignant clone is detectable.
- The analysis combines chromosome banding with fluorescence in situ hybridization (FISH) with spectral karyotyping and with comparative genomic hybridization.
- The cytogenetic abnormalities reflect the number of chromosomes (ploidy) and the structure of chromosomes (rearrangements).
- Translocation t(9;22) (BCR-ABL fusion protein) is present in 5% of children with ALL and is characteristic of a protein with tyrosine kinase activity with the ability to immortalize progenitors and is correlated with an unfavorable prognosis.

Cytometry

- Flow cytometry can measure the DNA and RNA content of individual cells.

  It provides:
  - The incidence of cells in different phases of the cell cycle
  - The determination of the DNA content of leukemic cells for prognosis (ploidy).
- The DNA index (DI) defines the cellular DNA content determined by flow cytometry (Table 27.2).

Table 27.2: DNA index

	DI (DNA Index)	
Normo-or pseudodiploid cells	1.0	Normal DNA content
Hyperdiploid	> 1.0	> 1.1:53 chromosomes/cell
Hypodiploid	< 1.0	

TREATMENT

- The treatment of ALL is subdivided into remission, induction, consolidation with CNS prophylaxis and maintenance phase.

Induction of Remission

- Remission means disappearance of all signs of leukemia in clinical examination and peripheral blood analysis; bone marrow analysis with less than 5% atypical cells and normal hematopoiesis established.
- Duration of induction treatment: 4-5 weeks.
- Regression of visceromegaly can be observed within the first 2 weeks.
- Rate of first remission in ALL: More than 90%.
- For prophylaxis of CNS leukemic disease intrathecal application of methotrexate before, during, and after remission has to be performed. The addition of preventive irradiation is probably necessary in children at high-risk of ALL as determined in most studies.
- Drugs commonly used in Induction phase: Prednisolone, Vincristine, Daunorubicin, L-Asparginase and Methotrexate.

Consolidation Treatment

- Without continuation of treatment leukemia will reappear within weeks or months.
- When remission with normal hematopoiesis is achieved further intensive chemotherapy is necessary to reach a complete eradication of leukemic cells.
- Combinations of different cytotoxic drugs reduce the number of remaining leukemic cells and the development of resistance against particular chemotherapies.
- Drugs commonly used in Consolidation phase: Cyclophosphamide, Vincristine, Cytosine Arabinoside and 6 Mercaptopurine.

Maintenance Treatment

- Duration of treatment is 1.5-2.5 years with daily 6-mercaptopurine and once weekly methotrexate, with or without reinduction treatment are commonly used
- A lifestyle as normal as possible as before the diagnosis has to be followed during maintenance treatment
- Drugs commonly used in maintenance phase: Prednisolone, Vincristine, Daunorubicin, L-Asparginase, 6 Mercaptopurine and Methotrexate.

DISCUSSION

DEFINITION OF ALL

- Greater than 25% replacement of bone marrow by malignant lymphoid precursors.
- If less than 25%, it is defined as Non-Hodgkin's lymphoma with marrow involvement.

PROGNOSTIC FACTORS

Prognostic factors	Favorable	Unfavorable
WBC	$<10 \times 10^9/l$	$>50 \times 10^9/l$
Age (years)	2-7	< 2 and >10 (especially in infants)
Response to steroid treatment	+	-
Response to treatment	< 4 weeks	> 4 weeks

Contd...

Time of relapse after treatment ends	>6 months	<6 months
Surface markers	Pre-B-ALL	T/B cell ALL
Cytogenetic characterization (DI) structure	Hyperdiploid	Hypodiploid, BCR-ABL fusion protein (translocation 9;22)
FAB	L1	L2/L3
Mediastinal enlargement	-	(+)
Visceromegaly	+ to + +	+ + +
LDH	Moderate	High

IMMUNOPHENOTYPING

CD stands for cluster differentiation. These are actually group of protein markers present on the surface of white blood cell. These markers are used to classify the lineage of the leucocytes and are used to establish international nomenclature standards. These markers are detected by immunophenotyping.

Immunophenotype Pattern of Various Leucocytes

Antigen	*Cell Lineage associated with*
CD1-CD 8	T cell
CD 10, 19, 20 to 23	B cell
CD 13 to 15, 33	Monocyte, macrophage
CD 16, 56	NK cell
CD 34	Stem cell and progenitor cell
CD 30	Activation markers
CD 45	All leucocytes

Immunophenotypic Pattern of ALL

ALL is of three 3 types and all the three types have different immunophenotypic pattern.

T ALL associated with - CD 2, CD 3, CD 5, CD 7

B ALL associated with - CD 19, CD 20, CD 22, CD 24

Null ALL

Immunophenotype Pattern of AML—M2

CD13, CD 33, CD 34

Immunophenotype pattern of AML—Mo

CD 13, CD 33

The type of acute leukemia's with immunophenotypic features of more than one cell lineage are referred to as acute leukemias of ambiguous lineage in new classification system proposed by World Health Organization.

Biphenotypic leukemia is a subtype of leukemia of ambiguous lineage in which the malignant cells population express markers of two different lineages—most commonly myeloid and either B lymphoid lineage.

MANAGEMENT OF COMPLICATIONS AND SIDE EFFECTS

- Dehydration, infection, anemia, bleeding and alteration of liver and kidney functions has to be continuously observed and corrected during the different treatment phases
- Anemia:
  - Support with packed red blood cell transfusion indicated when the hemoglobin level is less than 6 g/L.
- Bleeding:
  - Due to thrombocytopenia (decreased production, suppression by cytotoxic drugs).
  - Treatment: Platelet transfusion, substitution of coagulation factors, antileukemic treatment
- Infection:
  - Due to reduced humoral and cellular immune response
  - High risk of infection during induction treatment and during episodes of severe neutropenia with absolute neutrophil count (ANC) less than 0.5×10^9/l
  - Symptoms of infection may be atypical during phases of neutropenia
  - Procedure during fever and neutropenia (ANC less than 0.5×10^9/L): blood culture analysis and start broad-spectrum antibiotics

CNS LEUKEMIA

- CNS leukemia occurs in less than 10% of children, mostly diagnosed subclinically while analysis of cerebrospinal fluid.
- Definition of CNS leukemia: More than 5 leukemic cells/cm^3
- The CNS relapse occurs in isolation or in combination with bone marrow and/or testicular relapse.
- Treatment: Initially intrathecal chemotherapy until CNS and spinal irradiation and systematic chemotherapy continuation.
- Prognosis: Survival rate is 45% if relapse occurs less than 18 months from diagnosis, while survival is 80% if relapse occurs more than 18 months from diagnosis.

TESTICULAR LEUKEMIA

- Preventive biopsy of testes for occult testicular infiltration is not indicated because of side effects of biopsy; systemic treatment eradicates occult testicular leukemia
- Side effects: Sterility and sometimes reduced testicular function; in the latter case hormonal substitution may be necessary
- Patients with early relapse have an approximately 40% survival and patients with late relapse have an approximately 85% survival.

PROGNOSIS

- Approximately 80% of children with ALL survive without relapse with 7 to 10 years follow-up after diagnosis (long-term remission)
- In about 20% children a relapse of ALL occurs during maintenance treatment.
- A relapse within the first 6 months after stopping treatment indicates a poor prognosis
- A late relapse (more then 6 months after termination of maintenance treatment) usually has a better prognosis depending on the characteristics of the leukemic cells.

CHAPTER 28

HYPOTHYROIDISM

HISTORY

CHIEF COMPLAINTS

- Lethargy
- Prolonged jaundice
- Constipation
- Weight gain.

HISTORY OF PRESENT ILLNESS

History of Disease

- Fatigue, lethargy, sleepiness
- Difficulty in feeding—feeds poorly, choking spells during feeding in neonates while decreased appetite in older children
- Cold intolerance
- Hoarse voice (due to myxomatous infiltration of vocal cord)
- Blurred vision
- Muscle pain, joint pain, weakness in the extremities
- Cough, fever, noisy breathing, breathlessness (repeated LRTI)
- Delayed dentition
- Fullness in neck (goiter)
- Swelling over body (myxedema)
- Decreased hearing (myxedema/otitis media).

History of Risk Factors

- History in neighborhood: Endemic goiter (iodine deficiency)
- Drug intake
  - Ayurvedic medicines, cough suppressants/ expectorants (may contain iodine)
  - Antithyroid drugs or iodine intake in pregnancy.
- Surgery/irradiation: Destruction of thyroid tissue.

POSTNATAL HISTORY

- Delayed passage of meconium
- Prolonged jaundice
- Birth weight greater than average
- Hypothermia
- Poor feeding, hoarse cry, lethargy.

FAMILY HISTORY

- History in mother (hashimoto's thyroiditis, graves disease) and siblings (maternal antibodies).

DEVELOPMENTAL HISTORY

- In detail.

GENERAL PHYSICAL EXAMINATION

- Bradycardia
- Hypotension, diastolic hypertension
- Weight gain
- Edema (nonpitting)
- Dry skin
- Jaundice
- Pallor
- Coarse, brittle, straw like hair
- Loss of scalp hair, axillary hair, pubic hair
- Dull facial expression
- Coarse facial features
- Periorbital puffiness
- Macroglossia
- Goiter
- Hoarseness
- Decreased systolic blood pressure and increased diastolic blood pressure
- Hypothermia.

SYSTEMIC EXAMINATION

CARDIOVASCULAR SYSTEM

- Sinus bradycardia
- Pericardial effusion
- Congestive cardiac failure
- Cardiomyopathy.

CENTRAL NERVOUS SYSTEM

- Poor memory, mental confusion
- Slowed speech and movements
- Cranial nerves: Nerve deafness
- Hypotonia
- Hyporeflexia with delayed relaxation, ataxia or both
- Muscle stiffness.

DIAGNOSIS

——— year old with hypothyroidism; congenital/ acquired; etiology being———

DIFFERENTIAL DIAGNOSIS

Differential diagnosis will be dependent on presentation of disorder. Presentation is different at different ages.

Presentation	*Differential diagnosis*
At birth with lethargy	Inborn error of metabolism
First 6 weeks with hyperbilirubinemia	Criggler Najjar syndrome Breast milk jaundice
Delayed development milestones/ Mental retardation	Down syndrome Fragile X syndrome
Facial dysmorphism/ Short stature	Mucopolysaccharidoses

INVESTIGATIONS

Laboratory tests to determine thyroid function include:

- Plasma TSH estimation: Elevated
- Free T4 test is recommended over a total T4 test or other measurement because it is not affected by thyroid hormone binding proteins.
- If free T4 assays are unavailable, a free thyroxine index (FTI) is indicatior of the free hormone level. FTI is the product of the T3 resin uptake and total T4 levels.
- Evaluation of the presence of thyroid autoantibodies (antimicrosomal or anti-TPO antibodies) and antithyroglobulin (anti-Tg) to

determine etiology of hypothyroidism or in predicting future hypothyroidism.
- Plasma T3: Not of much help in diagnosis of hypothyroidism, required for diagnosis of T3 thyrotoxicosis.

Additional laboratory abnormalities may include:
- Low hemoglobin and low RBC count
- X-rays
  - X-ray bone age—Retarded bone age (absent distal femoral epiphysis in neonates)
  - X-ray skull—Large fontanelle, wide sutures, wormian bones, enlarged sella
  - X-ray chest—çardiac shadow enlarged due to cardiomyopathy or pericardial effusion
  - Deformity of vertebrae.
- ECG:
  - Sinus bradycardia
  - Low voltage complexes.
- Radioactive iodine uptake and thyroid scanning are not useful in hypothyroidism because these tests require some level of endogenous function in the hypofunctioning gland to provide information. Patients with Hashimoto thyroiditis may have relatively high early uptake (after 4 hours) but do not have the usual doubling of uptake at 24 hours suggestive of an organification defect.
- Fine-needle aspiration (FNA) biopsy: To evaluate suspicious nodules
- Thyroid scan: Look for agenesis/ectopic thyroid tissue
- Ultrasound of the neck and thyroid: Detects nodules and infiltrative disease. It has little use in hypothyroidism per se.

TREATMENT

Congenital Hypothyroidism

- Urgent treatment
- *L Thyroxine (the wonder drug and the only drug)*
- 10-15 μg/kg/day
- Follow-up: TSH 2 weeks later and then
  - 2 monthly for 1 year
  - 3 monthly for 3 years
  - Yearly after 3 years.
- At follow-up check for development, height, weight gain, overall well being and other clinical symptoms.
- Growth rate provides an excellent index of *adequacy of treatment.*
- *Overtreatment* leads to craniosynostosis and temperament problems.

Dosage in Older Children

< 6 months	– 6-8 μg/kg/day
6-12 months	– 5-8 μg/kg/day
1-5 years	– 4-6 μg/kg/day
5-12 years	– 3-5 μg/kg/day
12-18 years	– 2-3 μg/kg/day
18 years	– 1-2 μg/kg/day

- Radiologically bone age advance should be checked annually
- Treatment of complications
- Neonatal screening in next pregnancy after 72 hours of life.

Prevention

- Dietary iodide supplementation can prevent endemic goiter and cretinism, but not sporadic congenital hypothyroidism.
- Properly administered newborn screening programs have made diagnosis of infants with congenital hypothyroidism possible within the first 3 weeks of life. With early and adequate treatment, the sequel can be eliminated in most and minimized in the rest.

Prognosis

- Early diagnosis and treatment of congenital hypothyroidism prevents severe mental retardation and other neurological complications. Even with early treatment, some children demonstrate mild delays in areas such as reading comprehension and arithmetic.

- Infants with delayed bone age at diagnosis or a longer time to normalize thyroid hormone levels have poorer outcomes. Although continued improvement in IQ has been documented in treated patients through adolescence, some cognitive problems may persist. These may include problems in visuospatial, language, and fine motor function. Defects in memory and attention may also be present.

Patient Education

- Parents should be educated regarding their child's disorder, the potential problems associated with no treatment or inadequate treatment, and the benefits of early and appropriate treatment. This should include instructions on the proper administration of the medication and how and when to follow-up. Early childhood intervention programs, if available, should be encouraged.

CLINICAL FEATURES OF HYPOTHYROIDISM

- Increased head size due to myxoedema of brain
- Prolonged physiological jaundice, feeding difficulties in neonates
- Growth: Stunted (short limbs) with edema
- *Characteristic facies:*
  - Wide open sutures
  - Hypertelorism
  - Narrow palpebral fissures
  - Swollen eyelids
  - Depressed nasal bridge
  - Open mouth with thick broad protruding tongue
  - Delayed dentition.
- Neck: short, thick with deposits of fat above clavicles.
- Hypothermia
- Constipation
- Hair: Coarse, brittle with hairy forehead
- Skin:
  - Dry (little perspiration) and scaly
  - Edematous
  - Yellow complexion (due to carotenemia)
- Hands: Broad with short fingers
- Respiratory:
  - Nasal obstruction, noisy breathing, apnea (due to large tongue)
- CVS:
  - Bradycardia
  - Cardiomegaly
- Abdomen:
  - Distension
  - Umbilical hernia
- Delayed sexual maturation
- CNS finding:
  - Mental retardation, global retardation of milestones
  - Speech: Slow, sluggish and hoarse
  - Deafness
  - Muscle stiffness
  - Generalized hypotonia
  - Ankle jerk: Delayed relaxation of jerks.

DISCUSSION

SEQUALAE OF HYPOTHYROIDISM

- Spasticity
- Tremor
- Nystagmus

- Ataxia
- Mental retardation
- Behavioral abnormalities.

ANEMIA IN HYPOTHYROIDISM

- Lack of thyroxine: Normochromic normocytic anemia
- Myxedema associated with pernicious anemia
- Menorrhagia: Iron deficiency anemia.

CARDIOMEGALY IN HYPOTHYROIDISM

- Cardiac dilatation
- Pericardial effusion
- Cardiomyopathy.

EXCESSIVE DOSAGE OF L-THYROXINE THERAPY

- Benign intracranial tension
- Tremors, insomnia, hyperactivity
- Craniostenosis
- Osteoporosis.

AT RISK MOTHERS

- Maternal hypothyroidism
- Mothers on antithyroid drugs
- Maternal radioactive isotope treatment
- Recurrent fetal wastage.

PROGNOSTIC INDICATORS FOR CONGENITAL HYPOTHYROIDISM

- Prenatal onset
- High pretreatment TSH
- Delayed bone age
- Lower pretreatment T4
- Poor compliance and fluctuating T4 during 1st year.

TRANSIENT HYPOTHYROIDISM

- This accounts for 10% of cases and is usually related to either maternal medications, e.g. carbimazole or to maternal antibodies. In maternal thyroid disease IgG auto-antibodies can cross the placenta and block thyroid function *in utero;* this improves after delivery.

Management

- The aim of treatment is *early detection* and *early thyroid hormone replacement* to ensure that infants do not develop irreversible neurological disability.
- Thyroxine hormone replacement with L-thyroxine is given once daily and titrated to thyroid function tests.
- Transient hypothyroidism should be treated if low T4 and raised TSH persist beyond 2 weeks. Treatment is usually terminated after 3 to 5 months.

ETIOLOGY OF CONGENITAL HYPOTHYROIDISM

Transient Primary Hypothyroidism

- Transplacental transfer
  - Maternal antibodies
  - Antithyroid drugs.
- Maternal iodine deficiency
- Iodine exposure of fetus and newborn.

Permanent Primary Hypothyroidism

- Thyroid dysgenesis
- Dyshormonogenesis
- Maternal radioactive isotope treatment.

Permanent Hypothalamic—Pituitary Hypothyroidism

- Midline defects
- Asphyxia neonatorum

- Pituitary aplasia
- Gene mutation.

TIMING FOR NEONATAL SCREENING (TSH AND T4) FOR CONGENITAL HYPOTHYROIDISM

There is controversy regarding time and site of blood sample

- Cord blood should be taken on 1st day of life (Ghai and CPDT)
- Blood should be collected from heel pad on 4th day of life (Harrison) as there is TSH surge immediately following birth. This TSH surge can cause falsely positive neonatal screens for hypothyroidism. The level of TSH markedly decreases during first 48 hours of life and attains childhood levels by 2-4 weeks.
- Nelson does not mention anything about site and timing of blood sample.

SCREENING FOR THYROID DYSFUNCTION

I generally recommend that both a total T4 and a second generation TSH assay be used for screening in most patients. In those patients who are ill or taking medications known to interfere with thyroid binding globulin, screening should be done using both the second generation TSH and one of the estimates of free T4.

SERUM TOTAL T4 AND TOTAL T3 ASSAYS

The thyroid secretes mainly T4. Most of the serum T3 comes from conversion of T4 to T3 in the peripheral tissues although some is secreted by the thyroid. Virtually all of serum T4 (99.97%) is bound to thyroxine binding globulin (TBG). A smaller but still very high percentage of the T3 in the serum is also bound.

Normal range of total T4 is 4.6 to 11.2 μg/dL.

Normal range of total T3 approximately 75 to 195 ng/dL and tends to decrease with age.

The unbound or free T4 and T3 concentrations are the active forms that are available for uptake into cells. The bound hormone, on the other hand, represents a circulating storage pool that is not immediately available for uptake into cells.

SERUM TSH ASSAYS

First generation TSH assays have detection limits of about 5 to 10 mU/L. Since the normal range for TSH is about 0.5 to 5.0 mU/L, these assays often miss mild hypothyroidism (where the TSH is usually just above 5) and are totally inadequate for assessment of hyperthyroidism (where the TSH is usually below 0.5). As a result, first generation TSH assays are not used now.

Second generation TSH assays have a lower detection limit of about 0.1 mU/L. These assays distinguish normal from hypothyroid patients with a high degree of accuracy. These assays can also be used as screening tests to distinguish hyperthyroidism from normal thyroid function. Second generation assays are currently in wide use.

Third generation TSH assays have become available with detection limits of about 0.01 mU/L. Because of the considerably lower detection limit, these assays can reliably distinguish between normal and hyperthyroid patients. Because the distinction between normal and hyperthyroid patients is usually not a problem, these assays are not widely utilized.

MONITORING THYROID HORMONE THERAPY

Patients with primary hypothyroidism (failure of the thyroid) who are taking thyroid hormone therapy can be monitored with just the serum TSH. If TSH is high, the dose of thyroid hormone needs to be increased; if TSH is low, the dose needs to be reduced. In patients with secondary hypothyroidism (failure of the pituitary), the TSH cannot be used because these patients have impaired TSH release. One of the estimates of free T4 should be used in these patients.

APPROACH TO HYPOTHYROIDISM

If TSH levels are above the reference range, the next step would be to measure total T4 with a measure of binding proteins. Thyroxine is highly protein bound (99.97%). The levels of these binding proteins could vary by hormonal status, inheritance, and in various disease states.

Hence, free T4 assays are becoming popular as they measure unbound hormone. However, free T4 assays are unreliable in the setting of severe illness.

A free thyroxine index (FTI) serves as a surrogate of the free hormone level. Free thyroid hormone levels can be estimated by calculating the percentage of available thyroid hormone-binding sites (T3 resin uptake) or by measuring the concentration of thyroxine-binding globulin (TBG). The FTI is the product of the T3 resin uptake and total T4 levels.

Patients with primary hypothyroidism have elevated TSH levels and decreased free hormone levels. Patients with elevated TSH levels but normal free hormone levels or estimates are considered to have mild or subclinical hypothyroidism.

Primary hypothyroidism is virtually the only disease that is characterized by sustained, rising TSH levels. As the TSH level increases early in the disease, an increased conversion of T4 to T3 occur, this maintains T3 levels. In early hypothyroidism, TSH levels are increased, T4 levels are normal to low, and T3 levels are normal.

In patients with hypothalamic or pituitary dysfunction, TSH levels do not increase in appropriate relation to the low free T4 levels. Hence, when secondary or tertiary hypothyroidism is suspected, a serum TSH measurement alone is inadequate; a free T4 should be measured.

Evaluation of the presence of thyroid autoantibodies (antimicrosomal or anti-TPO antibodies) and antithyroglobulin (anti-Tg) may be helpful in determining the etiology of hypothyroidism or in predicting future hypothyroidism. Anti-TPO antibodies have been associated with a higher risk of infertility and miscarriage.

CHAPTER 29

Duchenne Muscular Dystrophy (DMD)

HISTORY

CHIEF COMPLAINTS

- Weakness
- Hypertrophy of calf muscles.

HISTORY OF PRESENT ILLNESS

History of Disease

- Weakness:
  - Age of onset
  - Pattern of involvement: Upper limb, lower limb or both
  - Weakness in proximal muscles (suggests proximal myopathy):
    - Raising arms above shoulders
    - Combing
    - Difficulty in climbing stairs
    - Getting up from sitting position.
  - Weakness in distal muscles (suggests distal myopathy):
    - Worsening of handwriting
    - Child not able to mix food by hand
    - Frequent falling of objects held in hand
    - Wearing slippers
    - Toe walking.
  - Upper limb involvement
    - Inability to button clothes,
    - Tie shoelaces.
  - Progression of weakness: Inability of patient to walk to distances which he initially could
  - Compare present activities with premorbid conditions when he could walk to school, play with his peer group, and perform physical training exercises.
- Hypertrophy of calf muscles
  - Onset
  - Progression
  - Associated atrophy of other muscles.
- Abnormal movements like
  - Rapid swinging of arms (chorea)
  - Fine, writhing movements of distal extremities (athetosis).
- Facial weakness:
  - Inability to smile, whistle
  - Fully close eyes
  - Squint/ double vision

- ❖ Drooping of eyelid
- ❖ Difficulty in chewing and swallowing
- ❖ Expressionless face.
- Sensory disturbances like twitching movements (fasciculation) (differentiates it from myotonia)
- Abnormal gait/tendency to fall
- Muscle cramps/stiffness
- Current problems
  - ❖ Disturbance in daily activities
  - ❖ Aids required
  - ❖ Solution adopted.
- Bladder/ bowel dysfunction (presence of these sensory symptoms suggest neurological involvement)
- Raised intracranial tension:Headache/nausea/vomiting
- Delay in motor milestones.

HISTORY OF COMPLICATIONS

- Breathlessness: Respiratory dysfunction
- Palpitation: Cardiac dysfunction
- Weight gain: Obesity
- Deformities/contractures (joint abnormalities)
- Severe acute pain in abdomen (dilatation of stomach)
- Scoliosis.

HISTORY OF DIFFERENTIAL DIAGNOSIS

- Difficulty in releasing objects after firm grasp (Myotonia)
- Mental retardation/frontal baldness/decreased vision (cataract) (Myotonia)
- Muscle pain, myalgia (polymyositis)
- Rash and photosensitivity (dermatomyositis)
- Similar illness on maternal sides (in maternal uncle)
- Constipation/lethargy (hypothyroidism)
- Reduced fetal movements (myopathy)
- Drug intake (steroids)
- Decreased urine output (uremia)
- Fever with rash (Mumps, measles, chicken-pox).

BIRTH HISTORY

- Fetal movements (Quickening)
- Oligohydroamnious
- Drug intake in pregnancy
- Labour: Normal/Cesarean section
- Cry activity and feeding problems in postnatal period.

FAMILY HISTORY

- Similar history in family
- Still birth and miscarriages
- Consanguinity
- Make detailed pedigree chart.

DEVELOPMENTAL HISTORY

Elicit in detail motor milestones.

GENERAL PHYSICAL EXAMINATION

- ❖ Vitals: Especially heart rate and respiratory distress
- ❖ Rash (SLE, dermatomyositis)
- ❖ Cataract (myotonic dystrophy)
- ❖ Dull expression
- ❖ Anthropometry
- ❖ Signs of hypocalcemia like latent tetany, Trousseau's sign
- ❖ Lordotic standing
- ❖ Wasting of deltoid, biceps, triceps, sternal head of pectoralis major
- ❖ Winging of scapula, internal rotation of femur
- ❖ Small thighs, prominent calves, equinovarus deformities of feet
- ❖ Spine: Scoliosis.

SYSTEMIC EXAMINATION

CNS EXAMINATION

- Cranial nerves
- Bulbar muscles
- Tongue (fibrillation)
- **Motor system:**
    - Wasting of muscles
    - Hypertrophy of muscles
      Calves/quadriceps/gluteus medius/deltoid/infraspinatus
    - Tone
    - Power—muscle charting.

Grading of Muscular Weakness

- Grade 0: Complete paralysis
- Grade 1: Flicker of contraction only (visible or palpable)
- Grade 2: Movements with elimination of gravity
- Grade 3: Movement against gravity but not against resistance
- Grade 4: Movement possible against gravity plus resistance but weaker than normal.
- Grade 5: Normal power
  Often, '+' or '–' symbols are used to improve the sensitivity of the grading.
- Test for muscle power in the different muscle groups as follows:

Hip Joint

Hip flexion: Ask the child to sit with his leg dangling, and then ask him to flex his thigh against resistance keeping the knee flexed (Femoral Nerve L2,3).

Extension for hip (*Glutei*): Patient lies supine; raise the patient's foot off the bed and ask him to push it down against your resistance. Knee must be kept extended (Gluteal Nerve L4,5).

Hip abduction: Ask the child to lie on the side opposite you want to test. Ask him to abduct the leg which is facing skyward. Now, offer resistance (L4, 5, S1).

Hip adduction: Ask the child to lie supine, and then abduct the hip you want to test. Now, ask him to adduct the abducted hip while you offer resistance (L2,3,4).

Knee Joint

Knee flexion: Ask the child to lie prone and flex the knee joint. Now, offer resistance (hamstrings L5, S1).

Knee extension (*Quadriceps*): Patient lies supine; first bend the knee and then ask the patient to straighten the leg when resistance is applied over the shin (L3,4).

Ankle Joint

Ankle dorsiflexion: Make the child sit with legs dangling and ask him to dorsiflex the foot at the ankle. Look for resistance. Inversion and aversion can also be tested in this position (peroneal nerve L4, 5).

Ankle plantar flexion (Gastroenemius): Patient lies supine with legs extended. Ask the patient to plantar-flex the foot against resistance (tibial nerve S1, 2).

Shoulder Joint

Shoulder flexion (Deltoid): Ask the child to sit and flex the arm at the shoulder against resistance (axillary nerve, C5).

Shoulder extension: Ask the child to sit and extend the arm at the shoulder against resistance.

Arm abduction: Ask the child to sit and extend his arm at the shoulder while you offer resistance.

Deltoid: First abduct the patient's arm to 30° and tell him to keep his arm in that position. Now ask him to abduct his arm upto 90° against your resistance (supraspinatus abducts the first 30°).

Latissimus dorsi: Palpate the posterior axillary folds from behind when the patient coughs. Compare the contraction on both sides.

Pectoralis major: Ask the patient to clap his hands together and you attempt to keep them apart. The contraction of pectoralis can be seen.

Elbow Joint

Flexion at elbow (Biceps): Ask the child to sit and flex the forearm at the elbow against resistance (musculocutaneous nerve, C5, 6).

Extension at elbow (Triceps): Ask the child to sit with the elbow flexed, and ask him to extend the elbow against resistance (radial nerve, C6, 7).

Infraspinatus: The patient is asked to tuck his elbow into his side with the forearm placed at right angle. He is now asked to rotate the limb outwards against your resistance (elbow will be placed against the side throughout the test).

Wrist Joint

Flexion at wrist: Ask the child to hold the palm skyward and keep fingers extended. Ask him to flex the hand at the wrist against resistance (C8).

Extension at wrist: Ask the child to hold the arm with the palm down and fingers flexed into a fist. Ask him to extend the fisted hand at the wrist against resistance (radial nerve C6, 7).

Hand

Finger flexors: Ask the child to squeeze your own fingers. Assess the power as he does so. The finger flexors are not graded (median nerve C8).

Intrinsic muscles of the hand: Ask the child to fan out his fingers and not allow you to reposition them. Normally, the child can keep his fingers fanned (ulnar nerve T1).

Neck

Neck flexion: With the child lying supine, ask him to flex his neck and see whether the flexors of the neck are weak.

Arm Drift Sign

Ask the child to extend both the arms in front of him as if he were carrying a book. Tell him to keep his eyes closed with arms in place and count to 10. Normally, the arms remain in place. The upper limbs will pronate and fall, if the muscle strength is poor. In psychogenic weakness, the limb falls without pronation.

Beevor Sign

Ask the child to raise his head and sit up from the supine, recumbent position. Keep his arms crossed across his chest, and apply resistance to the forehead with your hand. Bilateral lower abdominal paralysis results in upward deviation of the umbilicus.

Gower's Sign

When the patient is asked to stand from lying down position, he rises by first rolling over his body and then takes support successively on the ground, feet, legs, knees and waist and finally stands up. It seems that the patient is 'climbing up the legs' and it is known as Gowers' rising test or Gowers' sign.

Slip Sign

It indicates weakness of shoulder. When the child is picked up with hands under the arm, the arms go up and the child tends to slip through one's hand.

- **Reflexes:** Knee jerk is often lost (due to contractures) and ankle jerk is preserved

Grading of Deep Tendon Reflexes

0 Absent
1+ Sluggish or present only with rein-forcement
2+ Readily elicited

3+ Brisk without evidence of clonus
4+ Associated with clonus

- **Sensory system:** Look for fasciculations
- **Gait:** Waddling, Toe-walking.

CARDIOVASCULAR SYSTEM

- Cardiomegaly
- Palpitation, tachycardia, arrhythmia
- Myocardial failure.

RESPIRATORY SYSTEM

- Recurrent chest infection
- Cor pulmonale
- Restrictive lung disease
- Signs of respiratory failure.

DIAGNOSIS

Gradual onset progressive weakness of upper/lower limbs, proximal > distal with calf hypertrophy most probable diagnosis being Duchenne muscular dystrophy with/without complications.

DIFFERENTIAL DIAGNOSIS

DUCHENNE MUSCULAR DYSTROPHY

- Becomes apparent between ages 3 and 5.
- Male predilectation.
- Progressive loss of muscle strength with predilectation for proximal muscle group and neck flexors.
- Leg involvement more severe than arm involvement.
- Systemic involvement: Cardiomyopathy, intellectual impairment.

BECKER'S MUSCULAR DYSTROPHY

- Presents between ages 5 and 15, although late onset can also occur.
- Proximal muscles, especially of lower extremeties are prominently involved.
- Hypertrophy of calf muscles is prominent and early feature.
- Incidence of cardiac involvement and intellectual impairment is less as compared to DMD.

LIMB GIRDLE MUSCULAR DYSTROPHY

- Onset: Late in 1st decade to 4th decade.
- Progressive weakness of pelvic and shoulder girdle musculature.
- No intellectual impairment.
- Cardiomyopathy and respiratory insufficiency can occur.

EMERY DREIFUSS MUSCULAR DYSTROPHY

- Recognization in early childhood and teenage years.
- Development of contractures precedes muscle weakness.
- Muscle weakness affects humeral and peroneal muscles and then spreads to limb girdle musculature.
- Contractures persist throughout the course of disease, mainly at elbow and neck.

FACIOSCAPULAR HUMERAL

- Facial weakness initial manifestation, as inability to smile, whistle or fully close eyes.
- Arm elevation difficult due to involvement of shoulder girdle.
- Scapular winging.
- Biceps and triceps severely affected with sparing of deltoid.
- Wrist extensors more involved than wrist flexors, footdrop due to weakness of anterior compartment of leg.

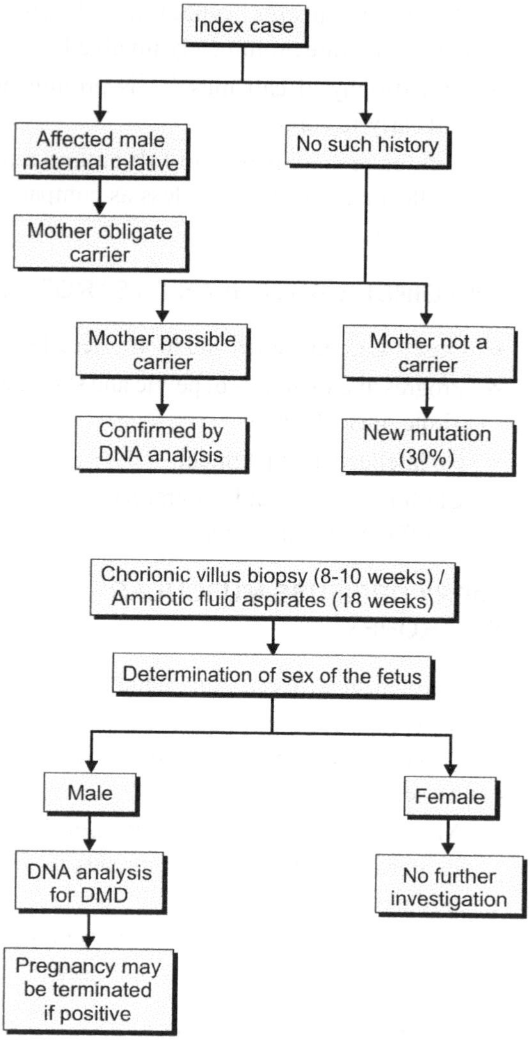

Fig. 29.1: Prenatal diagnosis

INVESTIGATIONS

- Serum creatinine kinase: Increased (Normal value 25-90 units/liter) in early stages, gradually declines with progression of disease.
- Aldolase and AST: Increased (Normal value 0-8 units/liter), less specific.
- X-ray chest to look for cardiomegaly and bronchopneumonia.
- ECG: Tachycardia, tall R waves in right precordial leads, deep Q waves in left precordial leads, bundle branch block due to cardiac involvement.
- Electromyography: Shows characteristic myopathic pattern (low amplitude, short duration, polyphasic motor action potentials).
- Nerve conduction: No evidence of denervation.
- Muscle biopsy: Diagnostic. Shows islands of muscular degeneration in the ocean of fibro-fatty tissue, without any cellular degeneration.
- Intelligence quotient.
- Dystrophin levels.
- Dystrophin gene mutation detection at DNA level by PCR and Southern blotting by DNA probes.

  Other tests for etiology as suspected:
  - ANA, LE cell in SLE
  - TSH (hypothyroidism)
  - Serum calcium, phosphorus, alkaline phosphatase (hypocalcemia).
- Genetic counseling:
  - Fetal blood sampling (16 weeks): Increased CPK levels.

MANAGEMENT

- Objectives:
  - Counselling
  - Prenatal diagnosis (Fig. 29.1)
  - Supportive care
  - Gene therapy
- Psychosocial:
  - Education of patient, parents and relatives
  - Social support
  - Financial assistance
  - Emotional support.
- Good nutrition:
  - Calcium supplementation
  - Obesity prevention.

- Physiotherapy
- Treatment of medical complications
- Genetic counseling if couple is further desirous of having child:
  - Carrier detection
  - Prenatal diagnosis
  - Pedigree analysis.
- Future therapy:
  - *Myoblast transfer therapy*: After multiplying normal cells in tissue culture, insert them into dystrophic muscles. The cells fuse inside muscle and introduce working copies of all their genes including the one which codes for dystrophin. In dystrophic muscle the muscle fibers produce dystrophin.
- *Gene therapy:* Minidystrophin gene is introduced into MDX mouse at a pre-embryonic stage. The mouse manufactures normal level of dystrophin.

Usually death occurs in second decade of life due to pneumonia, respiratory failure or cardiac failure.

DISCUSSION

DEFINITION

Myopathy is genetically determined abnormality characterized by progressive degeneration of a group of muscles without involvement of the nervous system.

In *Myotonia* relaxation is impaired following strong contraction.

CLASSIFICATION OF MYOPATHY

- Congenital
- Hereditary
- Mitochondrial myopathies
- Endocrine myopathies
- Ion channel muscle disease
- Drug induced—steroids/chloroquine/alcohol/emetine
- Immune myopathies—polymyositis/dermatomyositis/inclusion body myositis.

Congenital Myopathy

- Muscular dystrophy
- Ophthalmoplegias
- Myotubular myopathies
- Amyoplasia
- Central core disease
- Centrinuclear.

Hereditary Myopathy

- X-linked
  - Duchenne muscular dystrophy
  - Becker's muscular dystrophy.
- Dominant
  - Facioscapular humeral
- Recessive
  - Myotonic dystrophy
  - Emery Dreifuss.

Mitochondrial Myopathies

Defect lies in fatty acid oxidation and oxidative phosphorylation

- MELAS
- Leber's optic atrophy
- MERRF
- NARP (Neuropathy, Ataxia, Rhinitis, Pigmentosa).

Endocrine Myopathies

- Thyrotoxicosis
- Hypothyroidism
- Renal rickets
- Malnutrition
- Addison's disease.

Ion Channel Muscle Disease

- Hyperkalemic periodic paralysis
- Hypokalemic periodic paralysis
- Myotonia congenita.

IDENTIFICATION POINTS OF DMD

- Male child
- Wadding gait and positive Gowers' sign (ask the patient for demonstration)
- Pseudohypertrophy (principally the calf muscles) plus atrophy of muscles
- Proximal muscles weakness (ask the patient to get up from sitting position)

  Becker type is milder form of dystrophy starting between 5 and 25 years. Cardiac involvement is less often. The patients may survive up to 5th or 6th decade.

DIFFERENTIAL DIAGNOSIS OF GOWER'S SIGN

- Duchenne muscular dystrophy
- Becker's muscular dystrophy
- Kugelberg-Wilander syndrome (GMA—late variety)
- Drug induced: Steroid
- Polymyositis
- Uremic myopathy (proximal type)
- Inflammatory myopathy (proximal type).

TESTS TO DETECT EARLY MUSCULAR DYSTROPHY WHEN GOWER'S SIGN NOT COMPLETE

- Poor head control (weakness of neck muscles)
- Sitting up from supine position is difficult
- Difficulty in picking up fallen object (proximal muscles weakness)
- Positive Trendelenburg gait.

MUSCLES INVOLVED IN DMD

Upper Limb

- Supraspinatus
- Deltoid
- Latissimus dorsi
- Pectoralis
- Biceps
- Triceps
- Brachioradialis.

Lower Limb

- Glutei
- Quadriceps
- Sartorius
- Anterior tibial muscles
- Gastrocnemius.

DISEASES WITH LATE PRESERVATION OF ANKLE JERK

- Duchenne muscular dystrophy
- Werdnig-Hoffman's disease
- Friedrich's ataxia
- Kugelberg-Wilander syndrome.

DIFFERENTIAL DIAGNOSIS OF CALF HYPERTROPHY

- Physiological: Due to extensive use
- Duchenne muscular dystrophy
- Becker's Muscular dystrophy
- Kugelberg: Wilander syndrome
- Limb–girdle muscular dystrophy
- Polymyositis
- Myotonia congenita
- Hypothyroidism.

MUSCULAR DISORDERS WITH CARDIAC INVOLVEMENT

- Duchenne muscular dystrophy
- Becker's muscular dystrophy
- Carnitine deficiency
- Mitochondrial disease: MELAS, MERRF.

FEMALE PATIENTS OF DMD

Females can be patients of DMD in:

- Turner's syndrome
- Structural variation in X-chromosome
- Any condition causing lyonization.

DIAGNOSES OF CARRIERS OF DMD

- Muscle biopsy is diagnostic
- DNA analysis
- PCR Test
- DNA Probe
- Dystrophin levels.

COMPLICATIONS OF DMD

- Repeated respiratory tract infections/respiratory failure
- Cardiac failure/cardiomyopathy
- Contractures/scoliosis
- Obesity
- Mental retardation
- Acute stomach dilatation
- Behavioral problem.

DIAGNOSIS OF MYOTONIA

- Shake hand with the patient and then let it go suddenly: The patient's grasp is maintained for a moment, then released slowly and gradually.
- Percuss the thenar eminence by a hammer: It shows a peculiar movement of the thumb and a dimple of contraction appears on thenar eminence which relaxes very slowly.
- Percuss over the tongue: A dimple of contraction appears which relaxes very slowly.
- Ask the patient to close the eyes forcibly: Now ask him to open the eyes. The patient can not open the eyes promptly or opens it very slowly.

CLINICAL FEATURES OF MYOTONIA DYSTROPHICA

- Myotonia
- Ptosis with ophthalmoplegia
- Proximal muscles wasting
- Long facial structure (hatchet face and swan-neck due to atrophy of the temporalis and sternomastoid muscle respectively)
- Cataract
- Frontal baldness
- Mental retardation
- Testicular atrophy
- Alopecia
- Cardiac conduction defects, arrhythmias.

DRUGS USED IN TREATMENT OF MYOTONIA

- Quinine
- Phenytoin, and
- Procainamide.

CHAPTER 30

ATAXIA

HISTORY

CHIEF COMPLAINTS

- Frequent falls/inability to walk properly
- Abnormal movements.

HISTORY OF PRESENT ILLNESS

History of Disease

Inability to Walk Properly

- Age of onset
- Rate of progression
- Difficulty in initiation of movements
- Tendency to fall foreward, backward or sideways
- Impaired balance on turning
- Nature of ataxia on closure of eyes
- Associated with normal movement of upper limbs or not.

Abnormal Movements (Tremor)

- Most prominent in which part of body—limbs/tongue
- Proximal or distal
- Regular or irregular
- Frequency
- Can be controlled by voluntary movements or not
- Increased by emotional changes
- Disappear during sleep
- Response to drugs.

CNS Symptoms

- Impairment of higher functions
- Vomiting, headache, convulsions, focal neurological deficits (raised intracranial tension)
- Cranial Nerve palsies: Vision, hearing, speech, drooling of saliva and pooling of secretions
- Sensory deficits: Numbness, tingling, pain/burning, difficulty in feeling ground
- Regression of milestones
- Motor deficits
- Bladder/bowel complaints.

History of Complications

- History of fall
- Head injury
- Activities of Daily Living "DEATH", i.e. Dressing, Eating, Ambulating, Toileting, Hygiene.

HISTORY OF RISK FACTORS

- Fever with rash: Acute cerebellar ataxia (chickenpox)
- Head injury: Intracranial bleed
- Headache/nausea/vomiting/behavioral changes/convulsion/unconsciouness/altered sensorium (intracranial tumor)
- Contact with tuberculosis
- Drug ingestion (phenytoin)
- Ear discharge/tinnitus (labyrinthitis)
- Increase in head size: Dandy–Walker's syndrome or Arnold–Chiari malformation
- Diarrhea/bulky stools/malabsorption (abetalipoproteinemia)
- Similar complaints in siblings (hereditary ataxia)
- Birth asphyxia (ataxic cerebral palsy).

FAMILY HISTORY

- Consanguineous marriage: Autosomal recessive conditions (degenerative and metabolic)
- Similar illness in other family members autosomal dominant conditions (olivopontoce rebeller atrophy, Rousell-Levy syndrome)
- Make pedigree chart.

GENERAL PHYSICAL EXAMINATION

- Vitals
- Anthropometry
- Skull, spine for any deformity or tenderness
- BCG scar
- Eyes: Cataract, retinitis pigmentosa, cherry red spot
- Chronic otitis media, sinusitis (ataxia telangiectasia)
- Deafness (Refsums disease)
- Skin: Telangiectasia over face, acrodermatitis, alopecia
- Skeletal deformities (Friedreich's ataxia)
- Unusual body odor
- Xanthomas, Xanthelasmas (abetalipoproteinemia).

SYSTEMIC EXAMINATION

CNS EXAMINATION

- Mental retardation
- Cranial nerve examination
- Motor system
- *Abnormal movements:* Clinical evaluation of tremors
  - Distribution
  - Rate—No. of cycles per second
  - Amplitude—fine, coarse
  - Relation to movement:
    - Intentional (cerebellar)
    - Postural
    - Resting
    - End point tremor (finger nose test—cerebellum)
  - Relation to sleep and emotion
  - Response to drugs.
- Sensory system
- *Cerebellar signs* (above downwards)
  - Titubation
  - Nystagmus: Phasic horizontal with the fast component towards the side of lesion
  - Finger nose test: Demonstrates intention tremor
  - Speech: Scanning dysarthria
  - Dysdiadochokinesia
  - Oscillation of outstretched arms
  - Pendular knee jerk: Due to hypotonia
  - Heel knee test
  - Rhomberg's sign and truncal ataxia
  - Cerebellar gait
  - Broad based, irregularly placed feet
  - Tendency to fall on affected side
  - Inability to walk in tandem.

In *spinal ataxia* (lesion in posterior column), incoordination is seen only with closed eyes, but in *cerebellar ataxia* incoordination is present both with open and closed eyes.

CARDIOVASCULAR SYSTEM

- Cardiomyopathy (Friedreich's ataxia).

RESPIRATORY SYSTEM

- Bronchiectasis (ataxia telangiectasia).

GIT

Malabsorption syndrome: Vitamin E deficiency, abetalipoproteinemia.

DIFFERENTIAL DIAGNOSIS

Acute Ataxia (maximum deficit in less than 1 week)

- Acute postinfectious cerebeller ataxia: Coxsackie, Varicella, ECHO virus
- Drug induced: Anticonvulsants, Antihistaminics, Alcohol
- Intracranial tumors: Posterior fossa tumors, Intracranial infections, Hydrocephalus
- Miller-Fisher syndrome: Ataxia, Areflexia, Ophthalmoplegia.

Recurrent Ataxia (Two or More Episodes of Ataxia)

- Urea cycle defects
- Pyruvate dehydrogenase deficiency
- Basilar artery migraine
- Hartnup disease.

Chronic Static Ataxia (No Progression of Signs and Symptoms)

- Postencephalitis
- Agenesis of cerebeller vermis
- Hydrocephalus.

Chronic Progressive Ataxia (Signs and Symptoms Progress Over a Period of One Year)

- Posterior fossa tumor
- Ataxia telengiectasia
- Friedreich's ataxia.

ACUTE CEREBELLAR ATAXIA

- Generally affects children 1-3 years of age.
- The condition often follows a viral illness, such as varicella, coxsackievirus, or echovirus infection.
- The onset is sudden, and the truncal ataxia can be so severe that the child is unable to stand or sit.
- Fever and nuchal rigidity are absent. Horizontal nystagmus and dysarthria can be present.
- CSF is normal but pleocytosis of lymphocytes (10-30/mm^3) can be seen. Later in the course, the CSF protein undergoes a moderate elevation.
- The ataxia begins to improve in a few weeks but may persist for as long as 2 months.
- The prognosis for complete recovery is excellent; a small number have long-term sequelae, including behavioral and speech disorders as well as ataxia and incoordination.

ACUTE LABYRINTHITIS

- The condition is associated with middle-ear infections and intense vertigo, vomiting, and abnormalities in labyrinthine function, particularly ice water caloric testing.

ABETALIPOPROTEINEMIA

- Begins in childhood with steatorrhea and failure to thrive.
- A blood smear shows acanthocytosis and decreased serum levels of cholesterol and

triglycerides, and the serum β-lipoproteins are absent.

- Neurologic signs become evident by late childhood and consist of ataxia, retinitis pigmentosa, peripheral neuritis, abnormalities in position and vibration sense, muscle weakness, and mental retardation.
- Vitamin E is undetectable in the serum of patients with neurologic symptoms.

ATAXIA-TELANGIECTASIA

- Ataxia begins at about 2 years and progresses to loss of ambulation by adolescence
- Oculomotor apraxia of horizontal gaze (difficulty fixating smoothly on an object and therefore overshooting the target with lateral movement of the head, followed by refixating the eyes), strabismus and nystagmus are commonly seen.
- The telangiectasia is found on the bulbar conjunctiva, bridge of the nose, ears and exposed surfaces of the extremities.
- Skin shows a loss of elasticity.
- Abnormalities of immunologic function that lead to frequent sinopulmonary infections include decreased IgA and IgG levels.

FRIEDREICH'S ATAXIA

- The onset of ataxia is somewhat later than in ataxia-telangiectasia but usually occurs before age 10 years.
- The ataxia is slowly progressive and involves the lower extremities to a greater degree than the upper extremities.
- The Romberg test result is positive; the deep tendon reflexes are absent (particularly the Achilles), and the plantar response is extensor.
- Patients develop a characteristic explosive, dysarthric speech, and nystagmus is present in most children.
- Intelligence is preserved
- Loss of vibration and position sense caused by degeneration of the posterior columns and indistinct sensory changes in the distal extremities.
- Skeletal abnormalities, includes high-arched feet (pes cavus) and hammertoes, as well as progressive kyphoscoliosis.

INVESTIGATIONS

- USG skull (if anterior fontalle open)
- X-ray skull
- MRI: Preferred over CT scan since it gives better visualization of posterior fossa
- Mantoux test/chest X-ray (to rule out tuberculosis).

TREATMENT

Depending upon the diagnosis.

DISCUSSION

GAIT

It is the posture of the patient during walking (Decubitus means posture of the patient in bed).

ABNORMAL MOVEMENTS

- *Tremor:* Regular, rhythmic, repetitive oscillations of a part of a body around a fixed point, usually in one plane.
- *Athetosis:* Slow, involuntary, writhing movements more marked in distal extremity. It consists of alternate pronation and supination or flexion and extension of limbs (under cover of hypotonia), e.g.Wilson's disease, sequel to encephalitis.
- *Ballismus:* Sudden, violent flinging move-ment around proximal joints. Site of lesion is subthalmic nuclei.

- *Myoclonus:* Sudden jerk of limb or muscle group.
- *Chorea:* Sudden, jerky, involuntary, quassi – purposive, non-repetative movements. They increase by emotion and voluntary movement and disappear during sleep, e.g. Rheumatic chorea
- *Dystonia:* Transient abnormal posture due to simultaneous contraction of agonist and antagonist group of muscles.
- *Tics:* Stereotyped repetitive movement confined to particular muscle group. They are exacerbated by stress.

DIFFERENT TYPES OF GAIT

Hemiparetic gait: While the patient drags his foot, the foot is raised from the ground by tilting the pelvis and the leg is swung forward forming an arc. The affected arm is carried in a flexed position and does not swing naturally, e.g. hemiplegic patients (upper motor neuron lesion) after recovery.

Spastic paraplegic gait: The patient stands with crossed legs; each leg is advanced slowly and stiffly with restricted motion at the knee and hip. He steps one limb in front of the other in a semicircular fashion, e.g. spastic paralegia.

Stamping gait: The patient stands on a broad base, raises his feet suddenly to abnormally high level, jerks them forward and bring them on the ground with a stamp (the heel touches the ground first). Ataxia increases on closing eyes, e.g. posterior column lesion or sensory ataxia.

High stepping or equine gait: This is just like the gait of sensory ataxia where the patient elevates his legs to a high level and brings them on the ground with a slapping noise. As there is foot drop, toes touch the ground first (trophic ulcer is found in the ball of great toe), e.g. foot drop, peripheral neuropathy.

Waddling gait: There is exaggerated lumbar lordosis, patient walks on a broad base, tilting the pelvis abnormally downward.

Ataxic gait: The patient walks on a broad base with unsteady feet placed widely apart. Patient tends to fall or deviate to the side of cerebellar lesion. The ataxia is equally severe whether the eyes are open or closed, e.g. cerebeller ataxia

PRECAUTIONS TAKEN BEFORE EXAMINATION OF CEREBELLER SIGNS

- Assure the patient of his safety by your close presence.
- Expose legs and feet adequately.
- If patient is able to walk, examine his stance i.e. standing position taken before walking.
- Exclude the disease of joints and bone or surgical causes producing disorders in gait (osteoarthritis of the hip).
- The patient is asked to walk in a straight line and to turn back in the original position.
- Examine Tandem gait (heel to toe gait).

CHAPTER 31

MENINGOMYELOCELE

HISTORY

CHIEF COMPLAINTS

- Swelling at back
- Convulsions
- Inability to move lower limbs.

HISTORY OF PRESENT ILLNESS

History of Disease

- *Swelling:*
  - Duration: Since birth
  - Progression: Change in size of the lump
  - Exact site
  - Secondary changes like softening, ulceration, fungation
  - Ruptured or not
  - Any fluid leak
  - Nature of fluid.
- *CNS involvement:*
- Limb weakness
  - Onset: Sudden/acute
  - Progression: Static/increasing
  - Weakness of upper or lower limb.
- Degree and duration of paralysis:
  - Is patient able to stand with or without support
  - Able to walk with or without support
  - Noticed any abnormality while walking
  - Sensory symptoms
  - Cranial nerve involvement: Vision, hearing, speech, drooling of saliva and pooling of secretions
  - Involuntary movements
  - Sunsetting of eyes
  - Convulsions/unconsiousness
  - Increase in size of head (hydrocephalus).
    - Congenital/acquired
    - Onset
    - Progression.

History of Complications

- CSF leak (rupture of sac)
- Vomiting/convulsions/increasing head circumference/altered sensorium (raised ICT)
- Asymmetry of legs or feet
- Spinal abnormalities like scoliosis
- Fever/convulsions/unconsciousness/altered sensorium (meningitis)
- Bladder/bowel involvement

- Blindness/deafness
- Signs of brainstem herniation
- Dysphagia
- Poor feeding
- Recurrent aspiration
- Vocal cord paralysis
- Stridor
- Apnea
- Activities of daily living "DEATH", i.e. Dressing, Eating, Ambulating, Toileting, Hygiene.
- Older children may present with added features of:
  - Deterioration of gait
  - Change in urinary continence
  - Frequent urinary tract infection
  - Recurrent meningitis.

History of Risk Factors

- Maternal risk factors:
  - Malnutrition: Folic acid deficiency in diet
  - Drug ingestion: Valproate, carbamazepine
  - Irradiation during pregnancy
  - Maternal diabetes mellitus
  - Fever/rash/lymphadenopathy during pregnancy: Intrauterine infections
  - Antenatal screening: Ultrasound, α-feto protein.
- Abortions
- Mental retardation and other congenital anomalies: Trisomy 18
- Other siblings affected with similar complaints.

NUTRITIONAL HISTORY

- When were oral feeds started
- Who feeds the child
- How often
- How long does it take
- Associated problems like vomiting, constipation.

SOCIAL HISTORY

- Impact of illness on child and family.

GENERAL PHYSICAL EXAMINATION

- Anthropometry especially head circumference
- Assessment of general vigour (especially cry and sucking)
- Skull examination: Transillumination, fontanelles, separation of sutures
- Eyes: Strabismus, nystagmus.
- Neurocutaneous markers:
  - Facial nevus
  - *Adenoma sebaceum* (Multiple erythematous papules on the lower half of face-cheeks, nasolabial folds, sides of the nose and chin)
  - *Café-au-lait spots* (Pigmented macules (>1 cm) on the trunk)
  - *Subungual fibromas* (ulcerative lesions at base or corners of nails)
  - Neurofibromas
  - *Ash-leaf spots* (Hypopigmented macules generally 1 to 3 cm in size, multiple and discrete)
  - Axillary freckling
  - *Shagreen patch* (leathery plaques of subepidermal fibrosis, usually situated on the trunk).
- Examination of back:
  - Shape and size of defect
  - Health and laxity of the surrounding skin and soft tissue
  - Leakage from sac
  - Spinal deformity (kyphosis).

EXAMINATION OF SWELLING

Inspection

- Situation (level of lesion)
- Shape
- Size
- Surface
- Color
- Edge
- Number
- Pulsation
- Impulse on coughing
- Skin over the swelling.

Palpation

- Temperature
- Shape, size, surface and extent
- Edge
- Consistency
- Fluctuation
- Fluid thrill
- Translucency
- Impulse on coughing
- Relation to the surrounding structures.

Auscultation

- To exclude bruit.

SYSTEMIC EXAMINATION

CNS EXAMINATION

- Spontaneous activity
- Examination of cranial nerves.
- Motor examination:
    - Observation of muscle bulk
    - Spontaneous active movements
    - Movements in response to stimulation
    - Assessment of muscle tone by palpation
    - Reflexes.
- Response to sensory stimuli in all extremities
- Hydrocephalus
- Anal sphincter
    - Weakness of anal sphincter as demonstrated by:
        - Patulous anus
        - Absent anal reflex.
- Asses bladder function.

2 types of bladder dysfunction are seen:

A. LMN Lesion

- Constant dribbling of urine with palpable bladder

B. UMN Lesion

- Presence of urinary stasis
- Palpable bladder with dribbling
- In severe form, detrusor—sphincter dyssynergia occurs, leading to high pressure in bladder and vesicourethral reflux.

- Examine the infant for other malformations and syndromes
- Record muscle strength examination and sensory level
- Sensory level: A stimulus is applied to the lower extremities from distal to proximal until the infant grimaces
- Motor level: Stimulus is applied above the sensory level and the distal most voluntary movement is noted.

CVS EXAMINATION

- Congenital heart disease (incidence of congenital heart disease in meningomyelocele 40%).

RESPIRATORY SYSTEM EXAMINATION

- Chest wall deformity (kyphoscoliosis)
- Signs of aspiration pneumonia.

ABDOMEN EXAMINATION

- Scars, distension
- Palpate for kidney (hydronephrosis)
- Urine retention.

INVESTIGATIONS

- MRI: Study of choice for imaging neural tissue and for identifying contents of the defect
- CT scan: Allows direct visualization of the bony defect and detects the presence or absence of hydrocephalus and other intracranial anomalies
- Ultrasound is used antenatally for screening
- Urodynamics.
- X-rays:
  - Chest X-ray to look for pulmonary infection
  - Spine to look for extent of bony defect and abnormal vertebral bodies, posterior arches.

TREATMENT

Treatment of the Meningocele

- Position the infant in the side lying or prone position only; avoid pressure on the sac or nerves.
- Prophylactic antibiotics in ruptured lesions
- Cover the lesion with non-adhesive dressing wet with sterile saline (no povidone iodine)
- If unruptured: Elective surgery done at 48-72 hours of age
- If ruptured or a thin skin covering, prompt closure of defect to prevent meningitis.

Poor Prognostic Factors

- Gross hydrocephalus
- Marked paralysis of legs
- Thoracolumbarsacral lesions
- Kyphosis/scoliosis
- Associated birth injury
- Other congenital defects

  Surgery should be carried out in such cases only after a proper explanation of the prognosis
- Hydrocephalus—ventriculoperitoneal shunt before myelomeningocele closure (hydrocephalus is operated before because this reduces edema and it becomes easier to push sac during meningocele closure)
- Clubfeet requires casting
- Dislocated hips require operative procedure.

Supportive Therapy

- Regular catheterization of neurogenic bladder prevents urinary tract infection and reflux leading to pyelonephritis and hydronephrosis
- Bowel training with regime of timed enemas or suppositories for incontinence of fecal matter.

Later Management

- Physiotherapy
- Appliances depending upon level of lesion and motor deficit
- Orthopedic consultation
- Avoidance of pressure sores/charcot joints
- Maintenance of bladder function
- Avoid chronic constipation
- Sensory stimulation
- Developmental assessment at all visits
- Nutritional support
- Counselling of parents and child.

Antenatal Screening

- Serum alpha-fetoprotein (AFP) at 16-18 weeks of gestation

- Ultrasonography: Signs seen on ultrasonography.

Cranial Ultrasound

- Ventriculomegaly
- Small head size
- Elongated cerebellum with obliteration of cisterna magna from a Chiari II malformation (Banana sign)
- Scalloping of the frontal skull region (lemon sign).

Spinal Ultrasound

- Widening of the posterolateral spinal ossification centres
- Absence of the continuity of the skin over the spine
- Bulging sac past the dorsal skin line.
- Amniotic fluid acetylcholinesterase.

DISCUSSION

DEFINITIONS

Spina bifida occulta: Failure of neural arches to unite posteriorly but no protusion of cord or membrane is noticed.

Meningocele: Meninges protrude through the defect in the spine. It contains only cerebrospinal fluid.

Meningomyelocele: In addition to the protusion of membrane, normally developed spinal cord and cauda equine lie within the sac. It is differentiated from the previous condition by presence of dark shadows of the cord or nerves on transillumination.

Syringomyelocele: Central canal of the spinal cord becomes dilated and the cord lies within the sac and becomes adherent to the posterior part of the sac.

Myelocele: Central canal of the spinal cord opens on the surface and discharges CSF continuously.

Encephalocele: Protrusion of the brain.

Meningoencephalocele: Protrusion of meninges as well as the brain.

FACTS

- 80% patients with meningomyelocele have hydrocephalus, whereas patients with only meningocele rarely have hydrocephalus
- Generally, lower the deformity in neuraxis (e.g. sacrum), the less likely is the risk of hydrocephalus
- Incidence of meningomyelocele: 1/1,000 live births
- Risk of recurrence
  - After 1 affected child: 3-4%
  - After 2 abnormal pregnancies: 10%.

EMBRYOLOGY

Rostral end of neural tube closes on 23rd day and caudal neuropore closes by the 27th day of development before the time that many women realize that they are pregnant.

- Primary NTD
  - Failure of closure of neural tube at 17-28th day of gestation
  - Responsible for nearly 95% cases.
- Secondary NTD
  - Occurs after neural tube closure due to defects in mesoderm.

ETIOLOGY OF MENINGOMYELOCELE

Nutritional

Folates

Maternal periconceptional folic acid reduces the incidence of neural tube defects by at least 50%.

To be effective, folic acid should be initiated at least 1 month before conception and continued until at least 12 week of gestation.

Dose

- Those planning to become pregnant: 0.4 mg daily (primary prevention)
- Previous pregnancy with neural tube defect: 4 mg daily (secondary prevention).

Vitamin B_{12}

- Multiple studies reported vitamin B_{12} deficiency in pregnant females with NTD neonates.

Hyperhomocysteinemia

- Considered as integrated marker of folate and B_{12} status
- Studies suggest hyperhomocysteinemia in parents with NTD neonates.

Genetic

- Polygenic multifactorial inheritance
- Recurrence risk
  - 3-5% in 2nd offspring
  - 10-15% in 3rd offspring.
- Almost twice the risk of NTDs in consanguineous couples as compared to non-consanguineous couples.

CAUSES OF HYDROCEPHALUS IN MMC

Seen in 80-90% as per western data/60% incidence reported in Indian study.

Causes

- Aqueductal stenosis
- Meningitis
- Type II Arnold-Chiari malformation.

ARNOLD-CHIARI MALFORMATIONS

Chiari Malformation I

- Herniation of the cerebellar tonsils through the foramen magnum into the cervical spinal canal
- The cerebellar tonsils often elongated and peglike
- Caudal displacement of the medulla absent in type I
- Vermis cerebelli and the fourth ventricle are normal or only minimally deformed.

Chiari Malformation II

- Commonly (80%) associated with myelomening -ocele
- Includes downward displacement of the medulla, fourth ventricle, and cerebellum into the cervical spinal canal
- Elongation of the pons and fourth ventricle
- Small posterior fossa
- Hydrocephalus seen in atleast 80% patients.

Chiari Malformation III

- Rare
- Displacement of posterior fossa structures
- Cerebellum herniated through foramen magnum into cervical canal
- Often associated with encephalomeningocele
- Usually fatal.

Chiari Malformation IV

- Cerebellar hypoplasia
- No cerebellar herniation.

PROGNOSIS

- Aggressive treatment of MMC—mortality rate 10-15%
- Most deaths before 4 years of age
- Normal intelligence seen in 70% survivors
- Meningitis, ventriculitis adversely affect IQ.

SECTION–IV

MISCELLANEOUS STUDIES

CHAPTER 32

INVASIVE PROCEDURES

LUMBAR PUNCTURE (LP)

INDICATIONS

- As soon as possible on suspicion of meningitis.
- Repeat after 48 hours if the initial LP is traumatic. Traumatic LP is a common experience and still merits initiation of empirical treatment. Gram's stain, CSF sugar and cultures are still reliable in traumatic CSF.
- No response to treatment.

IN CSF ONE SHOULD LOOK FOR

- Opening pressure (high in acute meningitis)
- Gross appearance of the CSF (clear or turbid)
- Biochemistry sugar/(CSF: Sugar and proteins
- Cytology including total cell counts and differential counts, should be done within 30 minutes of doing a LP
- Giemsa staining is essential to determine DLC.

PRECAUTIONS BEFORE DOING LP

- Fundus examination to rule out papilledema
- There should be no infection at the site of LP procedure
- Bleeding diathesis should be ruled out.

PROCEDURE

- Blood sugar should be done 30 minutes before lumbar puncture
- Child should be held firmly in lateral position with head, knees and hip flexed so that the intervertebral spaces become prominent
- The site of LP is cleaned with spirit, betadine and spirit in that order and draped with sterile sheets
- A 24-gauge stilleted needle is generally used to perform a LP. The direction of needle should be perpendicular to spine and slightly cephalad.
- CSF is collected in sterile vials.

CHANGES EXPECTED IN CSF WITH TREATMENT

Cultures: Usually sterile within 24 hours of adequate therapy

Sugar: Normalizes by 48 to 72 hours

Cells: May increase initially.

- Neutrophilic predominance for first 24 to 48 hours beyond which lymphocytic predominance occurs.
- Persistance of neutrophils indicates poor response to therapy.

Protein: Proteins are not a good parameter for adequacy of therapy and may take longer time to normalize.

DURATION OF TREATMENT VARIES WITH VARIOUS ETIOLOGICAL AGENTS

- Seven days for *Meningococcus*
- Ten to fourteen days for *Pneumococcus* and *H. influenzae*
- Three weeks for gram-negative bacteria
- Four weeks for *Staphylococcus aureus.*

INTRAOSSEOUS CANNULATIONS

PROCEDURE

- Site: Anteromedial tibial surface, 1 to 3cm below the tuberosity.
- With all aseptic precautions, the needle is inserted through skin and bony cortex, directing it perpendicular to the bone using a gentle, twisting or drilling.
- A feeling of 'give way' is felt when the needle enters the bone marrow cavity.
- The stylet is removed and needle is flushed with 10 mL of saline. If this test injection is successful, secure the needle with plaster and bandage.
- Drugs delivered through this route should be followed by a saline flush.

POINTERS TOWARDS A SUCCESSFUL INSERTION

- 'Giving way' of resistance in introducing needle
- Needle remains upright without support
- Marrow can be aspirated and
- Fluid flows freely through the needle.

ADVANTAGES

- In certain emergency situations, intravenous access may be difficult to achieve
- Safe, rapid and reliable alternative to administer fluid and drugs
- Any intravenous drug or fluid required for resuscitation can be safely administered.

COMPLICATIONS

- Tibial fracture
- Skin necrosis
- Osteomyelitis.

HEEL PUNCTURE

PROCEDURE

- The heel is warmed by applying a warm towel for 5 minutes.
- Area to be punctured is cleaned with alcohol and allowed to dry.
- Heel is punctured perpendicular to the skin on the most medial or lateral portion.
- The puncture should not be more than 2.5 mm in depth.
- First drop of blood is wiped off and the subsequent flow is collected in a capillary tube.
- The heel should never be squeezed to increase the sample flow, as this may give erroneous blood gas values and high potassium and dextrose values.

USES

Most useful in neonates and infants for obtaining capillary blood sample for:

- Hematocrit estimation
- Glucose estimation
- Bilirubin estimation
- Blood gas analysis.

SUBDURAL TAP

The procedure is done in children with an open anterior fontanel, usually up to the age of 18 months.

PROCEDURE

- Scalp is shaved; the skin is cleaned aseptically and draped
- Assistant holds the head during the procedure
- The anterior fontanel is palpated and the lateral angles are marked
- 21-gauge needle is introduced at 90° to the scalp at the lateral most angle of the fontanel
- There is some resistance while the skin and dura are being entered but there is feeling of 'give way' after the dura is pierced. Insert needle slowly
- As the dura is pierced, the subdural fluid flows out and is collected in sterile vials
- Subdural fluid should not be aspirated with a syringe. After withdrawal of the needle, gentle pressure is applied and the entry point is sealed
- The same procedure is repeated on the opposite side.

USES

Subdural empyema or effusions.

BONE MARROW ASPIRATION

SITE

- Posterior superior iliac spine (children > 2 years of age)
- Upper third of the medial aspect of shaft of tibia (children < 2 years of age).

PROCEDURE

Aspiration from the posterior superior iliac spine

- The patient is placed in the prone position.
- Wear sterile gloves.
- The site is prepared, cleaned with an antiseptic (usually betadine) and draped, exposing only the biopsy area.
- The skin and the area down to the periosteum are infiltrated with 10 ml local anesthetic (1% xylocaine).
- A skin incision is made with a small surgical blade.
- The bone marrow aspiration needle, with a stylet in place, is inserted. Once the needle contacts the bone, it is advanced by rotating clockwise and counterclockwise slowly until the cortical bone is penetrated and the marrow cavity is entered. Usually, a sudden change in give is noted when the marrow cavity has been entered.
- Once within the marrow cavity, the stylet is removed, and, using a 20cc syringe, approximately 2-3 cc of bone marrow is aspirated for pathology slides.
- Process immediately; this avoids any cell morphologic artifacts. If additional marrow is needed for cytogenetics or flow cytometry, these subsequent specimens are obtained by attaching a separate syringe and aspirating additional marrow at a time to be placed in an anticoagulant-containing tube (EDTA (ethylenediaminetetraacetic acid) or heparin, depending on the situation).
- The marrow aspiration needle is removed, and pressure is applied to the site with gauze until bleeding has stopped.
- Following this procedure, a bone marrow biopsy usually is performed as well (see bone marrow biopsy).
- Several layers of gauze are applied to the site with a dynaplast on top to immobilize the gauze. The dressing is removed 48 hours later.

BONE TREPHINE BIOPSY

PROCEDURE

The patient preparation is the same as for bone marrow aspiration. Usually, the biopsy is obtained following the bone marrow aspiration.

- The needle is held with the palm and index finger, and the stylet is locked in place. Once the needle touches the bone, the stylet is removed.
- Using firm pressure, slowly rotate the needle in an alternating clockwise-counterclockwise motion and advance it into the bone marrow cavity to obtain an adequate bone specimen measuring approximately 1.5 to 2 cm in length.
- Rotate the needle along its axis to help cut the specimen, pull back approximately 2 to 3 mm, and advance the needle again slightly, at a different angle, to help secure the specimen.
- Following this procedure, slowly pull the needle out while rotating in an alternating clockwise and counterclockwise motion.
- Remove the specimen from the needle with the probe supplied, by introducing the probe through the distal cutting end.
- Place the specimen in formalin solution for histology processing.
- If the aspirate was a dry tap, the core biopsy may be used to make touch preparations prior to placing the specimen in formalin. A dry aspiration tap is seen in infiltrating bone marrow conditions (e.g. myelofibrosis, hematologic malignancies, metastatic malignancies).
- After the procedure, several layers of gauze are applied to the site with a dynaplast on top. The dressing is removed 48 hours later.

PROCESSING OF SPECIMENS

- Thinspread preparations on glass slides are prepared in a similar fashion to blood smears by selecting the marrow particles and avoiding dilution with blood.
- Squash preparations are prepared on glass slides by placing marrow particles on a slide and pressing the particles with another slide. These preparations are used to observe morphology because the architecture of the marrow unit is preserved.
- The samples are sent for wright or Giemsa staining and histopathological processing of the biopsy samples. Tests performed on biopsy and aspiration samples include flow cytometry, fluorescence-*in situ* hybridization (FISH) studies, and cytogenetics, when hematological malignancies and lymphoproliferative disorders are suspected; specialized cytochemistry, when the above are suspected; Prussian blue staining for iron when disorders of iron metabolism (sideroblastic anemias) are suspected; and fungal, acid-fast bacilli, and bacterial cultures when these conditions are suspected or a pyrexia of unknown origin is being investigated.

LIVER BIOPSY

- The disposable Tru-cut biopsy needle is usually employed. It consists of an outer hollow needle and inner solid needle with a gutter for biopsy tissue.
- Before biopsy, the degree of jaundice, prothrombin time, platelet count and blood group should be ascertained.
- The patient lies down supine on the edge of the bed with his arms behind his head. The liver is palpated in midaxillary line.
- The upper border of liver dullness is also percussed and marked. The skin (usually 10th space) is cleaned with spirit, draped and locally anesthetized.
- Tru-cut needle with the gutter closed by the outer needle is inserted medially through the lower intercostal space till it is felt to enter the liver.
- The inner needle is then advanced further into the liver by pushing the handle provided at the back. The outer hollow needle is advanced completely over the inner needle to close the gutter. The liver tissue is cut into as a whole.
- Tissue is removed from the gutter and put in to formalin.

- Vim-Silverman needle can also be used for liver biopsy but is more traumatic.

KIDNEY BIOPSY

- Heavy sedation may be required for kidney biopsy in infants and young children.
- The child is placed prone with his head turned to one side, arms abducted, and forearms beside his head with rolled up towel placed under the patient's abdomen.
- The bony landmarks for this are the dorsal process of lumbar spine and the lower border of 12th rib.
- A point about 2 cm below the lower border of the rib is usually chosen as the site for biopsy. The procedure should preferably be done under ultrasonographic guidance.
- Under all aseptic care, the skin is prepared and locally anesthetized. A 21-guage needle is used to explore the kidney.
- The needle is pierced through the skin and advanced slowly till the swinging movement with respiration is noticed. If patient is cooperative, he may be asked to hold his breath in inspiration when the needle is manipulated.
- After the kidney is located the needle is with-drawn and the track is locally anesthetized. Tru-cut disposable needle is used for biopsy.
- The skin is sealed with benzoin.

INSERTION OF NASOGASTRIC TUBE

- Wash hands properly.
- Insertion length is measured from *base* of the nose to *tragus* and further to *xiphisternum*. This distance may be marked with a piece of tape.
- The tube should be lubricated by dipping it in water or by applying water-soluble lubricant to the tube. Oil, gels or petroleum jelly should not be used because of the risk of aspiration and clogging of the tube.
- After slightly extending the neck of the child, tip of the tube is inserted into the nostril, guiding it towards the nasophrynx. No force should be used and if the tube is stuck or resistance is encountered, it should be slightly withdrawn and reinserted maintaining a medial and downward direction. As the tip of the tube reaches the nasopharynx, the head is flexed to facilitate the desired length to be gently pushed in.
- The tube should be immediately withdrawn if cyanosis or respiratory distress occurs, indicating that it may have entered the laryngeal opening.
- The tube should be fixed properly with adhesive tape, being careful not to block the nostril.
- The gastric contents should be aspirated and inspected to verify correct placement of tube. The placement can be confirmed by injecting air and auscultating over the epigastric area for gurgling sound. The final confirmation is obtained on X-ray.
- The end of the tube should be occluded with adapter or stopper. If continuous aspiration is required, the end of the tube needs to be connected to a container with an extension tube.

REMOVING THE TUBE

While removing it should be pinched with thumb and forefinger or gentle negative suction should be applied with syringe.

COMPLICATION

- Aspiration of gastric contents
- Reflex bradycardia
- Apnea
- Bleeding due to ulceration.

ABDOMINAL PARACENTESIS

Abdominal paracentesis of ascitic tap is the puncture of the abdominal wall with a needle for aspiration of peritoneal cavity fluid.

PROCEDURE

- Clean and sterilize a wider area around the puncture site
- The puncture is made on the umbilicoiliospinal line in right or left lumbar fossa, lateral to the lateral border of the rectus muscle when the patient is lying supine.
- A wide bore (18-20 G) needle is inserted, attached to a syringe at the desired site horizontally into the abdominal wall and then the direction is changed to put needle into the abdominal cavity through a zig-zag tract.
- A continuous negative pressure draws the fluid into the catheter or syringe, moment the abdominal cavity is reached.
- If upon entering the cavity, air is drawn then withdraw the needle immediately. Repeat the procedure with sterile equipment till free fluid comes out.
- The required amount of fluid is drawn and the needle is removed.
- The puncture site is sealed with tincture benzoin.

PRECAUTIONS

- Hypovolemia and hypotension, if large amount of fluid removed
- Avoid puncture around scars from previous surgeries, as there may be localized bowel adhesion in these areas increasing the chances of entering a viscus.

USES

- Confirm etiology of ascites
- Relieves respiratory embarrassment due to ascites.

PERICARDIOCENTESIS

Pericardiocentesis is technique of aspiration of fluid from the pericardial space.

INDICATIONS

Therapeutic

Cardiac tamponade

Diagnostic

Pericardial effusion

PROCEDURE

- After taking a proper consent and securing an intravenous line, the patient is given sedation (best omitted in emergency tapping).
- The patient is positioned with a 45-60° anti-Trendlenburg tilt of the bed or in supine position.
- The procedure is done under ECG or echocardio graphic guidance and continues pulse oximetry monitoring.
- ECG leads are placed with lead V of the ECG attached to the hub of the aspirating needle with alligator forceps.
- If the needle touches the epicardium, ST segment elevation becomes evident on the ECG monitor.
- Taking complete aseptic precautions, the part is painted and draped. Xylocaine is infiltrated at the site of puncture.
- The space can be approached between the left costal margin and xiphoid, near cardiac apex, 5th or 6th intercostals space at left sternal margin or 4th intercostals space at right sternal margin.
- The aspiration needle is attached to a 20 cc syringe with a three way and the needle is advanced with gentle negative suction till the time fluid is aspirated.

- If pericardiocentesis is being performed for tamponade, the fluid withdrawal is associated with relief of symptoms, decrease in CVP and increase in intra-arterial blood pressure.
- In case of hemorrhagic pericardial tap, a rough difference about the source of the blood can be made by the fact that pericardial blood does not clot while the blood from the ventricle clots. Also the hematocrit of the aspirated fluid can be compared with patient's to differentiate. It the needle goes in the ventricle, it should be withdrawn and patient monitored closely for vitals.
- If the amount of fluid is large, a small catheter may be left in the pericardial space to drain recurrent effusion or bleeding.
- The position of the tube is confirmed by chest roentgenogram. The collected fluid is sent for relevant investigations.

COMPLICATIONS

- Laceration of myocardium or coronary artery resulting in tamponade
- Dysrrythmia
- Pleural or intra-abdominal laceration
- Patient with previous cardiac surgery has higher chances of injury as the anterior margin of the heart may be adherent to the pericardium. Pericardiocentesis in such patient is best performed in operating room.
- Young and uncooperative children undergoing diagnostic centesis should also undergo the procedure in operating room under general anesthesia.

SUPRAPUBIC TAP

This procedure is feasible mainly in children below 2 years of age as the distended bladder is an intra-abdominal organ.

INDICATIONS

- To obtain urine for analysis and culture as part of sepsis workup in a neonate, and in small children with urinary tract infection.
- Relieving urethral obstruction, particularly in boys with tight phimosis.

PROCEDURE

- The child is put in a supine position. The bladder is palpated or percussed to confirm that it is full. The procedure may need to be postponed if urine has been passed in the preceding hour.
- Suprapubic area is cleaned with povidine-iodine and alcohol and draped. The site of tap is located as 1 to 2 cm above the upper edge of pubic symphysis in the midline.
- A 21 or 22 gauze needle attached to 10-20 ml syringe is inserted at 10-20° to the perpendicular, aiming slightly caudal towards the coccyx. Gentle negative pressure is maintained as the needle is advanced till urine is obtained, taking care not to enter beyond the depth of 2.5cm.
- 5-10 ml of urine is aspirated for examination. In case there is occlusion of the needle tip with mucosa, it needs to be rotated gently.
- After removal of the needle, the puncture site should be covered with sterile gauze piece or band-aid.

COMPLICATIONS

It is safe procedure in most infants.

- Transient microscopic hematuria
- Transient gross hematuria lasting less than 24 hours in 0.6 percent of patients.
- Improperly performed procedure carries as potential risk of intestinal perforation, peritonitis, hematoma, abdominal wall abscess and bacteremia.

CHAPTER 33

LEGAL ACTS

THE JUVENILE JUSTICE (CARE AND PROTECTION OF CHILDREN) ACT, 2000

1. "*Juvenile*" or "*child*" means a person who has not completed eighteenth year of age.
2. "*Juvenile in conflict with law*" means a juvenile who is alleged to have committed an offence.

COMMENTS

- The State Government has been authorized to constitute Juvenile Justice Board.
- The board shall consist of a Metropolitan Magistrate or a Judicial Magistrate of the first class and two social workers of whom at least one shall be a woman.
- A child in conflict with law can be produced before an individual member of the board when the board is not sitting.
- State Government is empowered to establish observation homes for the temporary reception of any juvenile in conflict with law during the pendency of any inquiry regarding them.

When a juvenile in conflict with law is apprehended by police, he has to be placed under the charge of the special juvenile police unit or the designated police officer who shall immediately report the matter to a member of the Board.

When any juvenile is placed in the charge of a person he shall have the control over the juvenile as he would have if he were his parents, and shall be responsible for his maintenance and the juvenile shall continue in his charge for the period stated by the competent authority, not withstanding that he is claimed by his parents or any other person.

When any person accused of a bailable or non-bailable offence and apparently a juveline is arrested or detained or appears or is brought before a Board, such person shall, notwithstanding anything contained in the Code of Criminal Procedure, 1973 or in any other law for the time being in force, be released on bail with or without surety; but he shall not be so released if there appear reasonable grounds for believing that the release is likely to bring him into association with known criminal or expose him to moral, physical or psychological danger or that his release would defeat the ends of justice.

When a person having been arrested is not released on bail, officer shall cause him to the kept only in an observation home in the prescribed manner until he can be brought before a Board.

When any juvenile is arrested, special juvenile police unit to which the juvenile is brought as soon as may be after the arrest, has to inform the parent or guardian of the juvenile about his arrest and direct him to be present at the Board before which the juvenile will appear.

No juvenile can be charged with or tried for any offence together with a person who is not a juvenile.

Newspaper, magazines, news-sheet or visual media have been prohibited to disclose the name, address or school or any other particulars calculated to lead to the identification of the juvenile in conflict with law.

If any person having the actual charge of or control over, a juvenile or the child, assaults, abandons, exposes or willfully neglects the juvenile months, or fine, or with both shall be punishable with imprisonment upto six months, or fine, or both.

State Governments have been empowered to constitute child welfare committees for exercising the powers and discharge the duties in relation to child in need of care and protection under the Act. For child produced in front of this committee inquiry has to be completed within four months of receipt of the order or within such shorter period as may be fixed by the committee.

After the completion of the inquiry, if said child has no family or ostensible support, it may allow the child to remain in the children's home or shelter home till suitable rehabilitation is found for him or till the age of eighteen years.

Restoration of child means restoration to:

- Parents
- Adopted parents
- Foster parents.

Child kept in a special home or children's home or shelter home or in an institution, is suffering from leprosy or unsound mind or addicted to any narcotic drug, the competent authority can order his removal to a leprosy asylum or mental hospital or treatment center for drug addicts or to a place of safety for being kept there.

State Governments have been empowered to create funds for the welfare and rehabilitation of the juvenile or the child. Such funds are to be administered by the State Advisory Boards.

THE PRENATAL DIAGNOSTIC TECHNIQUES (REGULATION AND PREVENTION OF MISUSE) ACT, 1994

An Act to provide for the regulation of use of pre-natal diagnostic techniques for the purpose of detecting genetic or metabolic disorders or chromosomal abnormalities or certain congenital malformations or sex linked disorders and for the prevention of the misuse of such techniques for the purpose of prenatal sex determination leading to female foeticide.

1. No genetic couseling center, genetic laboratory or genetic clinic unless registered under this Act, shall conduct or associated with, or help in conducting activities relating to prenatal diagnostic techniques;
2. Shall employ or cause to be employ any person who does not possess the pres-cribed qualifications;
3. No medical genetics, gynecologist, pediatrician, registered medical practitioner or any other person shall conduct any pre-natal diagnostic techniques at a place other than a place registered under this Act.
4. No prenatal diagnostic techniques shall be conducted except for the purpose of detection of any of the following abnormalities, namely;
   a. Chromosomal abnormalities;
   b. Genetic metabolic diseases;
   c. Hemoglobinopathies;
   d. Sex-linked genetic diseases;
   e. Other abnormalities or diseases as may be specified by the Central Supervisory Board;

5. No prenatal diagnostic techniques shall be used or conducted unless the person qualified to do so is satisfied that any of the following conditions are fulfilled, namely:
   a. Age of pregnant woman is above thirty-five years;
   b. Pregnant woman has undergone of two or more spontaneous abortion or fetal loss;
   c. Pregnant woman has been exposed to teratogenic agents such as drugs, radiation, infection or chemicals.
   d. Family history of mental retardation or physical deformities such as spasticity or any other genetic disease.
   e. Any other condition specified by the Central Supervisory Board.
6. No person being a relative or husband shall seek or encourage the conduct of any prenatal diagnostic techniques on her except for the purpose specified earlier.
7. No person referred shall conduct the pre-natal diagnostic procedures unless:
   a. He has explained all known side and after effects of such procedures to the pregnant woman concerned;
   b. Has obtained in the prescribed form her written consent in the language which she understands;
   c. A copy of her written consent is given to the pregnant woman.
8. No person shall communicate to the pregnant woman concerned or her relatives the sex of the fetus.
9. On and from the commencement of this Act— No genetic counselling center shall conduct prenatal diagnostic techniques including ultrasonography for the purpose of determining the sex of a fetus.
10. No person shall open any genetic counseling center, after the commencement of this Act unless duly registered separately or jointly under this Act.
11. Every genetic counseling center, genetic laboratory, genetic clinic engaged, either partly or exclusively, in counseling or conducting prenatal diagnostic techniques for any of the purposes mentioned earlier, immediately before the commencement of this Act, shall apply for registration within sixty days from the date of such commencement.
    - The appropriate authority after holding an inquiry and after satisfying itself that applicant has complied with the entire requirements grant a certificate of registration in the prescribed form.
    - Any person or center, who contravenes any of the provisions of this Act, shall be punishable with imprisonment for a term which may extend to three years and with fine which may extend to ten thousand rupees and on any subsequent conviction, with imprisonment which may extend to five years and with fine which may extend to fifty thousand rupees.

ADOPTION ACT

WHAT IS ADOPTION

Adoption is a process by which a child who has been abandoned or given up by his/her natural parents and is without any family, is given a safe, secure and loving family through legal process.

WHO CAN ADOPT

- A couple desirous of giving a child a family can adopt.
- Hindus, Buddhist, Jains and Sikhs can adopt under the *Hindu Adoption and Maintenance Act 1956*, whereas non-Hindus can take a child under the *Guardianship and Wards Act, 1890*.
- Adoption of destitute children has also been facilitated now under the new Juvenile Justice (Care and Protection of Children) Act, 2000.

- The adoptive parents should have a reasonable and regular source of income, which can support the needs of a child within a family.
- Neither of the parents should have a major illness that would come in the way of parenting.
- Neither of the parents should have a criminal record.
- The composite age of the adoptive couple should not exceed 90 years for adopting infants.
- Single parents can adopt too.
- The age difference between the adoptive parent and adoptive child should be at least 21 years.
- Additional family support is also required in case of single parents.

FROM WHERE CAN ONE ADOPT?

Any parent(s) desirous of adopting a child may contact the licensed recognized adoption agencies, the local Voluntary Coordinating Agencies, Sishu Greh or the Juvenile Justice Board.

- Do not adopt from unlicensed Agencies/Homes.
- Do not try adopting or taking children from Nursing Homes/Hospitals, as it is illegal.

PROCEDURE

Incountry Adoptions

- First prospective adoptive parents should register themselves with the local licensed Adoption Agency or Voluntry Coordinating Agency. The couple's interest in adoption and their decision to adopt is ascertained at this stage.
- A home study of the prospective adoptive parents is conducted by the social worker of the agency. To allay the fears, preadoptive counseling sessions are undertaken by the social worker during the process of home study. Assessing the ability of a couple to parent a child not born to them is of crucial importance in a successful adoption. Therefore, the couple's suitability to care for an unrelated child is ensured through this home study.
- Subsequently, the prospective adoptive parents submit the documents related to their financial and health status to the agency.
- A child is then shown to the parents. The agency takes care to match a child meeting the description, if any desired by the parents.
- Once a successful matching has been, the agency then files a petition in the court for obtaining the necessary orders under HAMA or any other relevant Act. In some cases, the child may also be placed in preadoption foster care with the adoptive parents.
- Fees, as prescribed will be charged by the licensed adoption agency for the cost of caring of the child and the legal procedures. Children under Sishu Greh Scheme shall be placed in adoption free of cost.
- The above process is normally completed in 6 to 8 weeks. Once the child has been matched with the parents, there are regular follow-up visits and postadoption counseling by the social worker till the child adjusts in his/her new environment.

THE INFANT MILK SUBSTITUTES, FEEDING BOTTLES AND INFANT FOODS ACT, 1992 (IMS ACT)

THE LAW TO PROTECT AND PROMOTE BREASTFEEDING

To control and monitor the marketing practices of companies manufacturing infant milk substitutes, infant foods or feeding bottles and to end the marketing practices that interfere with breastfeeding the Government of India enacted the Infant Milk Substitutes, Feeding Bottles and Infant Foods (Regulation of Production Supply and Distribution)

Act, 1992, which came in force on 1 August, 1993. This is a strong intervention to protect, promote and support breastfeeding.

OBJECTIVES OF THE IMS ACT

The main objectives of the IMS Act are to:

- Prohibit the promotion of infant foods, infant milk substitutes and feeding bottles.
- Educate pregnant women and mothers of infants about breastfeeding.
- Ensure the proper use of infant milk substitutes and infant foods.
- Define the role and responsibilities of health care institutions and health workers to ensure the proper use of infant milk substitutes, feeding bottles and infant foods.

THE KEY PROVISIONS OF THE IMS ACT

1. The Act bans advertising of infant milk substitutes (e.g. Lactogen 1, 2, Nestogen, Amul Spray, Milk Care, Lactodex and Dexolac, etc.) and feeding bottles and prohibits taking part in the publication of any such advertisement.
2. The Act prohibits promotion of infant foods (e.g. Cerelac, Farex, Weano and dexolac Rice, etc.) unless in accordance with the Act.
3. The Act prohibits all persons from giving incentives of any kind whatsoever to promote the use or sale of infant milk substitutes or feeding bottles.
4. The Act restricts donation of informational or educational material or equipment related to infant milk substitutes or feeding bottles.
5. It gives detailed guidelines about the information to be given on the label of every container of infant milk.
6. It provides to regulate the development and distribution of educational material: "Every educational or other material, whether audio or visual, dealing with prenatal or postnatal care or with the feeding or an infant and intended to reach pregnant women or mothers of infants shall include clear information relating to breastfeeding as prescribed....."
7. The Act prohibits all persons from promoting the use or sale of infant milk substitutes of feeding bottles or infant foods in the health care system, e.g. display of posters, placards, etc.
8. The Act prohibits producers, distributors and suppliers of infant milk substitutes or feeding bottles or infant foods, from promoting the use of these products by offering any financial inducement or gift, directly or indirectly, to a health worker or a member of his family.
9. The Act prohibits producers, distributors and suppliers or infant milk substitutes or feeding bottles or infant foods from offering commission or inducement to their employees for promoting sales of these products.
10. It also prohibits the employees of such persons from performing any function that relates to educating a pregnant woman or mother of an infant on prenatal or postnatal care of the infant.

Penalties for violations under the Act

Any persons who contravene the provision of section 3, 4, 5, 7, 8, 9, 10 of the IMS Act shall be punishable with imprisonment for a term which may extend to three years or with a fine which may extend to five thousand rupees or both. Any person who contravenes the provisions of this Act with regard to the label on containers of infant milk substitutes or infant foods (section 6) or the quality of infant milk substitutes or feeding bottles or infant foods shall be punishable with imprisonment which shall not be less than 6 months and which may extend to 3 years and a fine which shall not be less than two thousand rupees.

All health professionals must be aware of the IMS and its provisions and reporting to enable reporting agencies to take suitable action. The reporting is essential if the irresponsible marketing practices, which encourage mothers and health professionals to adopt article feeding, are to be stopped.

What You Can Do?

- Be aware of the provisions of the IMS Act.
- Question marketing of products under the scope of the IMS Act to be in accordance with the IMS Act.
- Report to suitable organization, if you think some one is violating the IMS Act: at bpni@bpni.org or acashorg@vsnl.com.

MEDICAL/LEGAL PITFALLS

Virtually all potential medicolegal problems in wards can be prevented with the following actions:

- Performing a complete history and physical examination
- Informing the parents about working diagnosis
- Take consent of parents before doing any invasive procedure
- Paying attention to the troublesome complications of disease
- Reassuring the parents and child at intervals
- Performing only the necessary examinations and discussing the results with family
- Developing a plan of follow-up care
- Keeping the family informed about the child's progress and how this progress relates to the diagnosis.

CHAPTER 34

TIMING OF SURGERY FOR COMMON PEDIATRIC CONDITIONS

CONDITIONS	TIMING OF SURGERY
I. Head and Neck	
• Hydrocephalus/spina bifida	At diagnosis
• Craniosynostosis/encephalocele	At diagnosis
• Cystic hygroma/thyroglossal cyst	At diagnosis
• Cleft lip	10-12 weeks
• Cleft palate	12-18 months
• Torticollis/sternomastoid tumor	After 15 months/earlier if causing facial hemihypoplasia
• Branchial cyst	After 6 months
• Brachial sinus	At diagnosis
• Tongue tie.	After 18-24 months.
II. Thoracic Conditions	
• Tracheoesophageal fistula	At birth (primary/delayed primary)
• Congenital diaphragmatic hernia	At birth after stabilizing hemodynamic and metabolic status
• Eventration of diaphragm/ congenital lobar emphysema/duplication of foregut	At diagnosis
• Foreign bodies/tumors	At diagnosis
• Pectus excavatum/carinatum	Early infancy/at diagnosis
• Gynecomastia (in males).	After puberty if persist.
III. Abdominal Conditions	
• Umbilical hernia	After 5 years unless very large or obstructed strangulated
• Umbilical granuloma	Conservative, chemical cautery

• Umbilical lesions (polyp, urachal cyst, Sinus, PVID, persistent urachus)	At diagnosis
• Congenital/encysted hydrocele	After 2 years
• Inguinal hernia	At diagnosis
• Undescended testis	After one year of age or diagnosis, earlier if associated with hernia
• Ectopic testis	At diagnosis
• Torsion testis	Immediate
• Omphalocele minor/major with ruptured membranes	At birth
• Omphalocele major associated with major birth defects	Conservative at birth, repair of ventral hernia at later age
• Anorectal malformations	
❖ Low anomalies	At birth
❖ Intermediate/high anomalies.	Sigmoid colostomy at birth; PSARP at 3 months/10 kg weight
• Hirschsprung's disease	a. Colostomy at diagnosis;definite surgery after 6-8 months b. Neonatal single stage surgery
• Infantile obstructive cholangiopathy	Earliest possible
• Idiopathic hypertrophic pyloric stenosis	At diagnosis after correction of metabolic status
• Neonatal intestinal obstruction (atresia, meconium ileus, malrotation)	At diagnosis after resuscitation, immediate if suspect volvulus
• Intestinal obstruction	At diagnosis after resuscitation.

IV. Urological Conditions

• Preputial adhesions	After 2 years, earlier if ballooning
• Labial adhesions	At diagnosis
• Neonatal circumcision	After 6 months if no hypospadias
• Hypospadias	6-18 months; complete before school going
• Exostrophy bladder	
a. Bladder closure	48-72 hours/at diagnosis
b. Epispadias repair	At one year
c. Continence/anti-reflux	3-4 years/> 60 ml capacity
• PUJ obstruction	At diagnosis
• Vesicoureteric reflux	After 1-2 years age
• Neoplasms (Wilms' neuroblastoma)	At diagnosis with/without preoperative chemotherapy.

CHAPTER 35

X-RAYS

RESPIRATORY SYSTEM

CHOICE OF VIEWS

A posteroanterior (PA) (or anteroposterior, AP) for children view (Fig. 35.1) is usually sufficient. If an abnormality is seen, a lateral view should then be added. However, the lateral view should only be taken when the PA view has been inspected.

Which lateral view? Take the left lateral view unless all the clinical symptoms and signs are on the right, in which case take the right lateral view.

Erect or supine: Whenever possible take the chest X-ray in the erect or sitting position, because many intrathoracic conditions (e.g. pleural fluid, pneumothorax, heart size, mediastinal width) are difficult to assess when the film is taken with the patient lying down.

Apical (lordotic) views are used only when the PA film shows a possible abnormality in the apical area of either lung. The additional views should only be taken after the routine film has been viewed, and when there is difficulty in interpreting an apical lesion.

Decubitus views are taken when there is strong clinical suspicion of pleural fluid but none can be seen on the PA or lateral films. The decubitus views are taken only after the routine PA and lateral projections have been viewed.

Rib oblique films are taken only for RIB abnormalities (e.g. local swelling) or when there is localized, unexplained pain in the chest, and only after the routine films have been reviewed. Even with good oblique films, rib fractures may not be seen.

An "expiratory" film is a chest X-ray taken in the PA or AP position with the patient in full expiration, breathing out. It is only taken when routine films fail to reveal a clinically suspected pneumothorax or an inhaled foreign body.

PLEURAL EFFUSION

- Costophrenic angle obliterated
- Homogenous opacity
- 'C' shaped concave upper border whose lateral edge is higher than the medial one
- Wide intercostal spaces
- Mediastinal shift to opposite side.

DIAPHRAGMATIC HERNIA

- Coils of air filled bowel loops are visible in hemithorax.

- Trachea and mediastinum grossly shifted to opposite side
- Both diaphragm are pushed downwards
- Gross displacement of liver downwards.

HYDROPNEUMOTHORAX

- Dense homogenous opacity
- Air-fluid level on the same side
- Costophrenic angle obliterated
- Shift of mediastinum to opposite side.

COLLAPSE OF LUNG

- Homogenous opacity with 'crowding' of bronchi and vessels and displacement of septa.
- Hyperlucency on same side
- Sparse bronchovascular markings seen on neighboring lung
- Shift of mediastinum to same side
- Cardiophrenic angle obliterated on same side due to superimposition by collapsed lung border
- Elevation of ipsilateral hemidiaphragm.

FIBROSIS OF LUNG

- Nonhomogenous, opaque, linear streaks which usually radiate towards the hilum of the lung
- Shift of mediastinum to ipsilateral side.

CONSOLIDATION

- Dense triangular homogenous opacity with its apex pointing towards the hilum.
- No mediastinal shift
- Costophrenic and cardiophrenic angle are clear
- Air-bronchogram (linear, lucent streak with-in opacity) may be visible due to presence of air within the bronchi, contrasted by the fluid filled alveoli.

EMPHYSEMA

- Increased radiolucency of lung (due to decreased interstitum, increase in air spaces and decrease in vasculârity)
- Hyperinflation

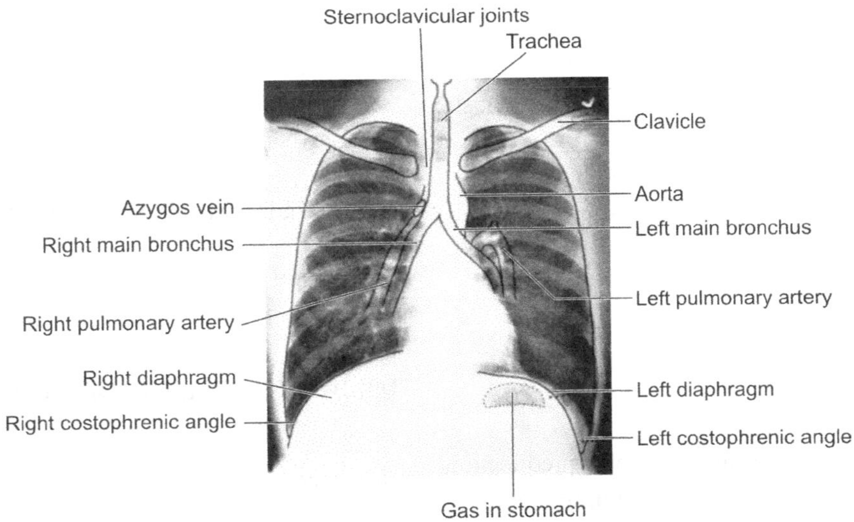

Fig. 35.1: Normal chest X-ray Posteroanterior view

- Flattening of the domes of the diaphragm.
- Small heart (tear-drop heart).

Causes

- Bronchial asthma
- Metabolic: Alpha-1-antitrypsin deficiency
- Infection: Bronchiolitis, miliary tuberculosis, cystic fibrosis
- Foreign body aspiration.

PNEUMOTHORAX

Erect View

- Hyperlucent lung field compared to opposite side
- Absence of the bronchovascular markings in the area of lucency
- Shift of the mediastinum towards the opposite side

If ventilated patients are imaged in supine position pneumothorax may be easily missed as it may be lying anterior to normal lung giving misleading appearance of lung markings on the radiograph. Supine pneumothorax should be considered if the following are seen:

- Hyperlucent lung field compared to opposite side
- Loss of clarity of diaphragm outline
- Deep sulcus sign, giving the appearance of inverted diaphragm
- A particular clear part of cardiac contour
- Lateral film may help.

LUNG ABSCESS

- While staphylococcal has no lobar predilection, *Klebsiella* is more common in upper lobe
- Characteristic feature is presence of thick wall and ragged inner lining.
- May be associated with effusion, empyema and pyopneumothorax.

BRONCHIECTASIS

- Multiple, small, cavities containing fluid (honeycomb appearance) in very severe disease
- Thickened bronchial markings
- Increased lung markings
- Compensatory emphysema.

Causes

- Infections: Measles, pertussis
- Bronchial obstruction: Foreign body, cystic fibrosis (mucus plugs)
- Congenital: Kartagener's syndrome
- Chronic aspiration

Bronchography and high resolution CT scan are diagnostic investigations of bronchiectasis.

TUBERCULOUS CAVITY

- Usually in the upper zone
- Exhibits "Tennis racket" appearance due to empty cavity communicating with a bronchus
- Infiltrates or enlarged or calcified lymph nodes elsewhere in the chest.

INFECTED EMPHYSEMATOUS BULLA

- Signs of emphysema seen
- Thin-walled cavities usually seen in lower zones.

MILIARY MOTTLING OF LUNG-FIELDS

Findings

- Bilateral uniform, fine, discrete opacities
- 0.5 to 5 mm in size

Causes

- Miliary tuberculosis
- Löffler's pneumonia (reticulogranular appearance)
- Bronchopneumonia (more confluent, not so well defined)
- Interstitial lung disease
- Tropical pulmonary eosinophilia
- Hemosiderosis (sharp, nonconfluent, smaller granules)
- Sarcoidosis (confluent)
- Histiocytosis.

D/D OF MEDIASTINAL MASSES (LATERAL VIEW)

- Finding: Homogenous opacity in mediastinum causing mediastinal widening.

Masses in Anterior Mediastinum

- Thymus
- Lymphoma
- Teratoma.

Masses in Posterior Mediastinum

- Neuroblastoma
- Neural crest tumors
- Neurofibromas.

Masses in the Middle Mediastinum

- Lymph nodes (enlarged)
- Cysts: Pericardial cysts, bronchial cysts.

HYALINE MEMBRANE DISEASE

- Fine granular pattern throughout both lungs
- Air bronchograms
- Obscured heart and diaphragmatic outlines in late stages
- May progress to 'complete white out'.

MECONIUM ASPIRATION SYNDROME

- Coarse linear and irregular opacities of uneven size
- Generalized hyperinflation
- Focal areas of collapse and emphysema.

TRACHEOESOPHAGEAL FISTULA

- Coiling of nasogastric tube in upper part of esophagus
- Distal end of esophagus remains a blind pouch
- Air is present in the abdomen
- Evidence of contrast media spilling into the right main brochus.

CALCIFIED SPOTS IN X-RAY CHEST

- Tuberculosis
- Hemosiderosis
- Fungal infection.

PULMONARY NODULES (ROUNDED PULMONARY OPACITIES)

- Multiple tuberculomas
- Multiple pyogenic abscesses
- Multiple fungal masses
- Secondaries—"Cannon-ball" metastasis
- Hydatid cysts
- Hamartomas.

RETICULOGRANULAR PATTERN IN X-RAY CHEST

- Meconium aspiration syndrome
- Hyaline membrane disease
- Pulmonary hemorrhage
- Pulmonary edema
- Congenital pneumonia.

D/D OF HILAR LYMPHADENOPATHY

- Tuberculosis
- Malignancy.

CARDIOVASCULAR SYSTEM

The Cardio-thoracic ratio (C-T ratio):
The Cardio-thoracic ratio =

$$\frac{\text{Maximum diameter of the heart}}{\text{Maximum diameter of the thorax}}$$

[The Maximum diameter of the heart is the sum of the distance of the farthest right border of the heart from the midline and the distance of the farthest left border of the heart from the midline.]

The normal C-T ratio should not exceed 0.5.

PERICARDIAL EFFUSION

- "Flask-shaped" heart on erect film which becomes globular on supine film
- Borders of heart are very sharp and well-defined (effusion masks ventricular wall movement) (Fig. 35.2)
- Acute angle between right heart border and right hemidiaphragm
- No recognizable chamber enlargement
- Lung-fields appears normal (neither plethoric, nor oligemic).

TETRALOGY OF FALLOT

- Typical appearance:" Boot-shaped heart"
- Right ventricular apex (clockwise rotation, horizontal heart)
- Pulmonary stenosis causes the pulmonary bay to become narrow
- Pulmonary oligemia.

VENTRICULAR SEPTAL DEFECT (LEFT TO RIGHT SHUNT)

- Cardiomegaly with left heart enlargement
- Prominent pulmonary conus
- Plethoric lung fields.

MITRAL STENOSIS WITH PULMONARY HYPERTENSION

- Cardiomegaly
- Straightening of the left heart border due to enlargement of left atrial appendage

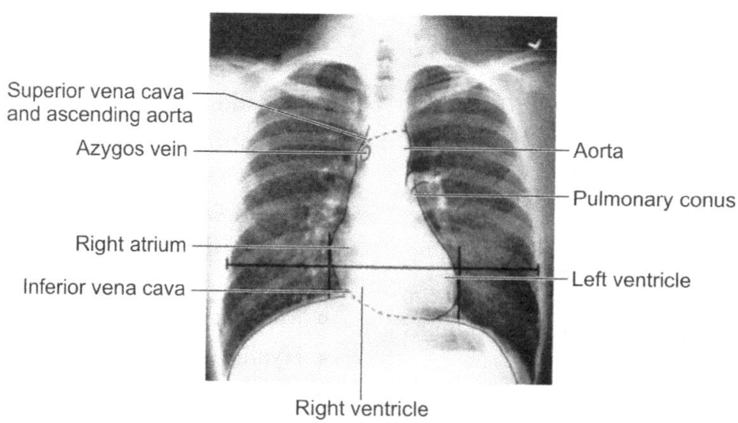

Fig. 35.2: Normal heart borders

- Prominent pulmonary conus due to enlarge-ment of pulmonary artery
- There may be prominent upper lobe veins—which are seen as arising from the pedicle of the heart— "Moustache sign"
- Double atrial shadow may be present
- Carinal widening to > 70° due to pushing up of left bronchus due to enlargement of left atrium.

COARCTATION OF AORTA

- Cardiomegaly with left ventricular enlargement (cardiac apex shifts downwards and outwards).
- Prominent ascending aorta and small descending aorta with intervening notch forming classic '3' sign (from above downwards) by:
  - Prestenotic dilatation
  - The coarctation narrowing
  - Poststenotic dilatation.
- Rib notching
  - Rib signs are unusual before 10 years of age
  - Notching of the inferior surface of ribs
  - Usually affects 4th to 8th ribs due to enlarged colaterals
  - Unilateral and right sided if lesion proximal to left subclavian artery
  - Unilateral and left sided if associated with anomalous right subclavian artery distal to coarctation.

EBSTEIN'S ANOMALY

- Cardiomegaly
- Right atrial enlargement
- Narrow pedicle of the heart
- Oligemic lung fields.

TOTAL ANOMALOUS PULMONARY VENOUS RETURN (TAPVR)

"Snowman appearance" (large supracardiac shadow along with the cardiac shadow which is produced by the dilated left SVC, left innominate vein and right SVC).

X-RAY SKULL

See Figure 35.3.

SILVER-BEATEN OR COPPER-BEATEN APPEARANCE IN X-RAY SKULL (AP VIEW)

- Widening of lambdoid and sagittal sutures (wide sutures—newborn >1cm, child >3 cm)

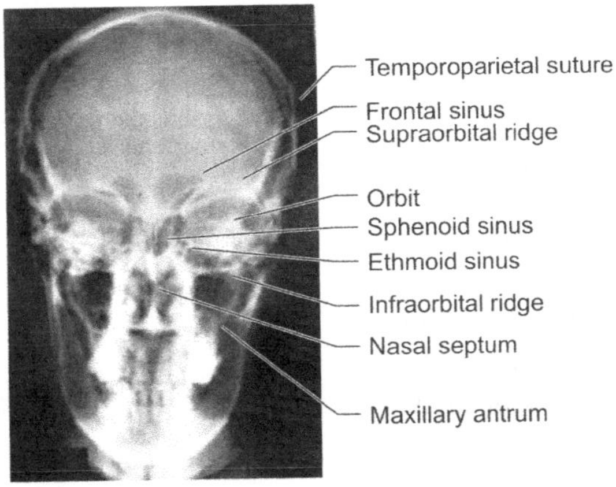

Fig. 35.3: X-ray skull

- Lacunae in the cranium
- Thinning of the bones of the vault of the skull
- Demineralization of dorsum sellae and the floor of the sella turcica followed by destruction of dorsum sellae
- Erosion of posterior clinoid process
- Progressive shallowness of the sella turcica.

Causes

- Raised intracranial tension
- Associated with meningomyelocele (this is not related to presence or absence of hydrocephalus).

HAIR-ON-END APPEARANCE IN SKULL

- Widening of diploic space with coarse trabeculae giving rise to hair on end appearance
- Thinning of the cortices of the bone
- Maxillary overgrowth
- Changes in the shape of the skull
- No signs of lytic lesion, bony erosion, calcification.

Suggestive

- Thalassemia
- Sickle cell disease
- Hereditary spherocytosis.

CALCIFIC SPOTS IN X-RAY SKULL

- Diffuse calcification with hydrocephalus: Toxoplasmosis
- Diffuse calcification with normal skull: Sturge-Weber syndrome (tram-track appearance)
- Periventricular calcification associated with microcephaly: CMV infection
- Calcification at base (suprasellar) associated with enlarged pituitary fossa: Craniopharyngioma
- Basal calcification associated with hydrocephalus (tuberculosis).

X-RAY BONES

CLASSICAL RICKETS (X-RAY WRIST) (FIG. 35.4)

- Widened growth plate
- Increased distance between the epiphysis and the metaphysis (loss of zone of provisional calcification) (Fig. 35.4).
- Metaphysis of reduced density
  - "Fraying" (margin of metaphysis become blurred)
  - "Splaying" (metaphysis becomes widened)
  - "Cupping" of the metaphysis.
- Osteoporotic changes (decrease in density of bone)
- Thin bony spur extending from metaphysics to surround uncalcified growth plate
- Indistinct cortex due to uncalcified subperiosteal osteoid
- Rickety rosary: Çupping of anterior ends of ribs
- Deformities: "Bending"of the bones or 'fracture'.

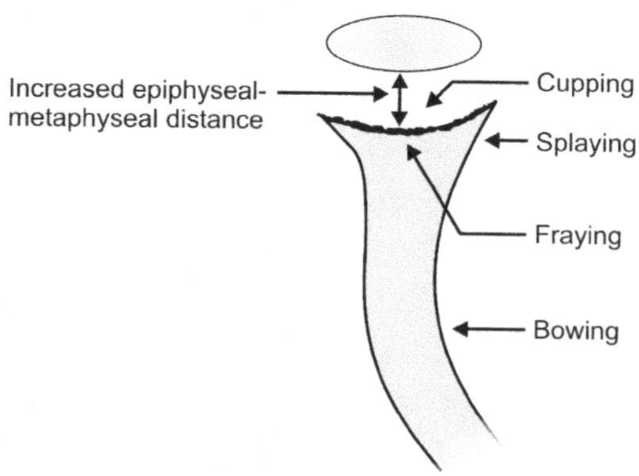

Fig. 35.4: X-ray wrist

HEALING RICKETS

- Dense white line of provisional calcification
- Decreased width between the epiphysis and metaphysis
- Increased density of bone.

SCURVY (X-RAY KNEE JOINT) (FIG. 35.5)

- Pencil thin cortex
- "Ground glass appearance" of shaft
- Epiphysis are small and have a very thin cortex—"Halo" sign of Wimberger.
- White line of Frankel (thickening of provisional zone of calcification at epiphyseal end)
- "Trummerfeld's zone" of rarefaction just below the while line of Frankel
- "Pelken spurs" (epiphysis extends as calcified line beyond limit of shaft)
- Calcified subperiosteal hemorrhages, resulting in areas of periosteum being lifted off the underlying bone.

CONGENITAL SYPHILIS

- Periostitis: Periosteal reaction due to infiltration by syphilitic granulation tissue
- Metaphysitis: White line due to callus formation at end of long bone. Proximal to it is a radiolucent zone
- Irregular metaphysic and metaphysial fractures may be seen
- Osteitis: Erosion on the surface of tibia
- Diffuse osteomyelitis may also be present.

ACUTE OSTEOMYELITIS

- Swelling of soft tissues and muscles
- Rarefaction and osteolysis of the metaphysis
- Periosteal reaction
- Sequestrum formation (more sclerotic than normal tissues)
- Involucrum formation

  Brodie's abscess (chronic osteomyelitis) is a well circumscribed, oval, radiolucent lesion with surrounding sclerosis (may or may not be associated with periosteal reaction) found at the end of a long bone (usually tibia).

EWING'S SARCOMA

- Osteolytic lesion in the shaft of long bone
- Periosteal reaction: "*Onion-peel appearance*" due to growth of periosteum in lamellar fashion around the diseased bone.
- Surrounding soft-tissue swelling may be present.

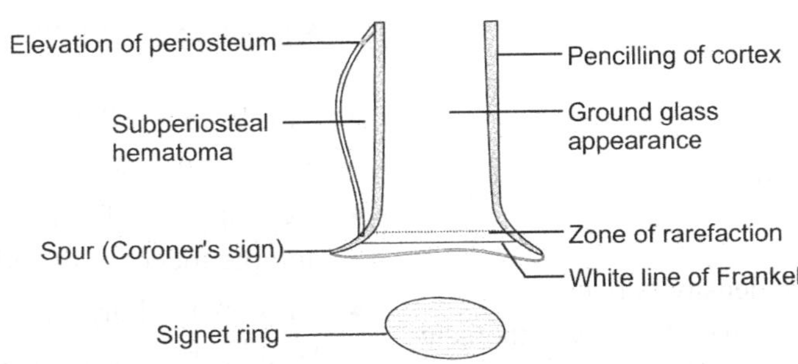

Fig. 35.5: X-ray knee joint

OSTEOGENESIS IMPERFECTA

- Thin bones (with cortical thinning) which are very fragile
- Multiple fractures
- Callus formation is abundant
- Dental abnormalities (dentigenous imperfecta)
- Wormian bones in skull may be present
- Pelvis may be deformed with protruded acetabulum.

BATTERRED BABY SYNDROME

- Multiple fractures involving the metaphysis
- The architecture of the bones is usually normal, i.e. these fractures are not pathological fractures
- Fractures of ribs are common.

OSTEOPETROSIS

- Generalized increase in bone density results in loss of differentiation between the cortex and the medulla. There is total absence of the medullary cavity
- "Bone within bone" appearance seen most markedly in the vertebral bodies
- Flask, shaped ends of long bones
- Rugger jersey spine
  (D/D of osteopetrosis—Fluorosis and Pyvno-dysostosis—both of which are extremely rare).

OSTEOPOROSIS

X-ray Thoracolumbar Region, Radius and Neck of Femur

- Decrease in mineral density in bone.
- Fracture (mostly seen in middle, lower thoracic and upper lumbar vertebral bodies). Upper dorsal spine fracture (above D4) suggests malignancy rather than osteoporosis.
- Collapse.
- The microfracture, expansion of intervertebral disc and biconcave-shaped vertebral body result in the so called 'codfish' vertebra.

ACHONDROPLASIA

- Skull:
  - Large calvarium
  - Short base
  - Small sella
  - Funnel-shaped foramen magnum.
- Thorax:
  - Thick stubby sternum
  - Short ribs with wide anterior ends.
- Axial skeleton:
  - Beaking in lumbar vertebrae
  - Decreased interpeduncular distance caudally in lumbar spine.
- Pelvis:
  - Square iliac wings
  - Champange glass pelvic cavity.
- Appendicular skeleton:
  - Rhizomelia (proximal bone is shorter than the distal one).
- Widened metaphysis.
- Trident-shaped hands (index and the ring finger diverge from each other, whereas the middle finger remains the same).

CONGENITAL HYPOTHYROIDISM

- X-ray bone age: Retarded bone age (absent distal femoral epiphysis in neonates)
- The epiphysis of femur may be stippled (have multiple foci of ossification)
- X-ray skull: Large fontanelle, wide sutures, Wormian bones, enlarged sella
- X-ray chest: Cardiac shadow enlarged due to cardiomyopathy or pericardial effusion

- Deformity of vertebrae: Beaking of the lower thoracic or upper lumbar vertebra.

GASTROINTESTINAL SYSTEM

PERITONITIS

- Gas under diaphragm with multipleairfluid levels
- Causes
  - Perforation of any part of the GI tract
  - Nectrotizing enterocolitis (in newborn).

INTESTINAL OBSTRUCTION

- Multiple air-fluid levels in intestine
- Causes:
  - Intussuception
  - Worms
  - Tuberculosis.

BARIUM-SWALLOW APPEARANCE OF ESOPHAGEAL VARICES

- Multiple filling defects due to dilated and tortuous veins
- Bunch of grapes or worms like appearance
- The site is most commonly the lower third of the esophagus.

BARIUM ENEMA APPEARANCE OF INTUSSUSCEPTION

- "Spring-coil appearance" (or the coiled spring appearance)
- "Claw sign" (due to the presence of barium in the intussuscipiens which is seen as a claw around the radiolucent shadow of the intussusceptum).

INVERTOGRAM

- Lateral film is asked
- Done after 18 hours of life
- Baby should be held in inverted position so that air reaches highest point in rectum. Then a radiopaque marker is placed on anal dimple.
- *High anomaly:*
  - Air column does not reach pubococcygeal line
  - Distance between air column and radio-opaque marker is more than 1.5 cm.
- *Low anomaly:*
  - Air column reaches the lower part of ossified ischium
  - Distance between air column and radiopaque marker is less than 1.5 cm.

PNEUMOPERITONEUM

- *Erect:* Free gas under diaphragm or liver can detect 10 ml of air
- *Supine:* Gas outlines both side of bowel wall appearing as white line
  In infants, round translucent area seen over central abdomen (due to gas collection)
  Curvilinear white line seen in right upper abdomen (falciform ligament outlined by free gas).

ASCITES

- Hazy appearance of entire abdomen
- Bowel gas floats centrally on supine film
- Bulging flank lines.

MECONIUM ILEUS

- Mottled lucencies due to gas trapped in meconium
- Few fluid levels (due to high viscosity)
- Bowel loops of various caliber

- Peritoneal calcification due to perforation occurring *in utero* is seen in 30%.

RETROGRADE PYELOGRAPHY

VESICOURETERAL REFLUX (VUR)

Gradations of a VUR

Grade I : Reflux occur in the distal portion of the ureter which is not dilated.

Grade II : Reflux occurs into the upper portion of the collecting system. There is no dilatation of the ureters.

Grade III : Reflux occurs into the upper collecting system. There is dilatation of the ureter which may or may not be accompanied by blunting of fornices.

Grade IV : There is reflux into the ureter which is hugely dilated.

Grade V : The ureter is dilated, tortous and there is effacement of the calyces. There is massive reflux.

CT SCAN

INDICATIONS FOR NONCONTRAST CT SCAN

- Head injury/ stroke
- Acute hemorrhage
- Subarachnoid hemorrhage.

HEMORRHAGE ON CT SCAN

- Acute hemorrhage < 48 hours: CT Investigation of choice
- Chronic hemorrhage > 48 hours: MRI Investigation of choice.

  Biconvex hyperdense: Extradural hemorrhage (Arterial)

  Concavo-convex: Subdural hemorrhage (Venous)

  The CT scan lesions are described as hypo or hyperdense and MRI lesions as hypo and hyperintense.

  Contrast CT scan can be identified by the falx-cerebri, which becomes white.

DIAGNOSIS OF HYDROCEPHALUS

- If the line joining the anterior horns of lateral ventricles is more than half of the same line touching the boundary of the skull then it is hydrocephalus.
- Normally the 4th ventricle is slit like, round and small. It is enlarged in communicating hydrocephalus and then other ventricles are also enlarged.

CHANGES IN CT SCAN IN C/O TBM

- Basal exudates
- Hydrocephalus with periventricular ooze
- Infarct
- Tuberculoma
- Calcification
- Cerebral edema
- Mild cerebritis
- Normal.

MRI

INDICATIONS FOR MRI CRANIUM

- Grey-white matter differentiation
- Structural lesion
- Infratentorial lesion.

IDENTIFICATION OF IMAGES IN MRI

The simplest way to identify is to look at CSF. It appears white in T2 and dark in T1 as in CT scan.

T1 Weighted Images

- Black CSF (i.e. hypointense CSF)
- Grey matter appears grey and white matter appears white
- Fat is hyperintense
- To look normal anatomy.

FLARE Images

- Black CSF
- To look for periventricular pathology.

T2 Weighted Images

- White CSF (i.e. hyperintense CSF)
- Grey matter appears white and white matter appears grey
- Fat is less hyperintense
- To look for abnormal findings.

Diffusion Weighted Images

- To see acute infarct within 30 minutes which appears as hyperintense (bright)
- If a lesion is hyperintense in diffusion weighted images and in ADC (acute deficient coefficient) mapping it is acute infarct
- If a lesion is hyperintense in Diffusion weighted images, but dark in ADC (acute deficient coefficient) mapping it is chronic infarct.

ROLE OF RADIATION

A radiation of 500 mrad for entire pregnancy is safe. Abortion is recommended if radiation dose exceeds 10,000 rads.

At an exposure of 1,000 to 3,000 mrad, no malformations occur and risk of malignancy is unknown.

Dose of radiation received by patient in radiological procedures:

Chest X-ray	1 mrad
Thoracic spine	11 mrad
Abdomen	221 mrad
Pelvis	210 mrad
Hips	124 mrad
Barium meal	171 mrad
Barium enema	903 mrad
IVP	588 mrad

CHOICE OF INVESTIGATION

- Head CT without contrast: To rule out bleed
- MRI with diffusion weighted imaging (DWI) and perfusion weighted imaging (PWI): DWI shows dying tissue and PWI shows 'penumbra' or tissue at risk of dying
- MR angiogram: To evaluate vessels, including the carotids and the circle of Willis
- Transesophageal echocardiogram: To evaluate cardiac thrombi and patent foramen ovale.

CHAPTER 36

ABG ANALYSIS

NORMAL VALUES

pH	7.35-7.45
pCO_2	35-45 mm Hg
pO_2	80-100 mm Hg
O_2 Saturation	95-100%
HCO_3^-	22-26 mEq/L
Base Excess	± 2

STEPS TO ABG ANALYSIS

1. Look at pH
2. Look at CO_2 levels
3. Look at HCO_3 levels
4. Match the CO_2 or the HCO_3 with the pH
5. Look whether CO_2 or the HCO_3 go the opposite direction of the pH
6. Look for pO_2 and the O_2 saturation.

Step 1: pH Analysis

The first step in ABG analysis is to look at the pH:

- Normal blood pH is 7.4, plus or minus 0.05, forming the range 7.35 to 7.45.
  - If blood pH falls below 7.35 it is acidic
  - If blood pH rises above 7.45, it is alkalosis.

Step 2: CO_2 Analysis

The second step is to examine the pCO_2:

- Normal pCO_2 levels are 35-45 mm Hg.
- Below 35 is alkalosis, above 45 is acidosis.

Step 3: HCO_3 Analysis

The third step is to look at the HCO_3 level:

- A normal HCO_3 level is 22-26 mEq/L.
  - If the HCO_3 is below 22, the patient is having acidosis.
  - If the HCO_3 is above 26, the patient is having alkalosis.

Step 4: Match the CO_2 or the HCO_3 with the pH

Next match either the pCO_2 or the HCO_3 with the pH to determine the acid-base disorder:

- If the pH shows acidosis, and the CO_2 is acidotic, then the acid-base disturbance is being caused by the respiratory system. Therefore, it is respiratory acidosis.
- If the pH shows alkalosis and the HCO_3 is alkalotic, the acid-base disturbance is being caused by the metabolic (or renal) system. Therefore, it will be a metabolic alkalosis.

Step 5: Look Whether CO_2 or HCO_3 go the Opposite Direction of the pH

- If CO_2 or HCO_3 go in the opposite direction of the pH, there is compensation by that system.
- If the pH is showing acidosis, the CO_2 is acidotic, and the HCO_3 is alkalotic. The CO_2 matches the pH making the primary acid-base disorder respiratory acidosis. The HCO_3 is opposite of the pH and signifies compensation from the metabolic system.

Step 6: pO_2 and the O_2 Saturation

Finally, evaluate the PaO_2 and O_2 sat. If they are below normal there is evidence of hypoxemia.

EXAMPLE

Parameter	Observed value	Interpretation
pH	7.31	Acidosis
pCO_2	55 mm Hg	Acidosis
pO_2	52 mm Hg	Hypoxia
O_2	Saturation 80%	Hypoxia
HCO_3^-	25 mEq/L	Normal

Step 1: The pH is less than 7.35, therefore is acidosis.

Step 2: The CO_2 is greater than 45, and is therefore acidosis.

Step 3: The HCO_3 is normal.

Step 4: The CO_2 matches the pH, because they both suggest acidosis. Therefore the imbalance is respiratory acidosis. It is acidosis because pH is acidotic, it is respiratory because the CO_2 matches the pH.

Step 5: The HCO_3 is normal, therefore there is no compensation. If the HCO_3 would have suggested alkalosis (opposite direction) then compensation would have been present.

Step 6: Last, the PaO_2 and O_2 saturation are low sindicating hypoxia.

The diagnosis for this ABG is: Uncompensated respiratory acidosis with hypoxemia.

ACID-BASE BALANCE

The mechanism by which the acidity and alkalinity of body fluids and kept in a state of equilibrium so that the pH of arterial blood is maintained at approx. 7.3 to 7.4. This is accomplished by the action of buffer systems of the blood and regulatory functions of the respiratory and urinary systems. Disturbance in acid-base balance results in acidosis or alkalosis. Figure 36.1 shows various disorders resulting from imbalance in acid and base in the body.

ACID-BASE DISORDERS

See Figure 36.1.

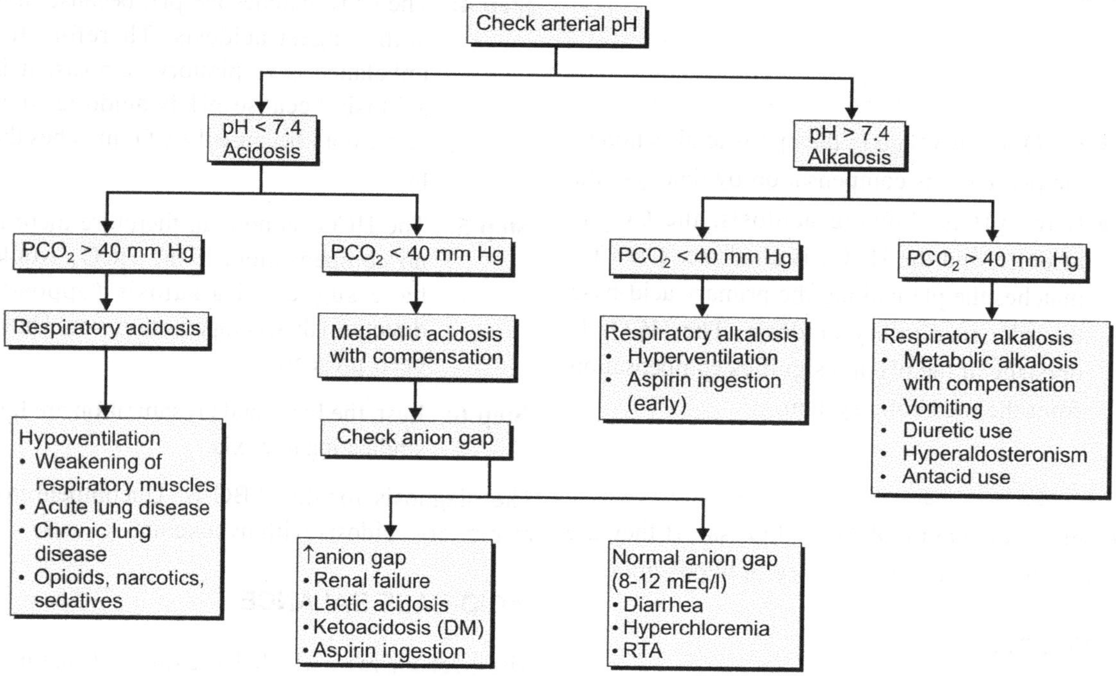

FIG. 36.1: Acid-base imbalance disorders

CHAPTER 37

SOCIAL PROGRAMS

NUTRITIONAL SUPPLEMENTATION PROGRAMS IN INDIA

NUTRIENT PROGRAMS

- Vitamin A prophylaxis program
- Prophylaxis against nutritional anemia
- Iodine deficiency disorders control programs
- Special nutrition program
- Applied nutrition program
- Balwadi nutrition program
- Mid-day meal program
- Integrated child development service scheme.

VITAMIN A PROPHYLAXIS PROGRAM

- *Beneficiaries:* 6 months to 5 years children
- Activities:
  - 1 lakh IU oral to infant (6-11 months)
  - 2 lakh IU oral to children (1 year to 5 years)
- Under Child survival safe motherhood program, 1st dose is given at 9 months along with measles vaccine and 2nd dose at 18 months along with booster dose of DPT.
- Evaluation: Reduction in prevalence of Bitot's spot by 2/3
- Reasons for inadequate coverage:
  - Short supply of vitamin A
  - Lack of supervision
  - Lack of nutrition education to beneficiaries.

PROPHYLAXIS AGAINST NUTRITIONAL ANEMIA

- *Beneficiaries:* Pregnant women and children (1-12 years)
- *Objectives:*
  - To assess prevalence of nutritional anemia in mothers and children
  - To supplement mother and children with iron and folic acid tablets
  - To monitor quality of iron—folic acid tablet
  - To assess hemoglobin level.
- *Activities:*
  - Promotion of regular consumption of food rich in iron
  - Provision of iron and folic acid supplement
  - Identification of severe anemia
  - Treatment of hook worm infection.

- *Iron Prophylaxis*
  - Pregnant women—1 tablet for 100 days of pregnancy (containing 60 mg of elemental iron and 500 µg of folic acid).
  - Children—1 tablet for 100 continuous days per year (containing 20 mg of elemental iron and 100 µg of folic acid after deworming).
- Treatment of anemia:
  - Pregnant women—2 tablets/day (containing 60 mg of elemental iron and 500 µg of folic acid)
  - Children—6 mg/kg of elemental iron for 3 months.

IODINE DEFICIENCY DISORDER CONTROL PROGRAM

- Initial survey to assess magnitude of Iodine deficiency disorder
- Resurvey to assess impact of iodized salt every 5 years.
- *Activities*
  - Iodization of salt in country by 1992
  - Banning use of noniodized salt.
- *Program Evaluation*
  - Irregular distribution
  - Lack of monitoring
  - No complete ban of noniodized salt.

SPECIAL NUTRITION PROGRAM

- *Beneficiaries:* Pregnant, nursing women and children < 6 years in slums and backward areas.
- It gives 300 kcal and 10-12 grams of protein per day for each child.
- Mothers receive 500 kcal and 25 grams of protein daily.
- Feeding is given for 300 days a year.
- Ministry of Social Welfare is in charge of this program.

BALWADI NUTRITION PROGRAM

- *Beneficiaries:* Children 3-6 years in rural areas
- Food supplements provide 300 kcal and 10 grams of protein/child/day
- It also provides primary education.

APPLIED NUTRITION PROGRAM

- *Objective:*
  - To make people conscious of their nutritional needs
  - Aimed at improvement in food production, distribution and nutrition education.
- *Beneficiaries:* Pregnant and lactating mothers, 3-6 years children
- *Activities:* Production of nutritious food by themselves by habit of having kitchen garden in houses, institutions and schools
- *Evaluation:* Could not generate sufficient awareness.

MID-DAY MEAL PROGRAM

- *Objective:*
  - To bridge the calorie gap among children belonging to low socioeconomic status
  - To attract more children to schools.
- *Principle*
  - It should be a supplement and not a home diet
  - Should supply 1/3rd of total energy and 50% of protein
  - Low cost/easily prepared / locally available food.

OTHER NATIONAL PROGRAMS

Many other programs contribute directly and indirectly to child welfare.

UNIVERSAL IMMUNIZATION PROGRAM (UIP)

- Initiated in India in 1985.
- It aims at 100% immunization of all infants against six major vaccine preventable killer diseases, namely, tuberculosis, diphtheria, pertussis, tetanus, poliomyelitis and measles, before 1 year of age.
- This program has helped to improve the immunization status of children.

CHILD SURVIVAL AND SAFE MOTHERHOOD (CSSM) PROGRAM

- Initiated in 1992 by integrating all the available services and resources into a new package to improve child survival.
- It has child survival and safe motherhood components.
- *Objectives:*
  - Universal immunization
  - Diarrhoea control and oral rehydration therapy
  - Control of acute respiratory infection
  - Existing vitamin A prophylaxis program to be universalized
  - Prophylactic iron and folic acid
  - Improving newborn and maternal care.

Services

- Children:
  - Essential newborn care
  - Immunization
  - Diarrhoea control and oral rehydration therapy
  - ARI control
  - Iron and folic acid supplementation.
- Essential newborn care:
  - Resuscitation
  - Prevent hypothermia
  - Prevent infections
  - Exclusive breastfeeding
  - Referral of sick newborn.
- Mothers:
  - Immunization
  - Prevention and treatment of anemia
  - Antenatal care
  - Deliveries by trained personnel
  - Institutional delivery promotion
  - Birth spacing.

MATERNAL AND CHILD HEALTH

- *Objective:*
  - To reduce maternal, infant and childhood mortality and morbidity
  - To promote reproductive health
  - To promote physical and psychological development of children and adolescents.

Package of Services

- Antenatal care:
  - Screening of anemia, eclampsia, multiple births
  - Measurement of hemoglobin, blood pressure and fundal height
  - Administer 3 doses of tetanus toxoid
  - Iron and folic acid tablet distribution.
- Intranatal care:
  - Delivery by trained birth attendant
  - Mother education about breastfeeding, immunization, family planning and hygiene.

- Child care:
    - Growth monitoring
    - Immunization
    - Treatment of common illness
    - Nutrition.
- At risk children:
    - Birth weight < 2.5 kg
    - Feeding difficulties
    - Single parent
    - Recurrent illnesses.

REPRODUCTIVE AND CHILD HEALTH (RCH)

Aimed at improving health status of women and children

- Components:
    - Child survival
    - Safe motherhood
    - Adolescent care.
- Child survival:
    - Breastfeeding and complementary feeding
    - Immunization
    - Vitamin A prophylaxis
    - Integral management of childhood illness strategy: ARI, diarrhea, anemia, worm infestation, vaccine preventable diseases
    - Referral services.
- Safe motherhood:
    - Antenatal care
    - Essential obstetric care
    - Emergency obstetric care
    - Postnatal care.
- Adolescent care:
    - Teenage counseling
    - Adolescent nutrition and anemia prophylaxis
    - Personal hygiene
    - Prevention of reproductive tract infection and sexually transmitted diseases.
- Community participation:
    - Safe abortion
    - Management of infertility
    - Contraception
    - Screening and management of cervical and breast cancer.

INTEGRATED CHILD DEVELOPMENT SERVICES (ICDS) SCHEME

- ICDS program was started in 1975.
- It is an excellent on going program aimed at total development of the child.
- *Objective:*
    - To improve nutritional and health status of children in age 0-6 years
    - To reduce mortality, morbidity, malnutrition in school dropouts
    - To provide optimum conditions for mental, physical and social development of the child.
    - To enhance capability of mother and nutritional needs of child through proper nutrition and health education
    - To achieve effective coordination of policy and implementation among various departments working for promotion of child development.
- The services are delivered through a network of Anganwadis (i.e. a community center). In project areas, one Anganwadi is established for every 1,000 population.
- The package of services available includes health check ups, immunization, referral service, supplementary nutrition, nonformal education for children (3-4 years), nutrition and health education for women, treatment of minor ailments and home visits.

- Growth monitoring is one of the major activities in the Anganwadi center. The Anganwadi teacher is expected to weigh all the children regularly and record it on the growth chart and thus show it to the mother. The Anganwadi teacher is also expected to report monthly, the data concerning the percentage of children with normal nutritional status and those with various grades of PEM. Growth monitoring can help only, if it is accompanied by appropriate interventional strategies.
- The average calorie intake among 1 to 5 years old children was estimated to be 810 calories per day as against the requirement of 1200 calories. Food supplementation is planned to bridge this calorie gap.
- In the ICDS, this is linked with nutritional supplementation. All children are expected to get around 400 calories per day and the severely malnourished are expected to get additional ration.
- The stimulation is mainly aimed at children above 3 years of age in the form of nonformal education. Lack of participation of the younger child is the main drawback in ICDS. The crucial period in child development, i.e. below 3 years, is not made use of in imparting stimulation. These children are not sufficiently reached and are difficult to reach. Often the food supplement is neither suitable for them nor available to them.
- Community participation is always expected as the Anganwadi teacher herself is a member of the community. But often the community remains a passive recipient. ICDS still remains a Government program rather than a community program.
- Active efforts are being made to integrate the program of sanitation and safe water supply with ICDS, to give more emphasis on family welfare services and economic uplift especially among women, with the help of the existing network. This program has helped to improve immunization status and nutritional status of children.

INTEGRATED RURAL DEVELOPMENT PROGRAM (IRDP)

- Composite program for rural development and economic uplift.
- This program has helped in providing self-employment.

ADULT LITERACY CAMPAIGN

- Adult literacy campaign has successfully implemented the first stage of adult education and also the second stage aimed at tribal and coastal population.
- The formation of family units and continuing education are planned in the third stage.

INDIA POPULATION PROJECT (IPP)

- Program aimed at population control and improved quality of life.

INTERNATIONAL PROGRAMS

- World Health Organization (WHO), United Nations International Children's Emergency Fund (UNICEF), World Bank, World Food Programme, Food and Agricultural Organization (FAO), United States Agency for International Development (USAID), CARE, etc. are some of the international agencies that initiate and support the child welfare programs, especially in the developing countries including India.
- These agencies provide financial and technical support to implement various educational and nutritional programs that help in child survival and child development.

Appendix

Neonatal Resuscitation: 2010 American Heart Association Guidelines

- *Initial steps:* Those newly born infants who do not require resuscitation can be identified by a rapid assessment of the following three characteristics:
  - Term gestation?
  - Crying or breathing?
  - Good muscle tone?

Approximately 60 seconds (the Golden Minute) are allotted for completing the initial steps, reevaluating, and beginning ventilation if required:

- The decision to progress beyond the initial steps is determined by simultaneous assessment of two vital characteristics: respirations (apnea, gasping, or labored or unlabored breathing) and heart rate (whether greater than or less than 100 beats per minute).
- Once positive pressure ventilation or supplementary oxygen administration has started, assessment should be by simultaneous evaluation of three vital characteristics: heart rate, respirations, and the state of oxygenation determined by a pulse oximeter. The most sensitive indicator of a successful response to each step is an increase in heart rate.
- *Clearing the airway*: When amniotic fluid is clear suctioning immediately following birth should be reserved for babies who have obvious obstruction to spontaneous breathing or who require positive-pressure ventilation.
- *Pulse oximetry* should be used when resuscitation can be anticipated, when positive pressure is administered for more than a few breaths, when cyanosis is persistent, or when supplementary oxygen is administered.
- Goal of *administration of supplementary oxygen* should be an oxygen saturation value in the interquartile range of preductal saturations measured in healthy term babies following vaginal birth at sea level and achieved by initiating resuscitation with air or a blended oxygen and titrating the oxygen concentration to achieve an SpO_2 in the target range using pulse oximetry.
- *Positive-pressure ventilation (PPV):*
  - If the infant remains apneic or gasping, or if the heart rate remains <100 per minute after administering the initial steps, start PPV.
  - Inflation pressure should be monitored; an initial inflation pressure of 20 cm H_2O may be effective, but $\geq$ 30 to 40 cm H_2O may be required in some term babies without spontaneous respiration.
  - Ventilation assisted ventilation should be delivered at a rate of 40 to 60 breaths per minute to promptly achieve or maintain a heart rate >100 per minute.
- *Endotracheal tube placement:* A prompt increase in heart rate is the best indicator that

the tube is in the tracheobronchial tree and providing effective ventilation. Exhaled CO_2 detection is the recommended method of confirmation of endotracheal tube placement

- *Chest compressions*:
  - Indicated for a heart rate that is <60 per minute despite adequate ventilation with supplementary oxygen for 30 seconds.
  - There should be a 3:1 ratio of compressions to ventilations with 90 compressions and 30 breaths to achieve approximately 120 events per minute to maximize ventilation at an achievable rate. Thus each event will be allotted approximately half second, with exhalation occurring during the first compression after each ventilation.
- *Medications*: If the heart rate remains < 60 per minute despite adequate ventilation (usually with endotracheal intubation) with 100% oxygen and chest compressions, administration of epinephrine or volume expansion, or both, may be indicated.
- *Postresuscitation care:* It is recommended that infants born at > 36 weeks gestation with evolving moderate to severe hypoxic ischemic encephalopathy should be offered therapeutic hypothermia.

INDEX

G

H

I

J

K